SECRETS OF TAI CHI

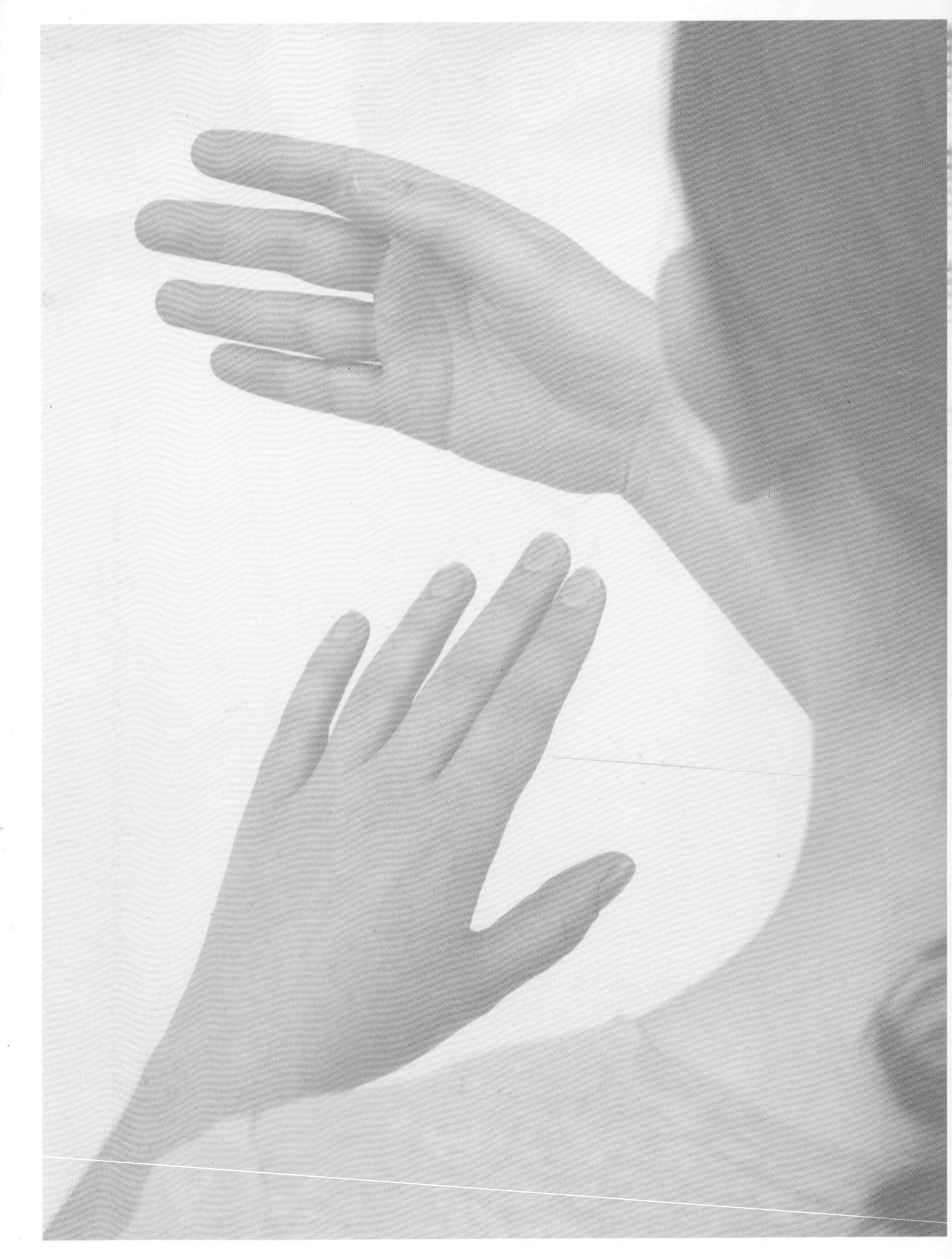

SECRETS OF TAI CHI

KIM DAVIES & SIMON ROBINS

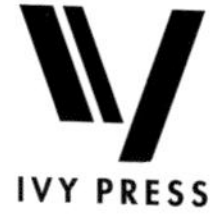

First published in the UK in 2018 by
Ivy Press
An imprint of The Quarto Group
The Old Brewery, 6 Blundell Street
London N7 9BH, United Kingdom
T (0)20 7700 6700 **F** (0)20 7700 8066
www.QuartoKnows.com

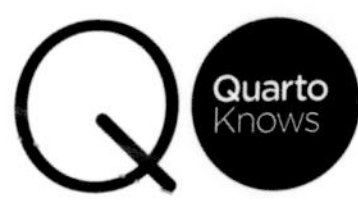

British Library Cataloguing-in-Publication Data
A catalogue record for this book is available from the British Library

ISBN: 978-1-78240-576-4

This book was conceived, designed, and produced by
Ivy Press
58 West Street, Brighton BN1 2RA, United Kingdom
Publisher: Susan Kelly
Creative Director: Michael Whitehead
Art Director: James Lawrence
Editorial Director: Tom Kitch
Designer: Ginny Zeal
Photographer: Neal Grundy
Models: Caroline Saul and Will Newmarch
Hair and Make-up: Justine Rice and Sarah Ellis

Printed in China

10 9 8 7 6 5 4 3 2 1

Note from the publisher
Although every effort has been made to ensure that the information presented in this book is correct, the authors and publisher cannot be held responsible for any injuries which may arise.

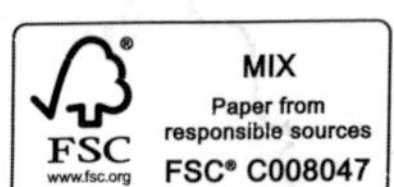

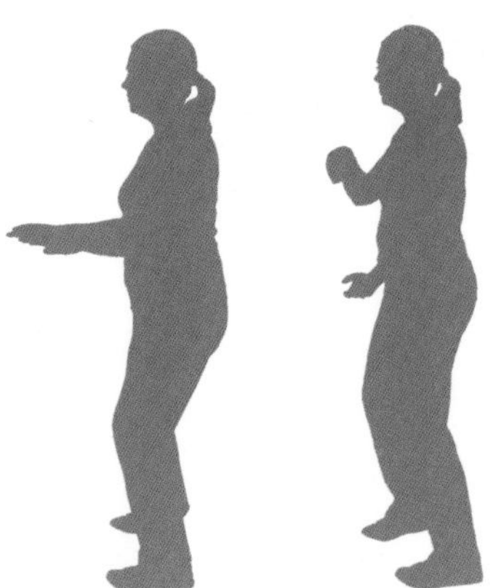

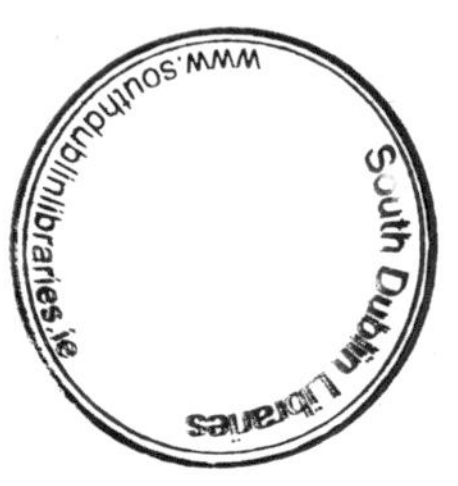

How to Use This Book 6

Introduction: What is Tai Chi? 8

The Worldwide Traditions of Tai Chi 10

Chapter 1: **Tai Chi Fundamentals** **16**

Chapter 2: **Getting Started** **42**

Chapter 3: **The Yang Short Form Part 1** **78**

Chapter 4: **The Yang Short Form Part 2** **120**

Chapter 5: **The Yang Short Form Part 3** **150**

Chapter 6: **The Yang Short Form Part 4** **178**

Glossary 218

Further Information 219

Index 220

Acknowledgments 224

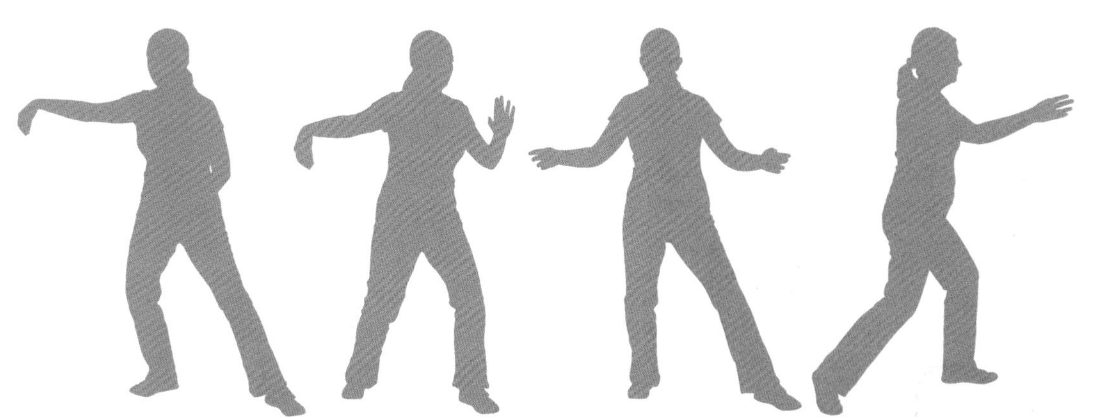

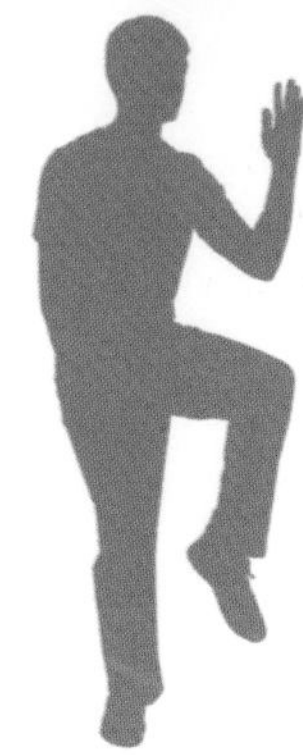

Body & mind

Tai chi is a martial art that serves as a mind-body system of exercise.

HOW TO USE THIS BOOK

Secrets of Tai Chi is a complete guide to the Yang Style Tai Chi, one of the most popular forms of the art. The book will serve as a useful introduction to the complete form for beginners, while those who are familiar with it already will find this an invaluable reference as they seek to master the art. As well as providing a fully-illustrated, step-by-step guide to the 37 postures in the form, this book covers the ideas and traditions behind tai chi that it is essential to understand in order to fully benefit from practicing it.

Important Notice

Although tai chi is a very gentle form of exercise, consult a physician if you have any physical health concerns or injuries, or if you have not exercised for a significant period of time.

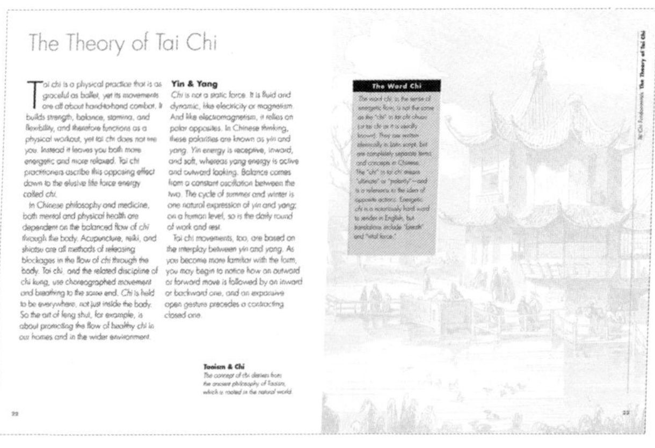

The Theory of Tai Chi

Tai chi is a physical practice that is as graceful as ballet, yet its movements are all about hand-to-hand combat. It builds strength, balance, stamina, and flexibility, and therefore functions as a physical workout, yet tai chi does not tire you. Instead it leaves you both more energetic and more relaxed. Tai chi practitioners ascribe this opposing effect down to the elusive life force energy called *chi*.

In Chinese philosophy and medicine, both mental and physical health are dependent on the balanced flow of *chi* through the body. Acupuncture, reiki, and shiatsu are all methods of releasing blockages in the flow of chi through the body. Tai chi, and the related discipline of chi kung, use choreographed movement and breathing to the same end. *Chi* is held to be everywhere, not just inside the body. So the art of feng shui, for example, is about promoting the flow of healthy chi in our homes and in the wider environment.

Yin & Yang

Chi is not a static force. It is fluid and dynamic, like electricity or magnetism. And like electromagnetism, it relies on polar opposites. In Chinese thinking, these polarities are known as *yin* and *yang*. *Yin* energy is receptive, inward, and soft, whereas yang energy is active and outward looking. Balance comes from a constant oscillation between the two. The cycle of summer and winter is one natural expression of yin and yang; on a human level, so is the daily round of work and rest.

Tai chi movements, too, are based on the interplay between yin and yang. As you become more familiar with the form, you may begin to notice how an outward or forward move is followed by an inward or backward one, and an expansive open gesture precedes a contracting closed one.

The Word Chi

The word chi, in the sense of energetic flow, is not the same as the "chi" in tai chi chuan (or tai chi as it is usually known). They are written identically in Latin script, but are completely separate terms and concepts in Chinese. The "chi" in tai chi means "ultimate" or "polarity"—and is a reference to the idea of opposite actions. Energetic chi is a notoriously hard word to render in English, but translations include "breath" and "vital force."

Taoism & Chi

The concept of chi derives from the ancient philosophy of Taoism, which is rooted in the natural world.

The story of tai chi

The book starts by describing the background to tai chi today, including what tai chi is, how it developed over time, and the main tai chi styles.

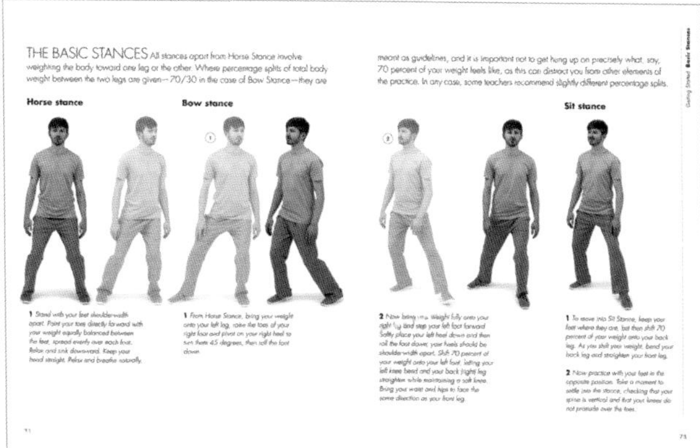

The basics

Physical and mental preparation exercises are provided to allow you to gain the most benefit from practicing tai chi.

The complete form

The bulk of the book takes you through the 37 postures that make up the Yang Short Form of tai chi. To aid continuity of movement, you will find the photograph of the current pose repeated when you turn the page.

STEP BACK TO RIDE THE TIGER In this sequence, you turn away and step backward—as if retreating from an opponent—before turning back to face him or her and bringing the right arm up as if to strike. Sink deeply into your right leg to help power the move, and make sure that your arm rises in conjunction with the waist turn.
TURN & SWEEP THE LOTUS In this complex sequence, you complete a 360-degree turn to the right followed by a sweeping kick. You begin by first turning left to help create the momentum for the clockwise turn, using the right foot as a pivot. Keep your waist relaxed as you turn.

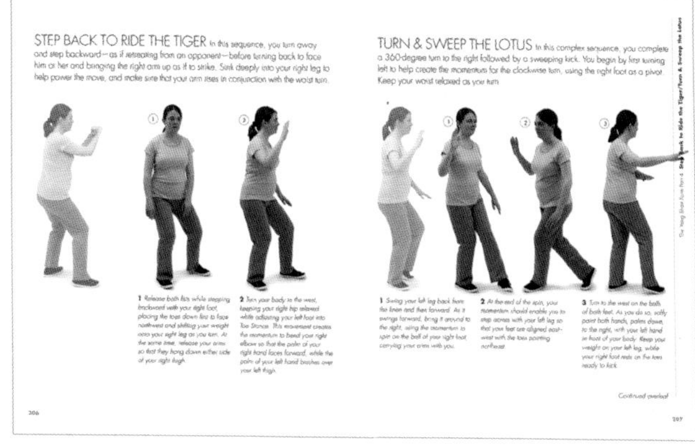

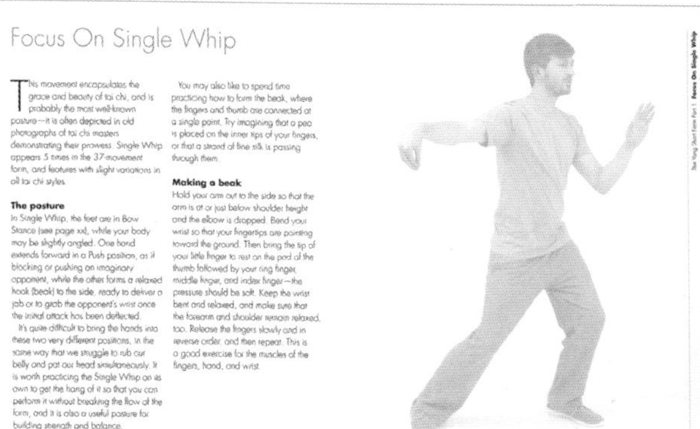

"Focus on" topics

Key movements in the form are covered in more detail to help aid your practice.

Introduction: What is Tai Chi?

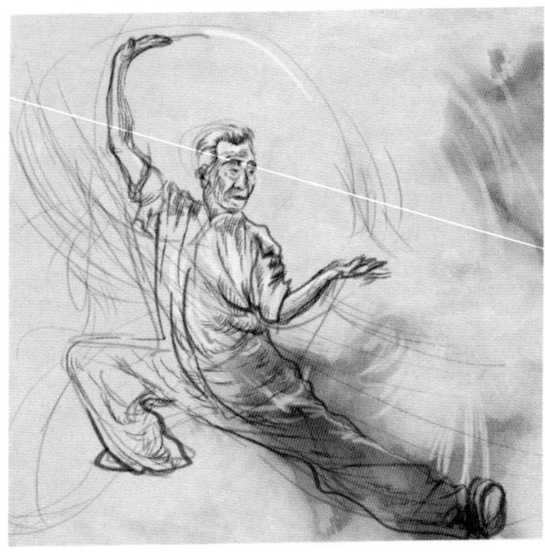

Awareness

Tai chi is a traditional martial art. However, unlike other forms of martial art, the focus is on softness and inner awareness rather than external force.

Tai chi, or *tai chi chuan* to give it its full name, is practiced as a slow and gentle mind–body system of exercise, but it is also a martial art. It originated in China, where to this day large groups of practitioners can be seen performing the movements outdoors. Over recent decades, tai chi has become popular in the West and other regions, and there are now millions of tai chi adherents worldwide.

Tai chi incorporates relaxed upright posture, slow rhythmic movements, deep breathing, and mental awareness. Each pose or sequence flows seamlessly into the next to create a graceful, dancelike progression that embodies the fundamental Chinese principles of health and movement. As such, tai chi is much more than simply a form of exercise. It is often described as "meditation in motion" and can be viewed as a complete system of self-development, wellbeing, and healing.

The Chinese approach to health and fitness is to store and regulate life energy (or *chi*) within the body, a principle that underlies other Chinese practices such as acupuncture (see page 22). Tai chi encourages us to align our bodies in a way that places minimum stress on its structures, to breathe deeply from the abdomen, and to perform relaxed movements that are designed to promote and conserve *chi*. Although tai chi is ancient in origin and is based on a fundamentally different approach from that of Western science, many research studies have confirmed its benefits. It is widely recommended by health professionals as an effective way to foster good mental and physical health.

Anyone is capable of practicing tai chi because the movements are generally very simple, and can be adapted to the particular abilities or physical health condition of the practitioner by a skilled teacher. All tai chi practitioners perform a set of movements called "the form." And although there are various styles of tai chi (see page 13), within each tradition the form is fixed and limited, with the same movements being repeated each time without any improvisation. As you gain more experience and mastery, you only go deeper into the form. In a sense, it is like being a musician who practices the same endlessly fascinating piece of music every day, always finding new nuances in it and better ways of performing it. Tai chi is easy to learn but takes a lifetime to master.

The Worldwide Traditions of Tai Chi

Usually translated as "supreme ultimate boxing," *tai chi chuan* stems from the Chinese philosophy of Taoism, which dates back at least to the third or fourth century BCE.

At the core of Taoist thought is the idea that humankind can and should live in harmony with the "Way" (*Tao* or *Dao* in Chinese). The Way cannot be apprehended intellectually because it is not a set of laws or a religious doctrine. It is something ineffable that must be lived, played out in daily life, and experienced holistically on its many levels. It is a kind of attitude, a mode of perception.

Tai chi (as tai chi chuan is generally called) is part of a physical outworking of Taoism, in particular of Taoist ideas about harmony and equilibrium. One of the central tenets of Taoism is the observation that the universe is composed of pairs of opposites: night and day; heat and cold; darkness and light; order and chaos; life and death; hardness and softness. In tai chi, these polarities manifest themselves as opposing actions, such as yielding and overcoming; advancing and retreating.

In one sense, this way of viewing the world is not so different from the scientific principle articulated by Isaac Newton, whose third law of motion states: "For every action, there is an equal and opposite reaction." But in Taoism and tai chi, the sense of duality is taken and opposites resolve into unity—"oneness is the essence," declares an ancient Tao text. In tai chi, as in life, we maintain balance by moving seamlessly between these opposites, and by recognizing that one cannot exist without the other.

The paradoxical juxtaposition of opposites and wholeness is expressed beautifully in the familiar *yin-yang* symbol where a perfect circle is both whole and divided, the black and white areas simultaneously wax and wane, and each contains the other at their core in the form of a small dot (see page 22).

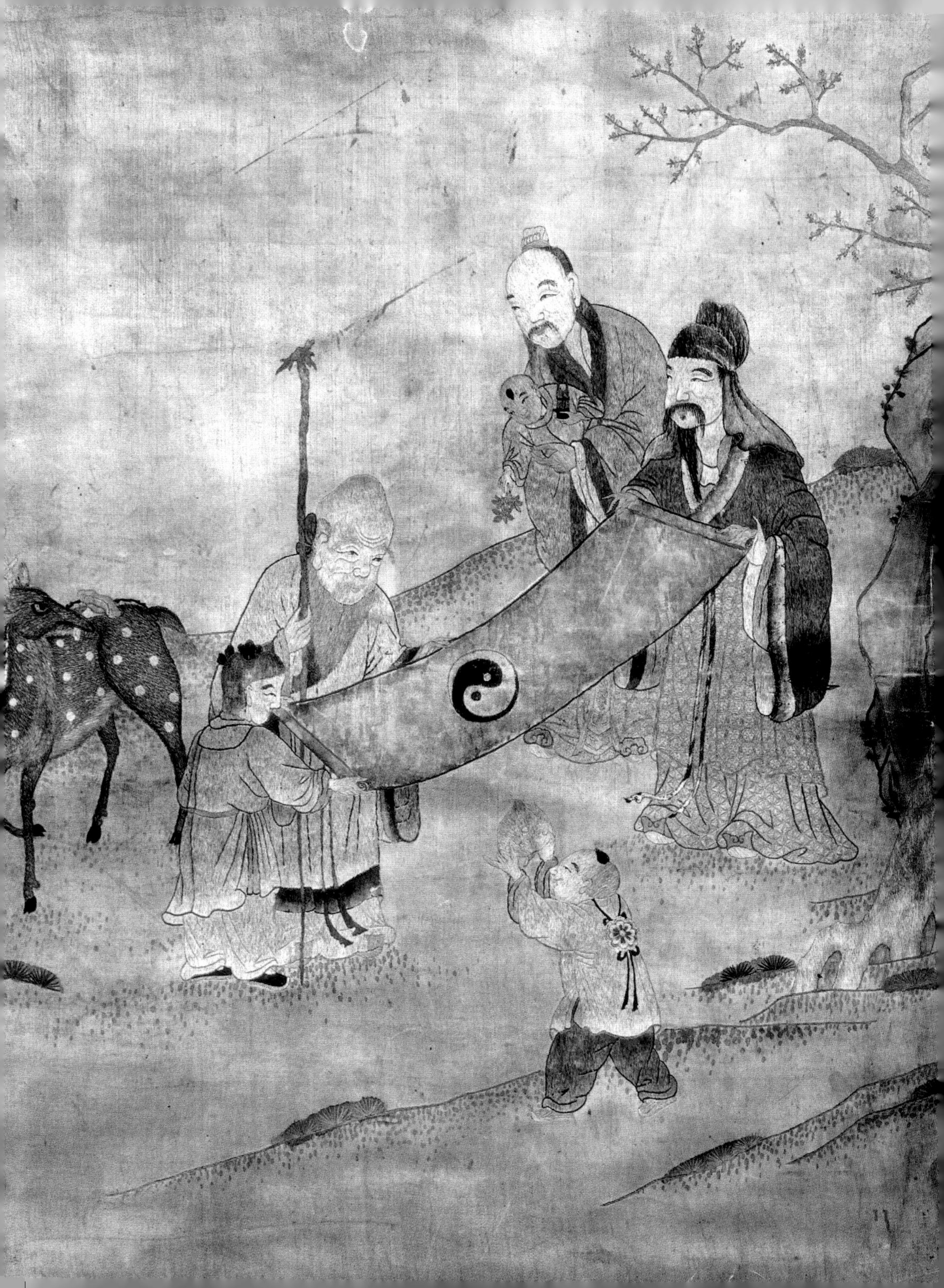

The origins of tai chi

We do not know how tai chi began, though there are various legends. These stories may not align with historical fact, but they still have something to tell us. One tale relates that a twelfth-century Taoist master named Zhang San Feng was walking in the mountains when he witnessed a fight between a crane and a snake. The crane was jabbing and lunging with its hard beak, but the snake was always able to curve and circle away using the flexibility of its body. Neither could overcome the other. Zhang took this contest as the inspiration for a new kind of martial art, one that absorbed the force of an opponent rather than countered it with an equal or greater force. This story is perhaps tai chi's respectful nod to the Taoist view of nature—a parable of sorts that teaches the required attitude to the art.

A verifiable record of tai chi does not appear until much later in time. We know for sure that by the seventeenth century the practice of tai chi was confined to one clan, the Chen, who lived in Henan Province, but it is unclear how this family came to be sole guardians of the knowledge. Here again there is a popular legend, which tells of a warriorlike Pied Piper figure who first defeated the best Chen fighters in combat, then generously shared his winning skills with the family. All modern styles of tai chi can trace their lineage back to the Chen family (see overleaf).

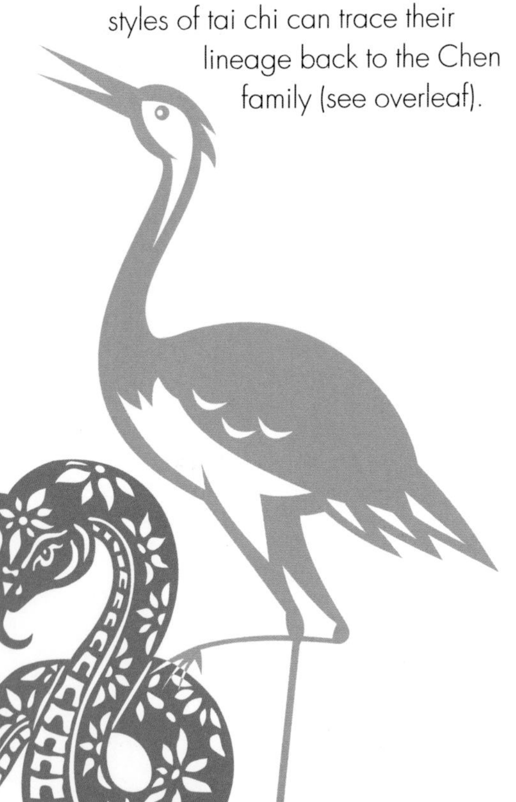

Styles of tai chi

There are five main styles of tai chi, each named for the person or family that originated it: Chen, Yang, Wu (Hao), Wu, and Sun. The most widely practiced styles are Chen, Yang, and Wu.

All tai chi styles use slow, circular movements, and emphasize the importance of a relaxed, stable posture. However, there are differences in both the pace at which the moves are performed and how expansive or compact the movements are. Tai chi continues to evolve, and even within one style there can be many variations. Some teachers practice a combination of styles, or adapt the movements to suit particular groups, such as people with arthritis.

Choosing a tai chi style

While each tai chi tradition has its idiosyncrasies and its advocates, the differences between them are less important than what the styles have in common and the benefits that they can deliver. Perhaps the key boon of all tai chi, especially for Western students, is that it facilitates wellbeing. It does this by promoting greater awareness of the body, focusing attention on the physical self and its connection to the mind and spirit.

This is something that tai chi shares with other Eastern practices such as yoga (though yoga's origins and philosophy are completely different), and it is a benefit that many of us in the West desperately need. You could say that the Western mode of thought is to divide, to isolate, and to analyze. This narrow focus, where we solve part of a problem, then the next part, and so on, is characteristic of our scientific methods and our wider culture, and it has often proved fruitful.

But somewhere along the way, we have lost sight of the wholeness and interconnectedness that is at the heart of Taoist thought. This is especially true when it comes to our bodies. So, for example, when we get a headache, we treat the pain instead of seeing the headache as the outward sign of an issue that has its roots in our entire being and therefore needs a whole-body solution. Tai chi is one way in which we can restore to ourselves our lost sense of oneness.

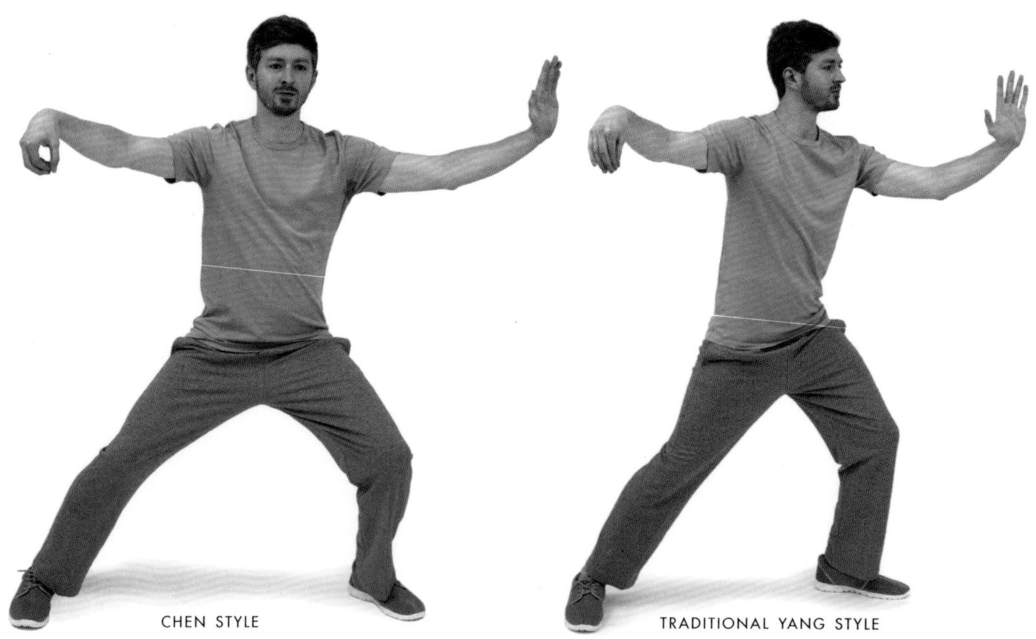

CHEN STYLE

TRADITIONAL YANG STYLE

Chen style

Chen-style tai chi is still widely practiced. It is more physically demanding than other styles, featuring broad movements and incorporating sudden bursts of speed, such as jumping kicks. These characteristics place the style close to its martial art origin—the world-famous Shaolin monastery where kung fu was born is not far away from the village of the Chen family—and make Chen style more difficult for a beginner to learn.

Yang style

One of the first people to take tai chi beyond the Chen clan was Yang Lu Chan. The story goes that Yang was a servant in the household of a Chen clan member. He was not privy to the practice, but picked it up by spying on his masters. One day he was caught, and under interrogation he was forced to demonstrate what he had seen. When Yang performed the moves perfectly, the Chen were so impressed that they invited him into their inner circle where he studied the practice for years. This tale serves to illustrate the basic tai chi principle not to counter an attack (in this case, Yang's prying), but instead to yield and absorb the aggressive act, defuse it, and own it.

Yang went on to teach the imperial guard in Beijing, and became known as "Yang the Invincible." His style of tai chi was passed down through his son

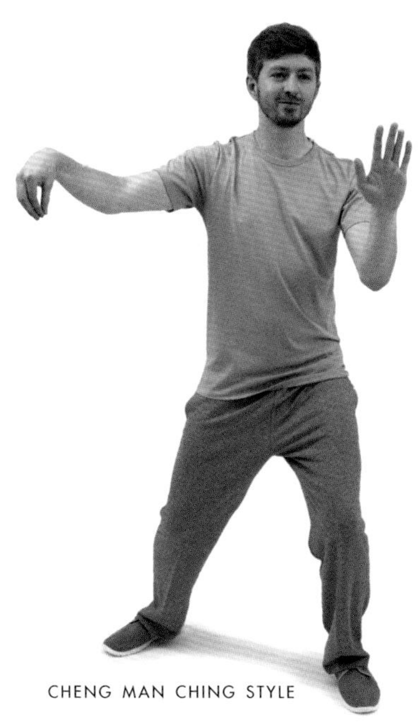

CHENG MAN CHING STYLE

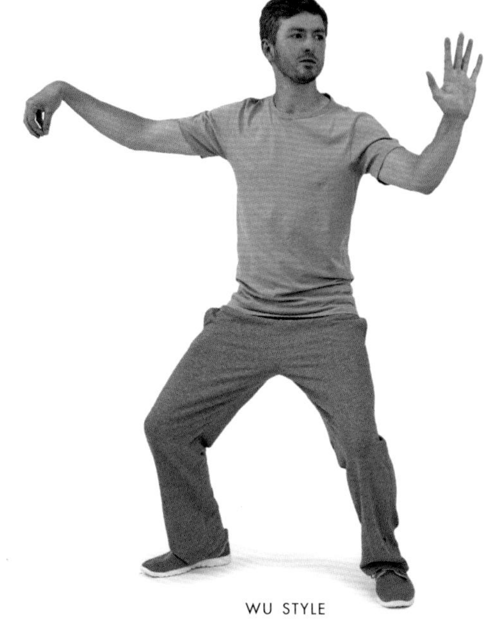

WU STYLE

and grandsons, one of whom developed a simplified system known as New Yang Style. A pupil of that grandson, Cheng Man Ching, was one of the first to bring tai chi to the West in the early 1960s. He developed a much shorter form of 37 postures that he called Yang Style Tai Chi. This form is often called Yang Short Form, and is the form described in this book.

In Yang-style tai chi, the movements are expansive and the entire form is executed at a uniform slow, fluid pace, with kicks and hand strikes performed in the same stylized, dancelike way as the rest of the form. It has become the most commonly practiced style of tai chi worldwide. Cheng Man Ching was also a physician and used tai chi to aid his recovery from tuberculosis, and his form emphasizes the health-giving benefits of tai chi.

Wu style

Other styles came into being after Yang had been established, and Wu style is the most important of these, which was founded by a guard at the imperial court in Beijing, where Yang Lu Chan was teaching his style of tai chi (see above). It is sometimes said that the Wu style—characterized by smaller, less expansive movements and a more emphatic planting of the feet—was influenced by the fact that it was designed to be performed in restrictive military uniforms. Certainly there is an element of contained power or restrained force to this style, which is one of the most popular after Yang style.

TAI CHI FUNDAMENTALS

Tai chi is very different from Western forms of exercise and from other Eastern practices such as yoga. Before you begin to learn tai chi, you need to understand some of the essential principles behind tai chi movement. This chapter introduces you to them, and demonstrates some simple exercises to put them into practice. It also includes ways to develop a tai chi attitude, which you can bring to other aspects of your daily life.

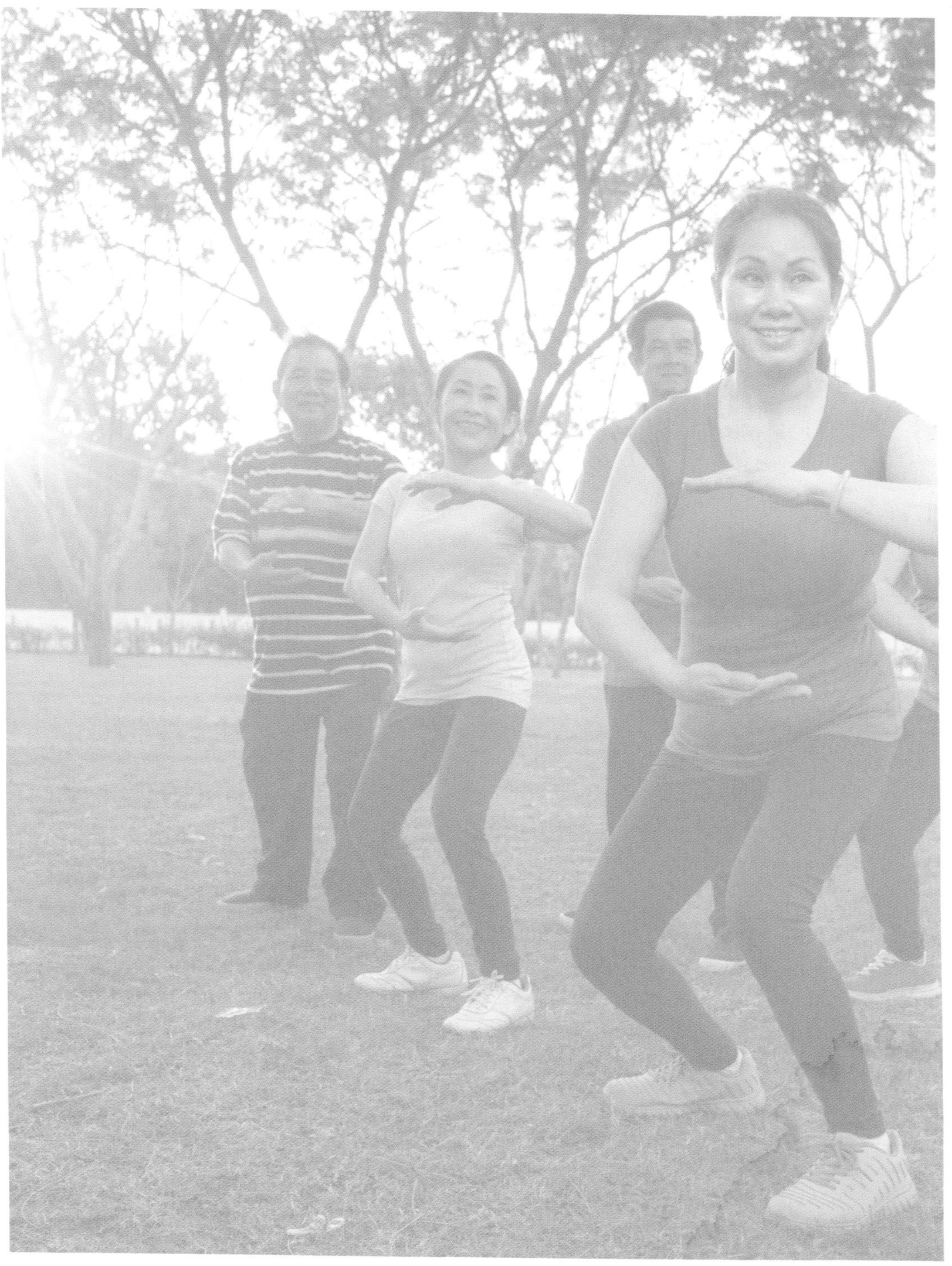

The Benefits of Tai Chi

Tai chi is a noncompetitive martial art that is widely practiced as a form of meditative movement. Millions of people practice tai chi for its health and relaxation benefits, and countless studies attest to its effectiveness. Tai chi is much gentler and slower than most forms of exercise, but it offers many of the key gains that more intense workouts offer. These include:

Balance In tai chi, you continually shift your weight from one leg to the other while maintaining a stable base. This helps to improve everyday balance skills. Tai chi also promotes proprioception—the ability to sense one's own movement and position of the body—which is something that naturally declines with age. Studies have consistently shown that elderly practitioners of tai chi are far less likely to suffer a fall.

Strength and endurance Tai chi increases muscle tone, primarily in the knees and legs, but in the upper body and arms, too.

Flexibility The range of movements increases general mobility. And because tai chi is a low-impact form of exercise, it does not place undue strain on the joints.

Better breathing Tai chi involves deep (abdominal) breathing, which improves cardiac and respiratory fitness, though you will probably need to do a more aerobic form of exercise as well. Some studies have found that tai chi can reduce high blood pressure.

Posture Maintaining a vertical spine is integral to tai chi. Many practitioners notice an improvement in their day-to-day posture after practicing tai chi regularly. Better posture reduces back pain and encourages the body's organs to work more efficiently.

Reducing stress

Tai chi helps with relaxation, and is a useful antidote to the high-pressure, high-tech world in which we live. A review of 40 studies concluded that tai chi was associated with improved psychological wellbeing and feelings of self-esteem. And a 2016 study at the University of California, Irvine found that practicing tai chi increased the number of neurons in the area of the brain that regulates the emotions (the hippocampus), helping to suppress the stress response.

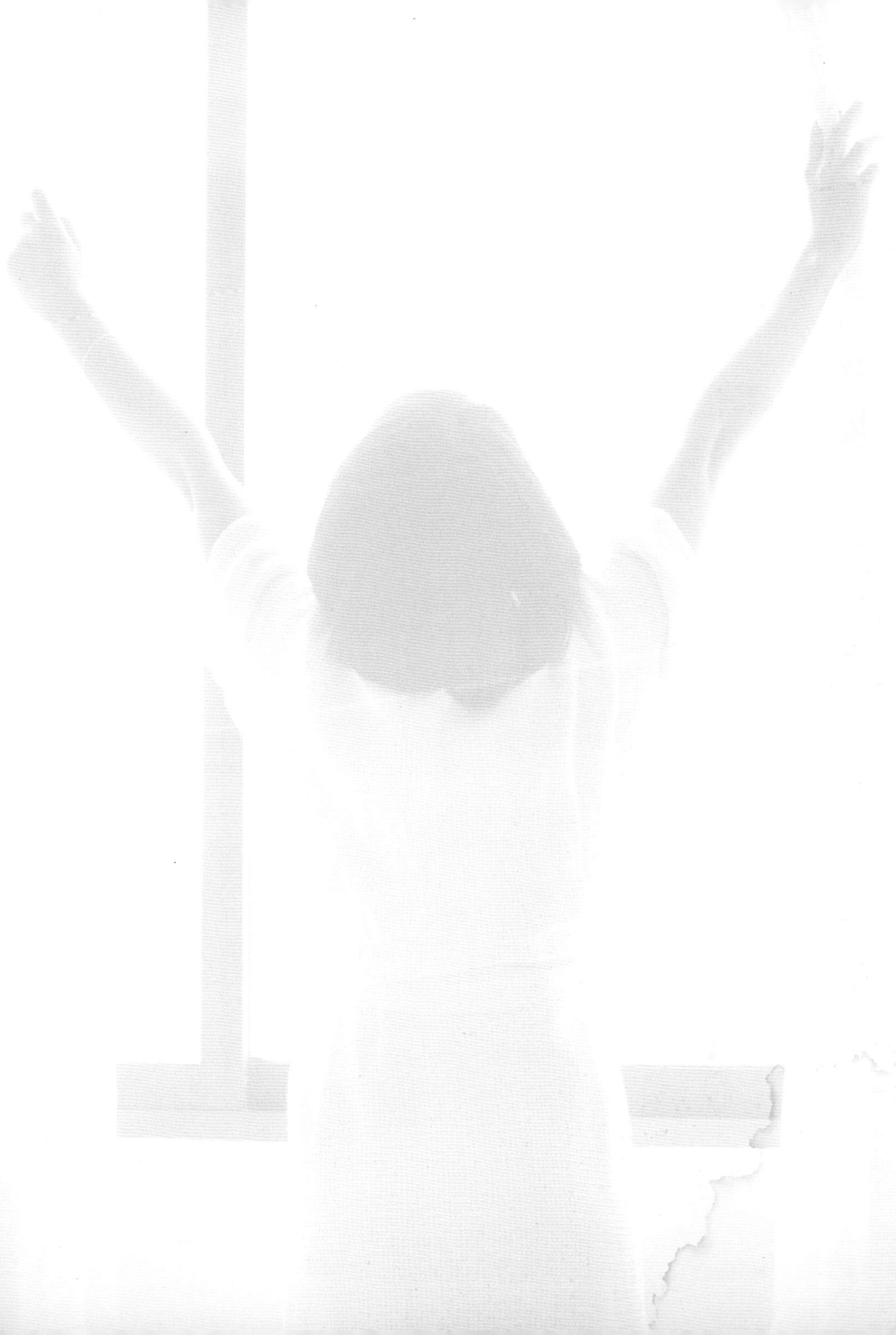

BREATHING FROM THE BELLY

Slow, deep breathing is integral to the practice of tai chi. The breathing is natural and comes from the belly—abdominal or diaphragmatic breathing. This is the relaxed and efficient breathing that we do as

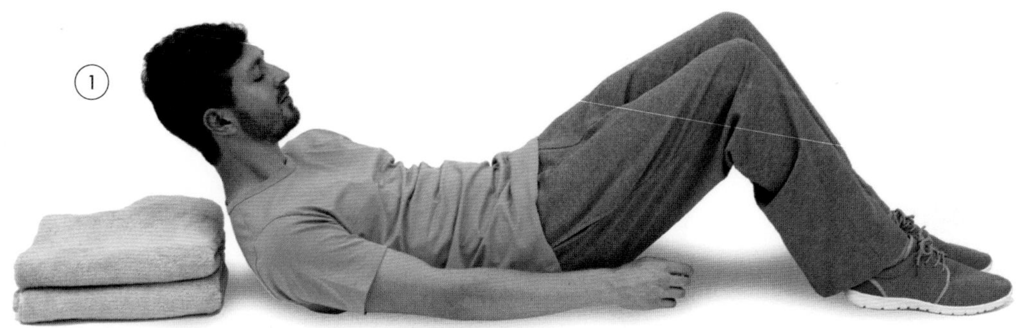

Focus & Movement

It can be helpful to place a book on your belly to help focus your mind and also enable you to feel the movement of your abdomen more easily.

1 *Lie on the floor with your legs bent at the knee and your feet flat on the ground. Lift your head and look down the length of your body to check that it is straight. Then place the back of your head on the ground (or on a soft cushion).*

babies, but in adulthood many of us develop a habit of shallow breathing, often due to stress or poor posture. Try this abdominal breathing exercise lying down, which is also a useful relaxation exercise that you can use.

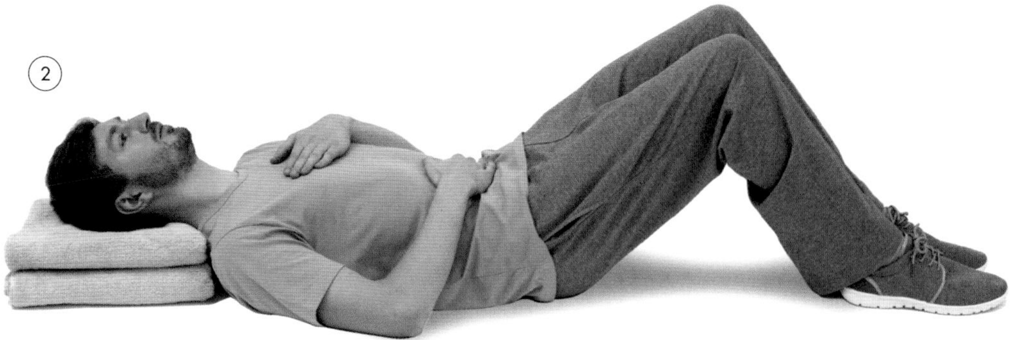

2 *Place one hand on your belly, under the navel, and one on the top of your chest. Close your mouth and take a long, slow, deep breath in through the nostrils. The lower hand should move as you breathe, while the upper hand should remain still.*

3 *If you find that your top hand moves, then you are breathing from the chest rather than the belly. Try this: As you take a breath, visualize it traveling through your nostrils, down the back of your throat, past the lungs, and into your belly. Let your lower abdomen relax and expand as the breath arrives. Then as you breathe out, imagine that the breath begins in your lower abdomen and travels upward through your body.*

4 *Once you feel you are breathing from the belly, continue in this way for several minutes.*

The Theory of Tai Chi

Tai chi is a physical practice that is as graceful as ballet, yet its movements are all about hand-to-hand combat. It builds strength, balance, stamina, and flexibility, and therefore functions as a physical workout, yet tai chi does not tire you. Instead it leaves you both more energetic and more relaxed. Tai chi practitioners ascribe this opposing effect down to the elusive life force energy called *chi*.

In Chinese philosophy and medicine, both mental and physical health are dependent on the balanced flow of *chi* through the body. Acupuncture, reiki, and shiatsu are all methods of releasing blockages in the flow of *chi* through the body. Tai chi, and the related discipline of chi kung, use choreographed movement and breathing to the same end. *Chi* is held to be everywhere, not just inside the body. So the art of feng shui, for example, is about promoting the flow of healthy *chi* in our homes and in the wider environment.

Yin & Yang

Chi is not a static force. It is fluid and dynamic, like electricity or magnetism. And like electromagnetism, it relies on polar opposites. In Chinese thinking, these polarities are known as *yin* and *yang*. *Yin* energy is receptive, inward, and soft, whereas *yang* energy is active and outward looking. Balance comes from a constant oscillation between the two. The cycle of summer and winter is one natural expression of *yin* and *yang*; on a human level, so is the daily round of work and rest.

Tai chi movements, too, are based on the interplay between *yin* and *yang*. As you become more familiar with the form, you may begin to notice how an outward or forward move is followed by an inward or backward one, and an expansive open gesture precedes a contracting closed one.

Taoism & Chi

The concept of chi *derives from the ancient philosophy of Taoism, which is rooted in the natural world.*

Chi

The word *chi*, in the sense of energetic flow, is not the same as the "chi" in *tai chi chuan* (or tai chi as it is usually known). They are written identically in Latin script, but are completely separate terms and concepts in Chinese. The "chi" in tai chi means "ultimate" or "polarity"—and is a reference to the idea of opposite actions. Energetic *chi* is a notoriously hard word to render in English, but translations include "breath" and "vital force."

ACCESSING THE *DANTIEN*

Chi flows through the body via a series of interconnected channels or meridians. There are also said to be three main energy centers—the upper, middle, and lower *dantiens*—which serve as a focal point for meditation and for energetic practices such as tai chi. The lower *dantien* is in the belly, and is held to be the body's physical center, so it is the most important for the purposes of tai chi. Tai chi practitioners direct their movements from this spot in order to unlock their inner power and create fluid movement. Try this breathing exercise to connect with the lower *dantien*, referred to in the rest of the book as "the *dantien*" for simplicity.

1 *Take a comfortable seated or standing position. Sit or stand up straight, as if there were a cord attached to the top of your head pulling you upright. Lower your chin slightly. Take a deep breath, and as you exhale, let your body relax but maintain your upright stance.*

2 *Place one hand gently on the other on your belly, just under your navel. Don't press. Breathe in and out, being aware of the gentle rising and falling of your hands.*

3 *Imagine that you are breathing in energy from the atmosphere and directing it to a point about two to three thumb widths below the navel and two to three thumb widths inside the body (this is the location of the dantien). As you breathe out, relax and empty the whole of the chest—imagine you are breathing out through a straw, which will make your lower muscles become taut around your center.*

4 *Keep breathing in and out of your dantien for 5 to 10 minutes, gently directing your attention back here whenever you notice you have become distracted. Don't worry about whether you feel an energetic connection or not; this takes time.*

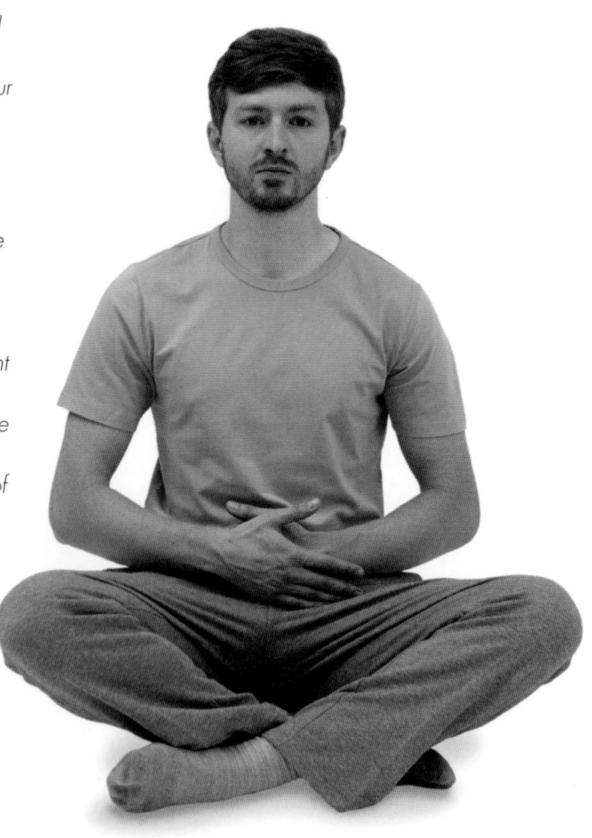

The *dantiens*

The three *dantiens* are sited along the midline of the body: One is between the eyes, the next in the middle of the chest, and the third —the lower dantien—is in the lower abdomen.

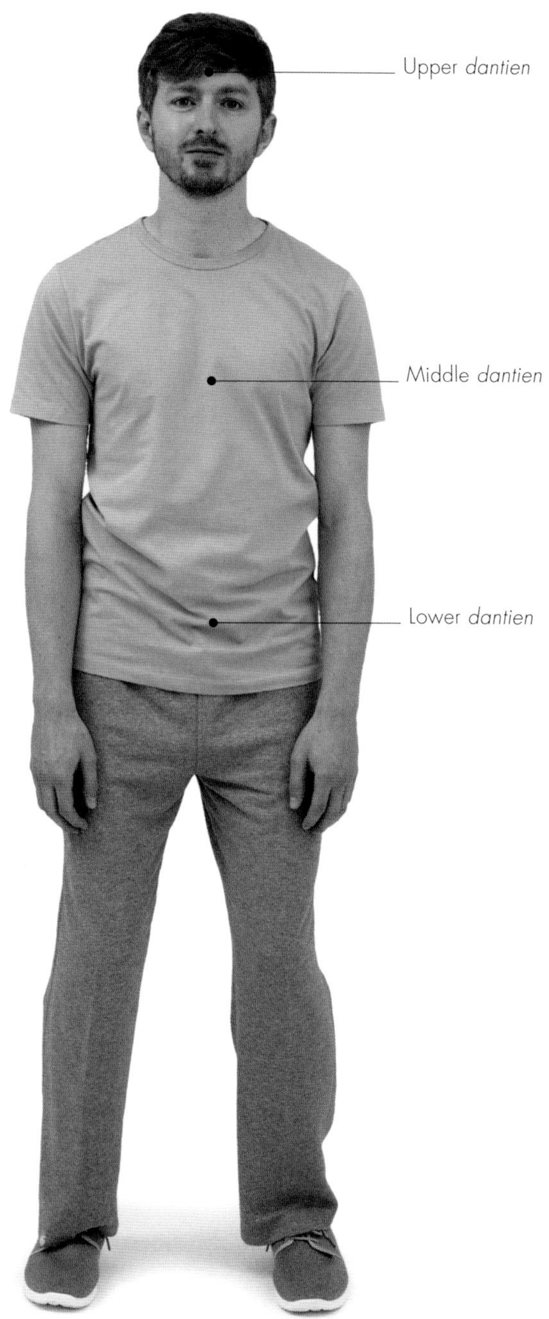

Foundation Principles of Tai Chi

Cheng Man Ching, tai chi master and the originator of the 37-movement tai chi form followed in this book (see page 15), identified five principles or universals that apply to all tai chi movements. They are intended to promote the flow of *chi* through the body and develop inner power.

Relaxation/sinking

This is the core principle of tai chi—there is no forcing and no tension. When we relax the muscles, we are able to sink into the correct posture. We also sink the body closer to the ground by bending the knees. The legs and feet feel stable and well connected to the ground. The upper body, meanwhile, is light and flexible, with the shoulders relaxed, the elbows dropped, and the chest slightly sunk inward. All the joints are loose and soft, never locked.

Straight spine

The spine is straight, with the tailbone tucked in; the neck and head are in alignment with the spine, with the chin tucked in. This pose elongates the spine and places the minimum amount of stress on it, enabling greater ease in movement.

Moving from the waist

In tai chi, the waist denotes the area extending from the hips to the lower ribs above, so it incorporates not only the *dantien* but also the lower back. When you direct your movements from this area, the whole body is involved in the movement, and power is transferred from the lower body into the upper body and out through the hands and fingers.

Separating weight

In tai chi, weight is not equally balanced between the legs. Except at the very start of the form, the weight is always on one leg or the other. The continual shifting of weight creates the fluidity of movement that is a characteristic of tai chi. When all your weight is on one leg, it is termed "full"; the weightless leg, meanwhile, is termed "empty."

Beautiful hands

In tai chi, the hands are always held in a relaxed position, with the fingers naturally curved rather than rigidly straight. The hands form a straight line with the arm, which improves the flow of *chi* through them. Cheng Man Ching called them "beautiful lady hands."

Encouraging relaxation

The sense of relaxation from beautiful hands should permeate through the arms and into the rest of the body.

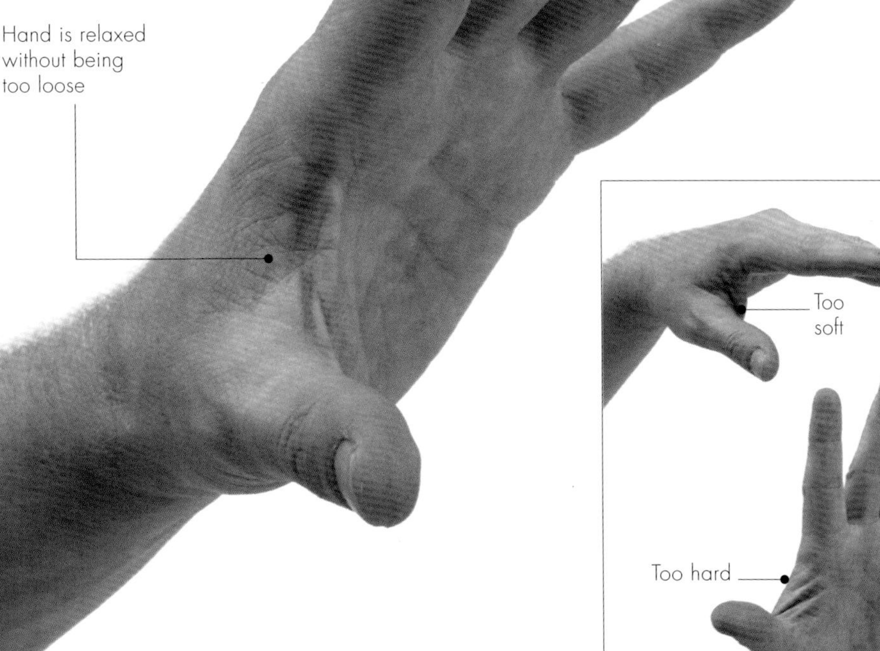

TAI CHI POSTURE

Practice this simple standing exercise daily to perfect your tai chi posture. Do it barefoot, or wear thin, flexible-soled tai chi shoes or sneakers.

1 *Stand tall with both feet flat on the ground, hip-width apart, facing forward.*

2 *Note where the soles of your feet make contact with the ground. Shift your weight onto the balls of your feet and back to your heels a few times before coming to a position that feels equally balanced.*

3 *Shift from the inside to the outside of your soles a few times to find the same balance laterally. The entire foot should be in contact with the ground.*

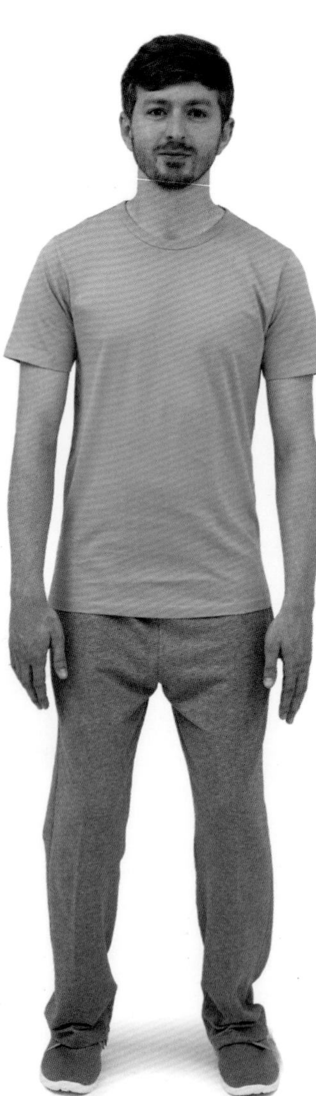

4 *Softly bend your knees, as if about to sit down. Make sure that they face directly forward, like the toes. To avoid strain, do not push the knees out farther than the toes.*

5 *Imagine that a weight on a cord is attached to your tailbone pulling it downward. This has the effect of tucking in the tailbone, which helps to lengthen the spine.*

6 *Imagine that a similar cord is attached to the top of your head from which you are suspended. Pull the chin slightly back and down. This helps elongate the upper spine. Relax the shoulders, letting them drop down and slightly forward.*

7 *Bring the arms away from the body slightly, making a space in the armpits. Round your arms—do not lock the elbows. Keep your hands softly relaxed with the fingers apart.*

8 *Place your tongue on the hard palate above your front teeth (try saying "l-l-l-l" to find the right position). Close your mouth and relax your jaw. Breathe naturally through your nostrils.*

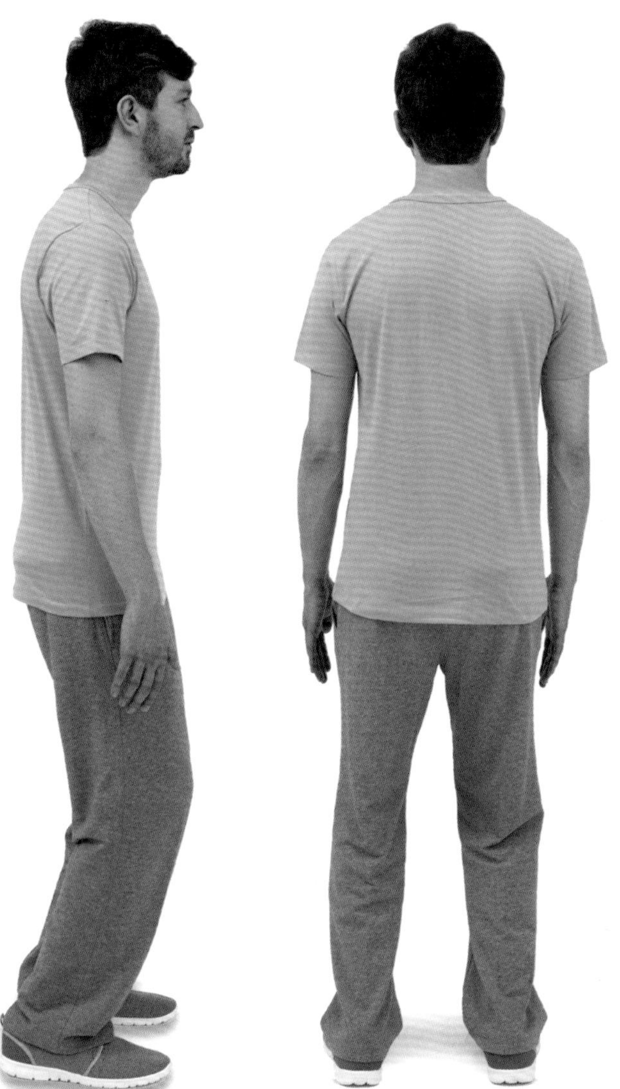

TRANSFERRING WEIGHT

In tai chi, your body weight is always loaded toward one leg or the other. You must be able to transfer your weight easily between them, as if pouring sand from one tall jar to another.

1 *Stand with your feet parallel and hip-distance apart. Take some time to run through the checklist for tai chi posture on pages 28–29. Breathe naturally through your nostrils. Make sure that you "sit into" your legs by bending the knees and imagining the spine dropping downward.*

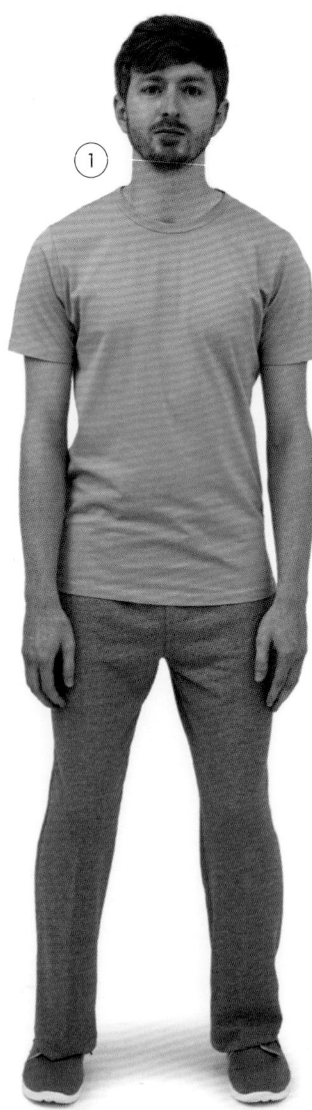

2 *Focus on your right foot, bringing all your attention to the contact that it makes with the ground. Slowly transfer your weight onto this foot, bending your knee to facilitate it. Make sure that your right knee stays in line with the foot and does not extend past the toes. Imagine that your inward breath is traveling through your body and out through the sole of your foot, rooting it into the ground. Notice that your weight comes into the right hip and all the way down the leg, while the left hip softens and relaxes.*

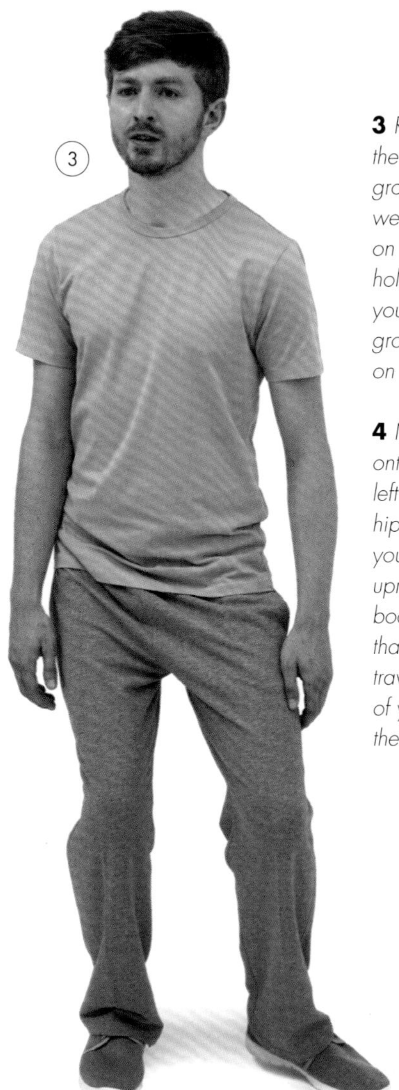

3 *Raise your left heel, leaving the ball of your foot on the ground without holding any weight there. Keep your focus on your rooted right foot and hold for a few moments. Roll your left foot back onto the ground, keeping your weight on your right foot.*

4 *Now slowly shift your weight onto your left foot, bending your left knee and noticing your right hip relax as the weight shifts to your left. Keep your spine upright and watch that your body does not rise up. Imagine that your inward breath is traveling out through the sole of your left foot, rooting it into the ground.*

5 *Once your weight is on your left foot, raise your right heel, resting on the ball. Keep your focus on your rooted left foot and hold for a few moments before bringing your weight back to the center.*

Weight Testing

To check that your weight is fully loaded onto the supporting foot, raise your "empty" foot to see if you wobble. Your balance will improve with regular practice.

Further Principles

There are some supplemental principles that complement Cheng Man Ching's five constants. It is helpful to bear these in mind and integrate them into the tai chi movements.

Take it slow

Tai chi movements are performed very slowly and evenly. It helps to imagine that you are moving against some invisible force such as water (tai chi is often described as swimming in air). But at no point in tai chi do you come to a standstill—let each movement flow seamlessly into the next.

Think circles

There are no corners or straight lines in tai chi. The knees and elbows are softly bent so that the limbs are curved. This promotes smooth movement and the unimpeded flow of chi through the body.

Rooting

In tai chi, strength and stability come from rooting yourself in the ground like a tree. The physical relaxation/sinking (see page 26) is part of it, but rooting is also a mental process. Imagine that your body weight is in your belly and legs rather than your upper body.

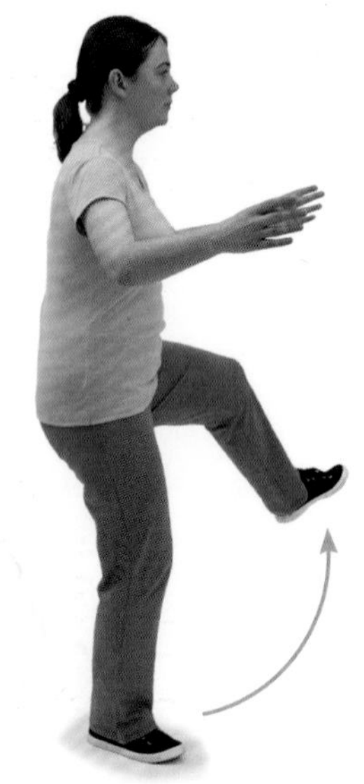

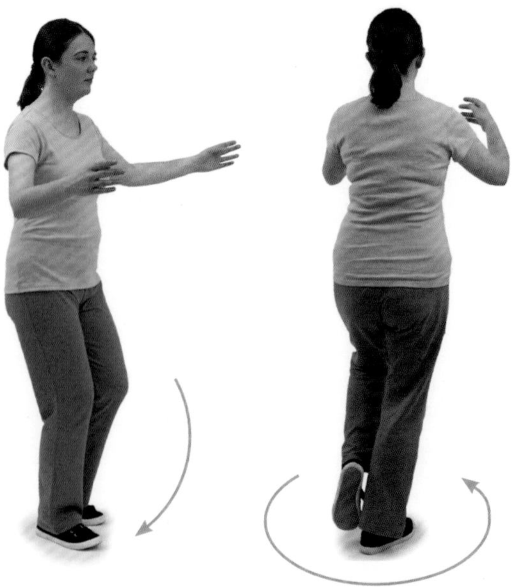

Whole-body movements

In tai chi, every movement begins from the feet, which are rooted in the ground. After that, the motion flows upward through the body, transferring smoothly and fluidly from one part to the next—from the legs to the waist, from the waist to the spine, and then to the chest, the arms, and the hands. It is as if the energy were literally a kind of liquid, rising like a spring and issuing through your fingertips.

Relaxed attitude

You cannot practice tai chi while thinking about something else. The mind must be calm and fully conscious of the body, setting the intention to move before the movement itself unfolds. Tai chi is mindfulness in motion—you are conscious of the present moment, neither thinking of the previous action nor looking forward to the next one. This also helps you to be patient with yourself and treat your body with kindness. A relaxed mind encourages a relaxed body, and vice versa.

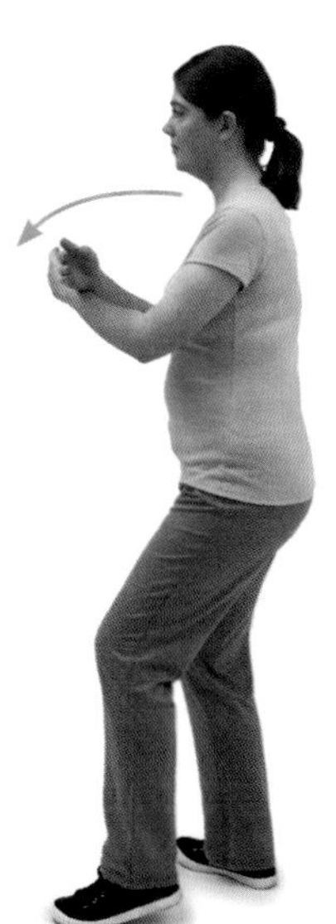

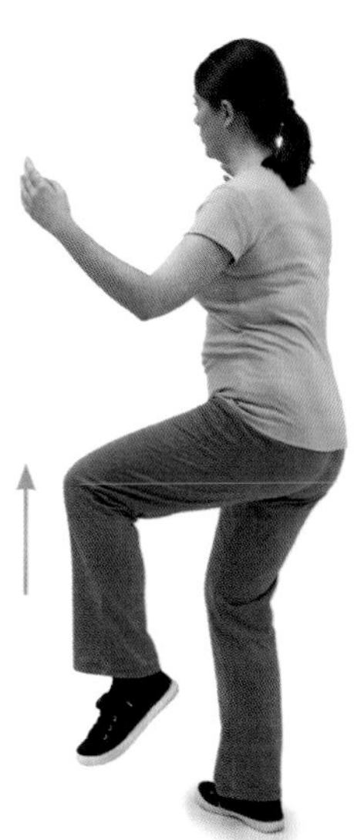

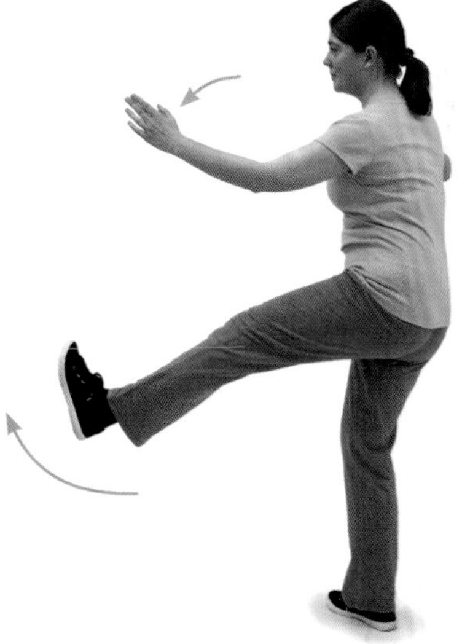

TAI CHI WALKING

This wonderfully meditative exercise quietens the mind, and is a good way to start integrating the elements of tai chi movement. You will need a clear area that is at least 33 ft. (10 m) long and free from obstacles—a grass area or a corridor perhaps.

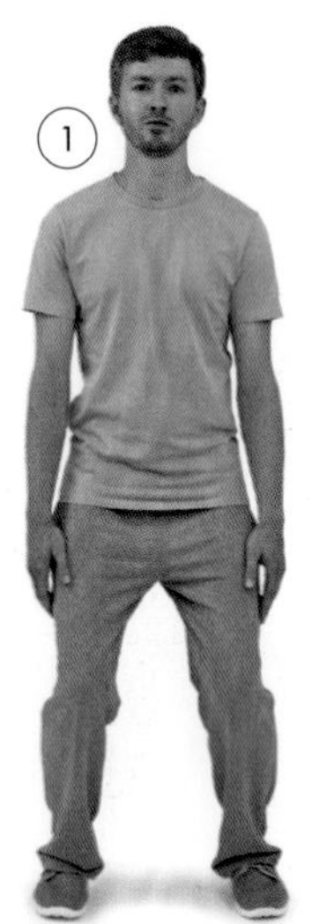

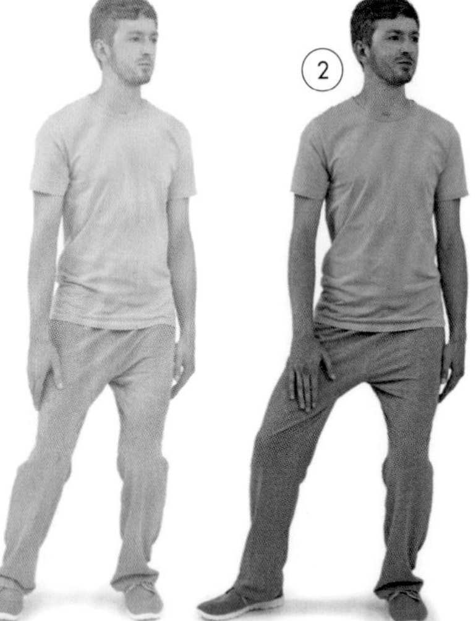

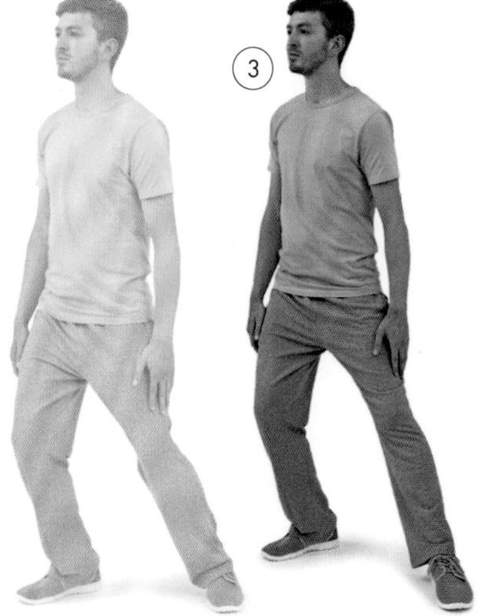

1 *Stand at one end of the walkway, feet shoulder-width apart, knees bent, and your weight sunk downward in tai chi posture* *(see page xx)**.*

2 *Shift your weight onto your left leg, then lift your right toes off the ground. Pivot on your right heel to turn your toes out by 45 degrees, keeping your weight on your left leg.*

3 *Then shift your weight fully onto your right foot. Bring your left heel off the ground. Take a step forward and out with your left leg. Put the heel down first before rolling down the rest of the foot, toes pointing directly forward.*

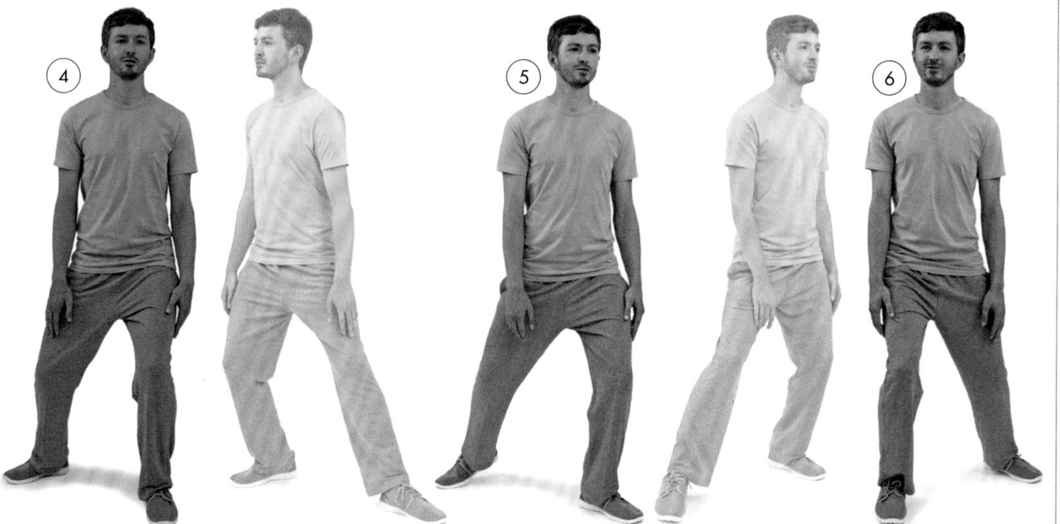

4 *Shift your weight onto your left leg.*

5 *Then bring your weight back onto the back (right) leg. Raise the front (left) toes off the ground and pivot on your heel to turn them out by 45 degrees. Roll down your left foot and bring your weight fully onto your left leg again.*

6 *Now take a step with your right leg in exactly the same manner as you did with the left, placing your heel first, shifting the weight, and then pivoting. Continue stepping in this way the length of the walkway, keeping focused.*

Developing a Tai Chi Attitude

The practice of tai chi encourages us to align our bodies in a way that places least stress on them, and to breathe deeply from the abdomen. Both the alignment and the breathing are part of the natural way—it is what we are designed to do. We can incorporate these principles and the other fundamentals of tai chi into our lives on a much wider level, as well as when performing the tai chi form itself.

Chi walking

The ancients instinctively understood that spending time outdoors rejuvenated the mind and body, and countless scientific studies have confirmed that taking a walk in a park or spending time in a garden relieves stress and improves wellbeing. Try to walk in natural surroundings, where *chi* is powerful, every day—20 minutes outdoors is enough to increase feelings of vitality. As you walk, practice deep abdominal breathing (see page 20). Try to imagine that energy is traveling up the spine as you breathe in, and then down the front of your spine to the pubic bone as you breathe out.

It can be helpful to have reminders of nature around you when you are inside too—research shows that just looking at natural images can give you a boost. For example, office workers who have a view of nature are less stressed than those who do not. Even looking at images of natural phenomena has been shown to give a wider perspective on life.

Embrace the yin

Our ancestors rose with the sun and retired as it went down. They were naturally in tune with the daily *yin-yang* cycle of work and rest. But technology means that our world is now disconnected from that—we can be on the go any time of day or night. So give priority to resting as well as to activity. It is helpful to work out what time you need to go to bed in order to get the required amount of sleep (most adults need at least seven hours a night), then to set a winding-down alert a couple of hours before bedtime. Make a point of avoiding high-energy or screen-based activities after this time and focus on gentle, relaxing ones. If possible, dim the lights to start priming your body for rest.

TAI CHI MOMENTS We all need to find spaces in our frenetic lives when we can slow down. Tai chi practice can help us to do this, and you can also find other ways to introduce a slower pace into your day. Try leaving your home five minutes earlier so that your journey to the station or the office can be done in a less hurried way. Treat this time as an opportunity to be aware of yourself as you move through your surroundings. Here are some other ways to introduce a tai chi attitude into your routine.

Sink into the ground

When standing while using public transportation, bend your knees and sink your weight downward. You will find that this gives you better stability, which makes it easier to keep your balance on a jerky journey.

Waiting in line is a good place for tai chi standing, and also to practice shifting weight from one leg to another (see pages 30–31). In fact, you can do this in any idle spare moment—for example, when waiting for the computer to boot up.

Sit like a tai chi master

When you sit at a desk, take a moment to put your spine in a perfectly erect position, with your head and neck aligned. Bring to mind once more the imaginary cord that is attached to the top of the crown (see page 28). Feel it gently pulling you upward, or imagine that your crown is touching the sky. Create a stable base by having both feet flat on the floor and thinking about the other point of contact—where your buttocks rest on the chair. Check that they are level. Sit near the front of the chair so that you are not tempted to lean back, and place your knees slightly lower than your hips, because this encourages an upright spine. This is the ideal position in which to practice meditation or breathing exercises—take three deep breaths into the abdomen before you start.

Check & sink

Make a habit of checking in with yourself at regular points through the day, wherever you are and whatever you are doing. Check your alignment—are you twisting awkwardly or in discomfort? Run through the principles of tai chi posture (see page 28), take one deep breath into the *dantien* (see page 24), and sink into a better posture.

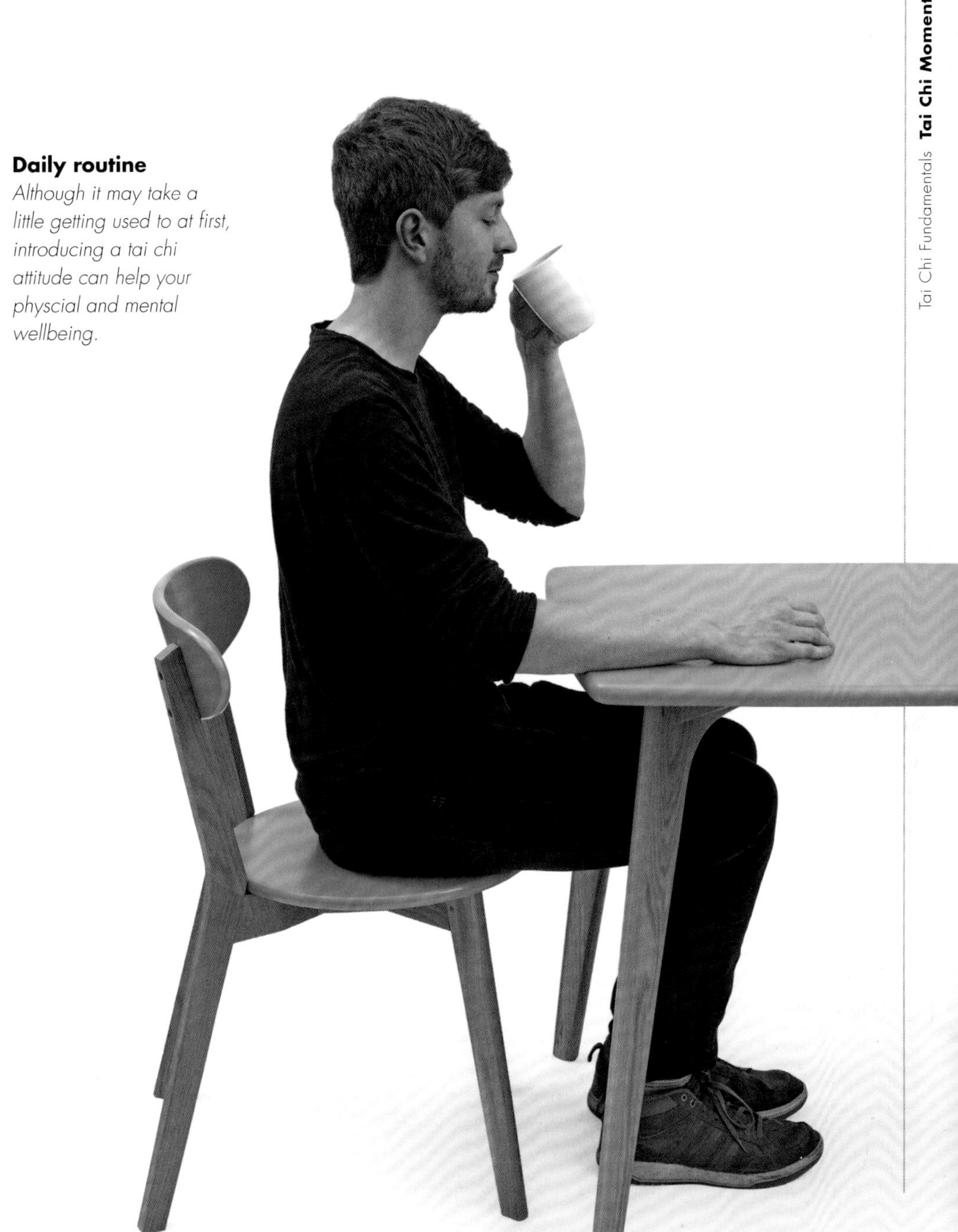

Daily routine

Although it may take a little getting used to at first, introducing a tai chi attitude can help your physcial and mental wellbeing.

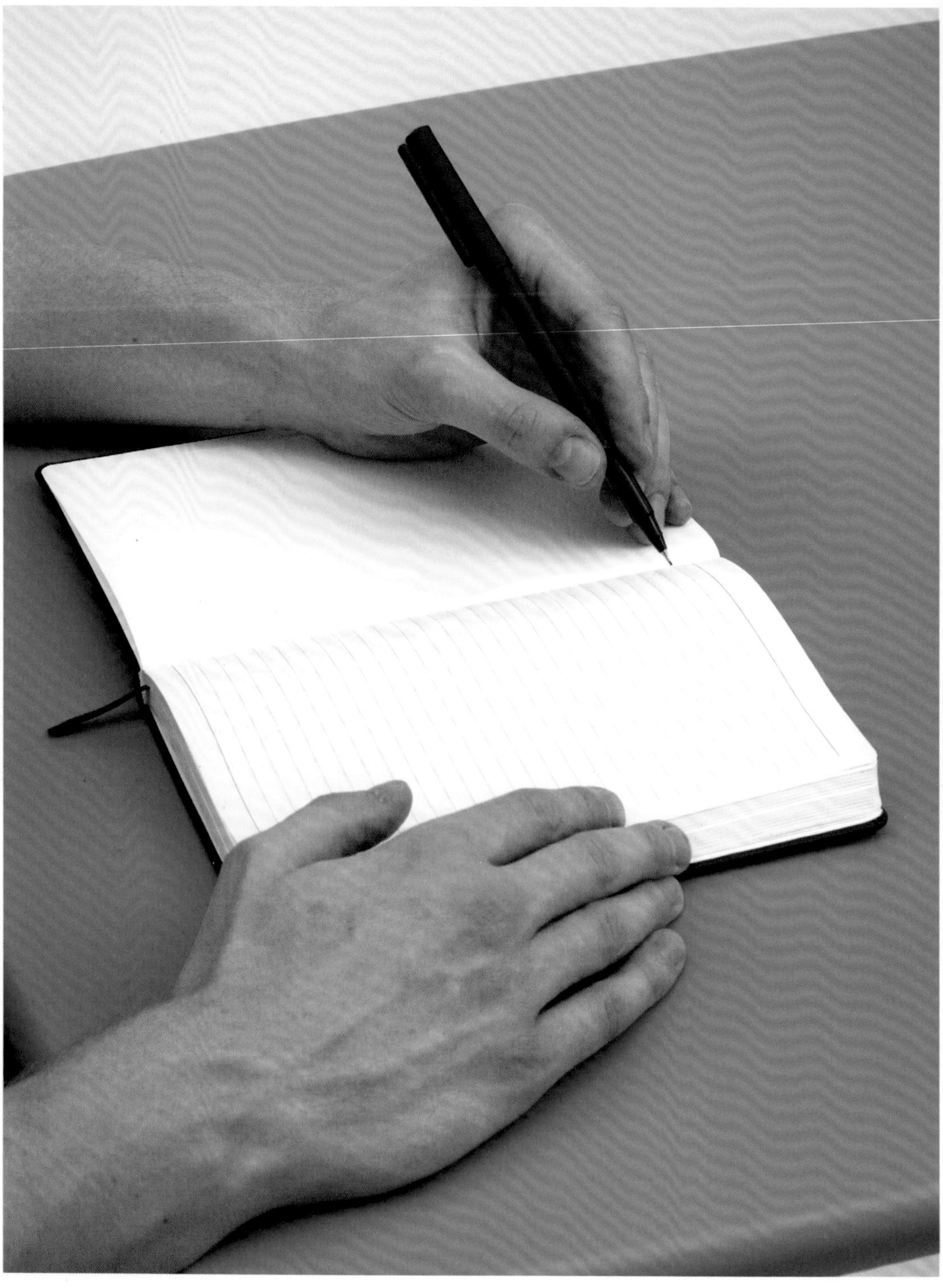

Minimum effort

Most of us put superfluous energy into small daily action. So, for example, we might grip the steering wheel so hard that we cause tension in our arms and shoulders. Tai chi teaches us that strength is not the same as brute force. Paradoxical as it may seem, true strength requires softness and flexibility. Try bringing greater softness into daily activities—if you are cleaning your teeth, try to hold your brush as softly as possible; when writing, explore the extent to which you can reduce the tension in your hand while still being able to control the pen. This may help reveal the unnecessary exertion that you invest in routine activities.

Integrated movements

Tai chi teaches us that the whole body is involved in physical tasks, or should be. Pick a task to practice working with the whole body rather than just your arm or hand. Ironing might be a good one to try—check that you are firmly rooted and see if you can move from the waist instead of the shoulder. Remain focused on your movements as you work. You can also do this when stepping forward to open a door. As your hand grasps the handle, shift your weight onto your back leg so that the backward movement of your body helps bring the door toward you with minimal effort in the hand and arm.

And breathe . . .

When you get up in the morning, try sitting on the edge of the bed and practicing breathing into the *dantien* (see page 24). It's a great way to start the day (or to end it). You can rest one palm on the other just under the navel and keep your attention on the movements of your belly as you breathe in and out, just as you do in standing posture (see page 28).

Or try bending your arms so that your hands are at *dantien* height, palms facing in. Then as you breathe in, open the forearms out, as if your hands were the leaves of a double door as it opens. As you breathe out, bring the arms back toward you. Play with the idea of drawing energy inward as you inhale, and releasing it outward as you exhale.

Staying soft

Bringing softness into common activities such as writing or typing may help to reduce the stress you are constantly putting on your joints.

GETTING STARTED

You need very little in terms of facilities and kit to start practicing tai chi, and this chapter guides you through the essentials. It also gives advice on how to develop an effective home practice, as well as how to find a good teacher of tai chi. Although tai chi is very gentle, nevertheless it is a form of exercise that will test your body in perhaps unfamiliar ways. Preliminary exercises and stretches are included to help you warm up before you begin the tai chi form, and ensure that you get the most from your practice.

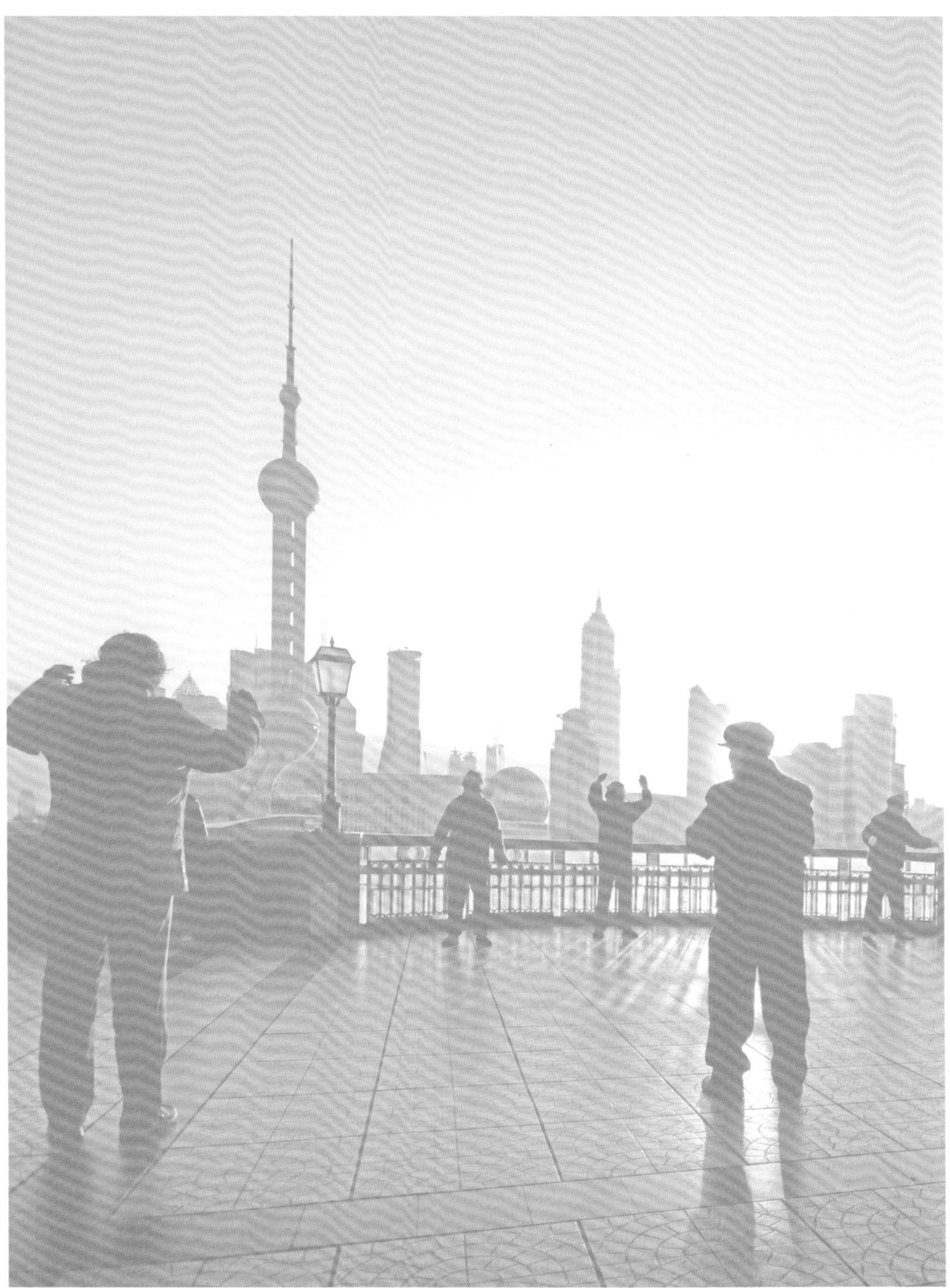

When & Where to Practice

To practice tai chi, use any space that is clear from obstacles and large enough to enable you to progress through the complete form as you step from side to side and back and forth. It is often said that tai chi is best practiced outdoors, in a tranquil natural space where the chi flows freely. Many people like to practice their tai chi in a park or other public space—it is a common sight in China to see groups of people doing tai chi in public areas. However, when you are first learning tai chi, you will probably feel more comfortable in a private space where you are not observed. If you want to practice outside, then an area of backyard would be suitable.

When practicing inside, it's more pleasurable—and more conducive to a relaxed practice—if the room is clean and free from clutter. Make sure that it is well aired and, if possible, naturally lit. You may like to make a point of having houseplants or flowers in this space or other items that help you to feel peaceful. Some people like to practice tai chi to soft music, or to play a recording of the sounds of nature.

What to wear

You don't need any special clothes to practice tai chi, but you do need to be comfortable and warm, and able to move freely. So wear jogging pants or leggings, and a loose top. Go barefoot, as long as the ground is suitable, or invest in a pair of flexible, thin-soled tai chi shoes or sneakers.

When to practice

Tai chi should be practiced regularly, at least four times a week and ideally every day. Traditionally, tai chi is practiced in the morning, because at sunrise the yin energy of the night shifts to the yang energy of the day, and again at sunset, when yang gives way to yin once more. If you are able to do this, it is a wonderful way to start and close the day. But the best time to practice tai chi is really when it suits your schedule. You are much more likely to maintain a regular practice if there are no conflicting demands on your time.

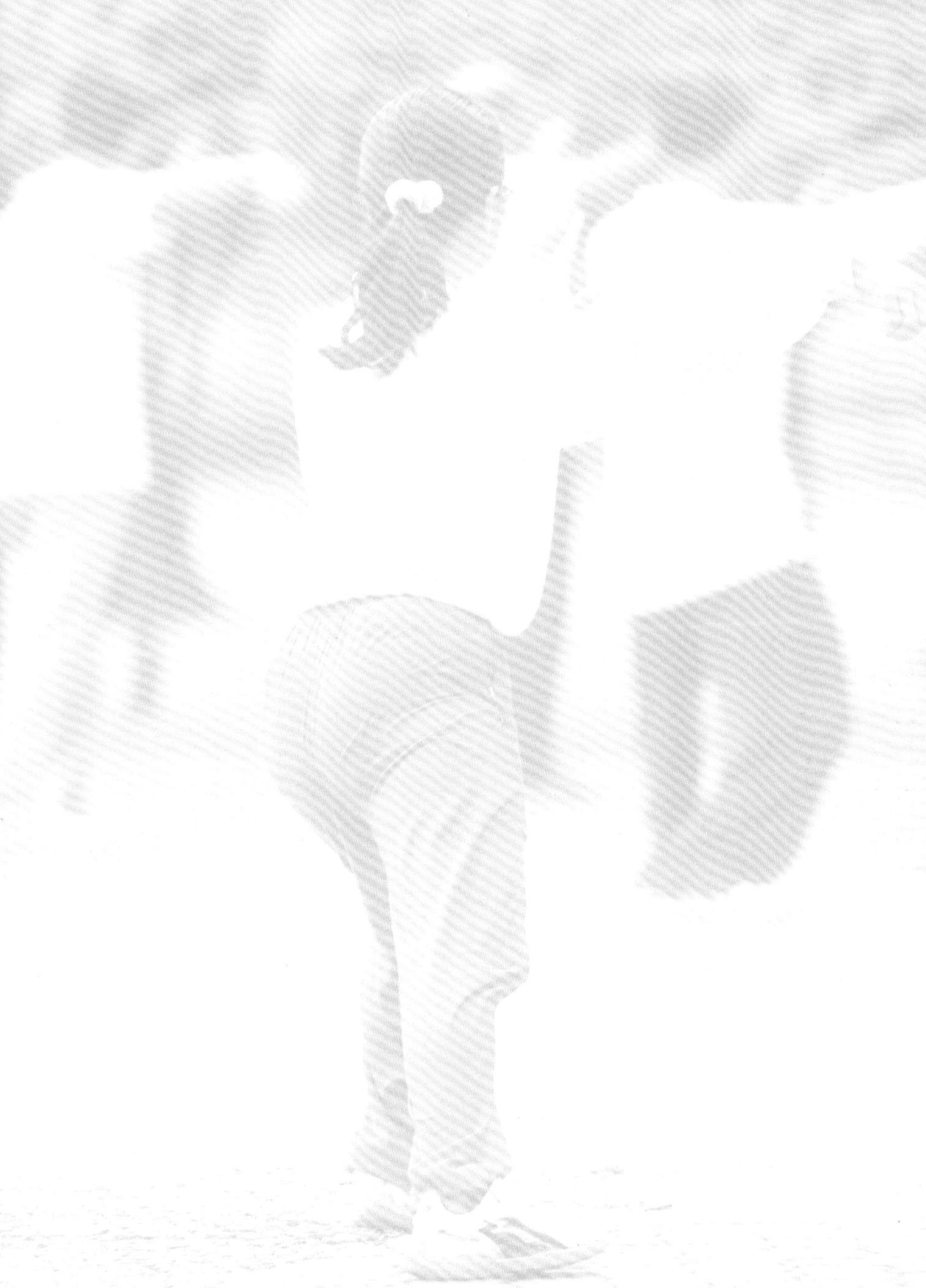

IS TAI CHI FOR ME?

It is worth considering why you want to do tai chi and what benefits you expect to gain. This will help you to remain motivated and provide a baseline against which you can judge your progress.

You may find that your answer is very clear. Perhaps you want to improve your strength and flexibility, or maybe you are bored going to the gym. Or you might want to explore an interest in Eastern practices, or feel the need to try something new. These are all valid reasons.

Your health level

Think, too, about your current state of health. If you are young and fit, great. If you are older and less fit, also great—tai chi is suitable for anyone who can walk, and is recommended for older people who want to increase their activity levels in a gentle and safe way. Specialist teachers can even adapt the exercises so that they can be done sitting down or in a wheelchair.

Note your answers to the following questions:

- **Do you have any health issues?**
- **Are you taking medication?**
- **Are you recovering from an injury?**
- **Do you have foot or joint problems or stiffness?**
- **Are you very overweight?**
- **Has it been a long time since you last exercised?**
- **Are you elderly or unsteady on your feet?**

If you answer yes to any of the above, then check with your physician that tai chi is suitable for you. It may be advisable to learn from a specialist teacher, for example, or to limit yourself to a few minutes a day.

Caution

Tai chi is usually a safe form of exercise for healthy pregnant women, but check with your healthcare provider first.

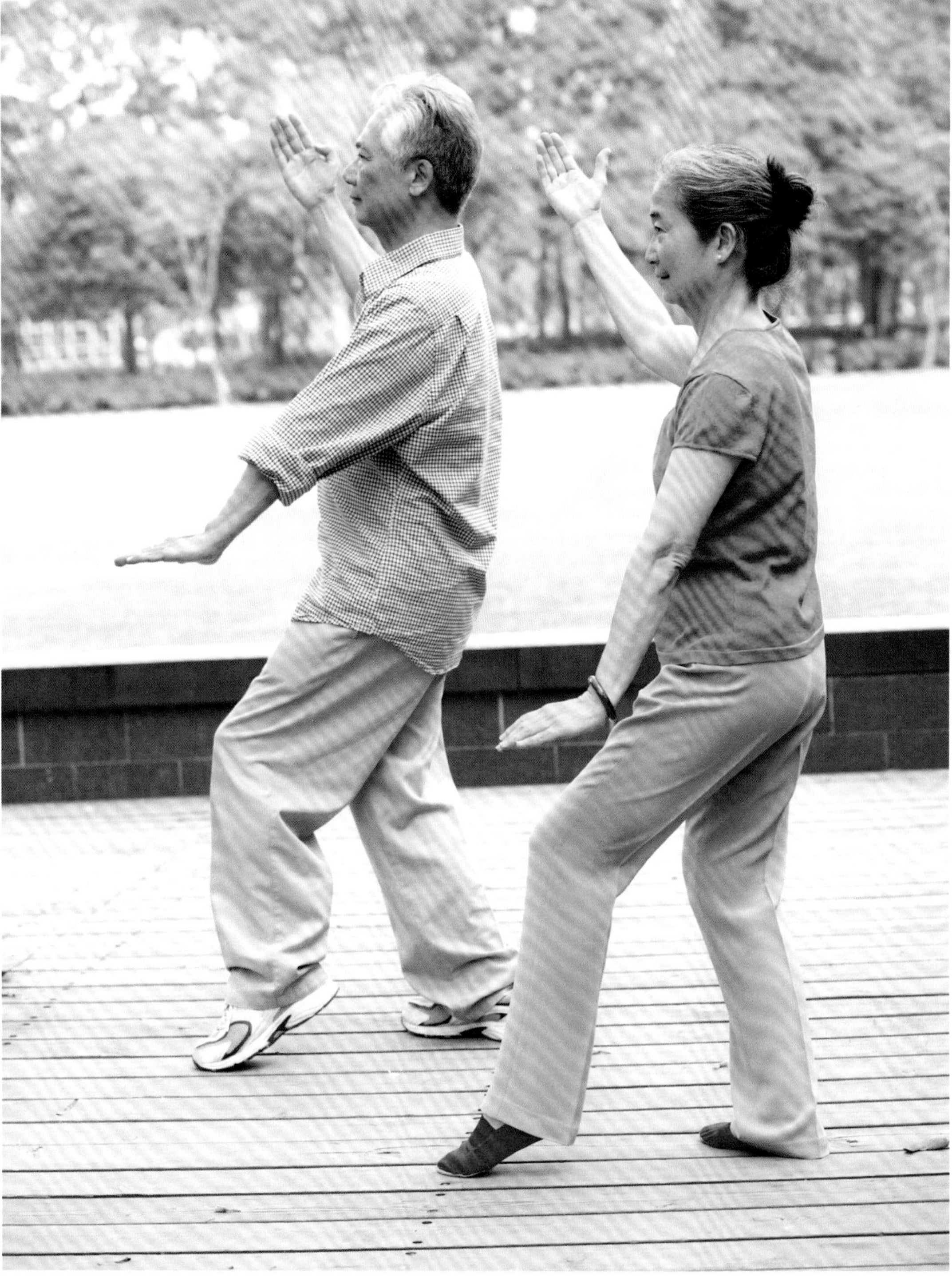

THE ART OF DISCIPLINE

All tai chi teachers agree that it is better to practice for ten minutes a day than for an hour a week. Here are some ways of disciplining yourself to do regular practice.

- **Book it in** If you have a to-do list, add tai chi to it. Better still, put it at the top of the list.
- **Commit to doing it** It takes time for any activity to become a habit. Make a promise to yourself to do tai chi for at least a month.
- **Establish a routine** Do your practice at the same time each day.
- **Do it whatever your mood** If you don't feel like doing tai chi, don't let that stop you.
- **Make it the first thing you do** Getting up earlier and doing your tai chi gets the day off to a positive start.
- **Have a reason** Remember why you are doing tai chi. You may like to write your underlying motivation on a sticky note and put it somewhere you will see it.

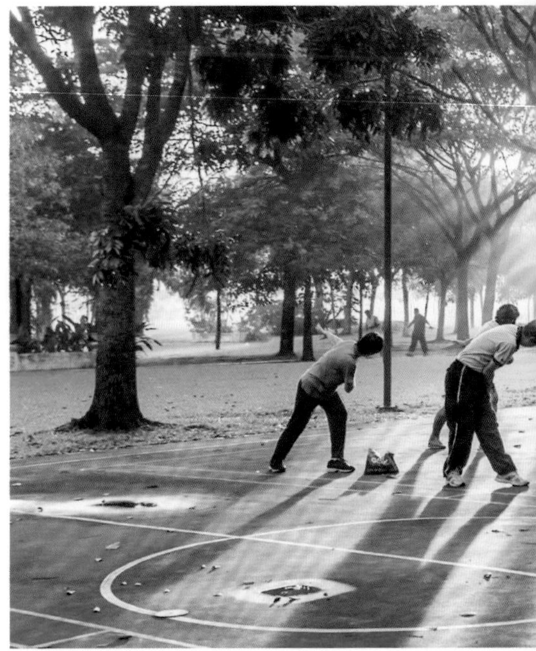

- **Tie it to something else** One of the best ways to start a new habit is to tether it to something you already do. So try doing your tai chi after your morning shower, or after walking the dog.
- **Be proud** Take pleasure in having done your practice, however short.

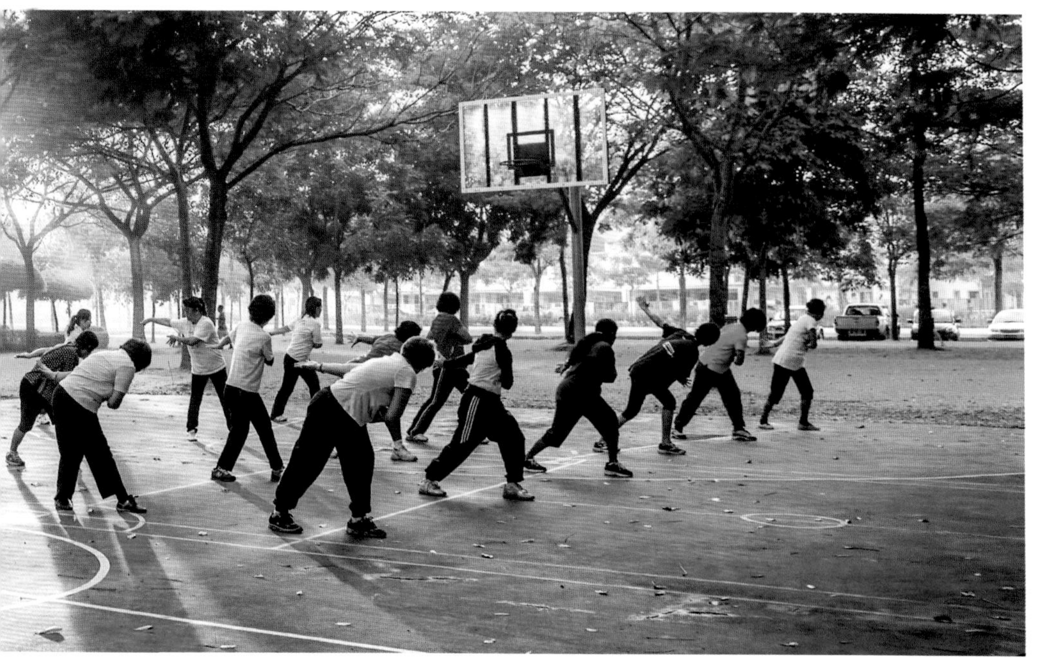

- **Have everything ready** If you practice tai chi in a particular area of the home, make a point of keeping it tidy so that all you need to do is get there.

- **Have a group** Tai chi is commonly practiced in groups, so see if friends want to join you. Or go to a class.

Group effort
There are many benefits to practicing tai chi in a group, including making it a social acitivity and also providing additional encouragment to undertake it regularly.

GOING TO A CLASS

It is always best to learn tai chi from an experienced and skilled teacher as well as practicing on your own at home. Watching a teacher go through the form will enlighten your own practice, and help you to practice safely and effectively. A good teacher can show you precisely how to break the moves down, how to adapt them to the particular needs of your body, and explain where you are going wrong and what to do to make improvements. And working in a group brings great energy to your practice.

Think location Look for a class that is close to where you live. You are more likely to attend a class if it is easy to get to than if it is a long distance away.

Check the style Your class must teach the same style that you practice at home.

Ask around Word of mouth is usually the best way to find a teacher. If you don't know anyone who practices tai chi, contact a national tai chi association (see the Further Information section on page 219).

Try it out Most tai chi teachers will let you observe or sample a class before making a commitment. You can get a good sense of a teacher by watching him or her demonstrate the form—are the movements fluid and beautiful to watch?

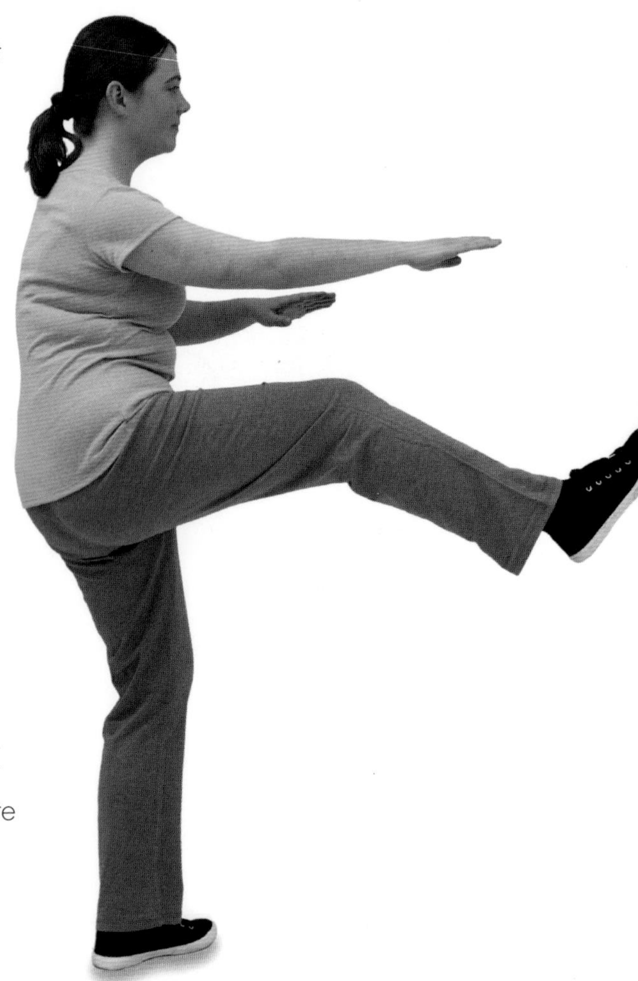

Ask questions Ask who the instructor learned from—tai chi has traditionally been passed down from master to student. Ideally, go for someone who has been practicing for ten years or more. Check that they are registered and insured.

Reserve judgement Tai chi can feel different from other forms of exercise, so it may take a few sessions before you feel comfortable with it. Do not expect instant progress—you may simply learn some preparatory movements rather than practicing the form.

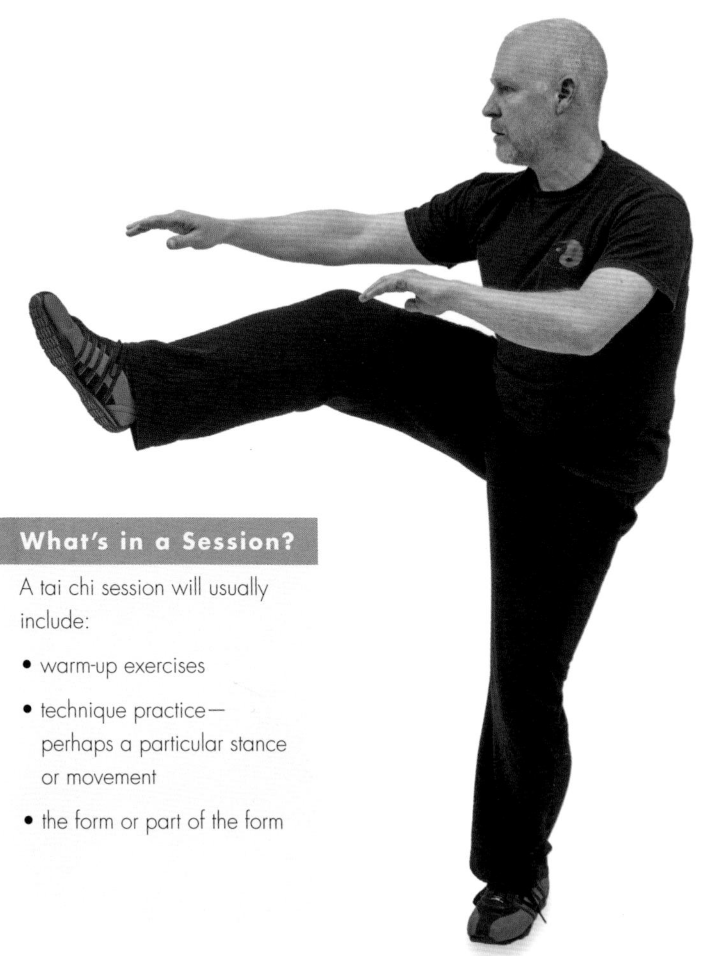

What's in a Session?

A tai chi session will usually include:

- warm-up exercises
- technique practice—perhaps a particular stance or movement
- the form or part of the form

Warming Up

You should warm up before any exercise session. Though tai chi is a very gentle form of movement, it will likely work your legs and body in unfamiliar ways, so a warm-up is just as necessary as with more vigorous activities. The warm-up is also an opportunity for your mind to shift its focus away from day-to-day activity, and to prepare for the meditative movements of the form. And warm-up time gives you the chance to start practicing the deep breathing that is an essential part of tai chi.

For some experienced practitioners, the warm-up might take the form of moving slowly through the form itself. This can be done if the practitioner already has a high level of flexibility and has a good understanding of the body's capability. Beginners, however, should certainly adhere to a warm-up routine.

Working with your body

Some of the exercises on the following pages are simple stretches that you may already be familiar with; others may be new to you and are intended to encourage the whole-body attitude that is integral to tai chi. Respect the needs and capabilities of your body, and never exercise to the point of discomfort, either in the warm-up or when practicing tai chi. At the start of each of the sequences, do not exceed 60 percent of your normal range of movement. You can always progress as you repeat the movement, but you should never push yourself to the limit of your capability. Breathe naturally and deeply throughout.

The Danger of "Loosening the Knees"

There is a common tai chi warm-up exercise called "loosening the knees" that involves standing with your feet together or hip-width apart, bending the knees, leaning down with your hands to cup the knees, and then circling the knees. Avoid doing this. The knee is a hinge joint and therefore should not be rotated, which means that "loosening the knees" carries a risk of injury. Instead, try the hip circling and ankle circling on page 66. You can also rub your hands together and massage the knees to help warm them up.

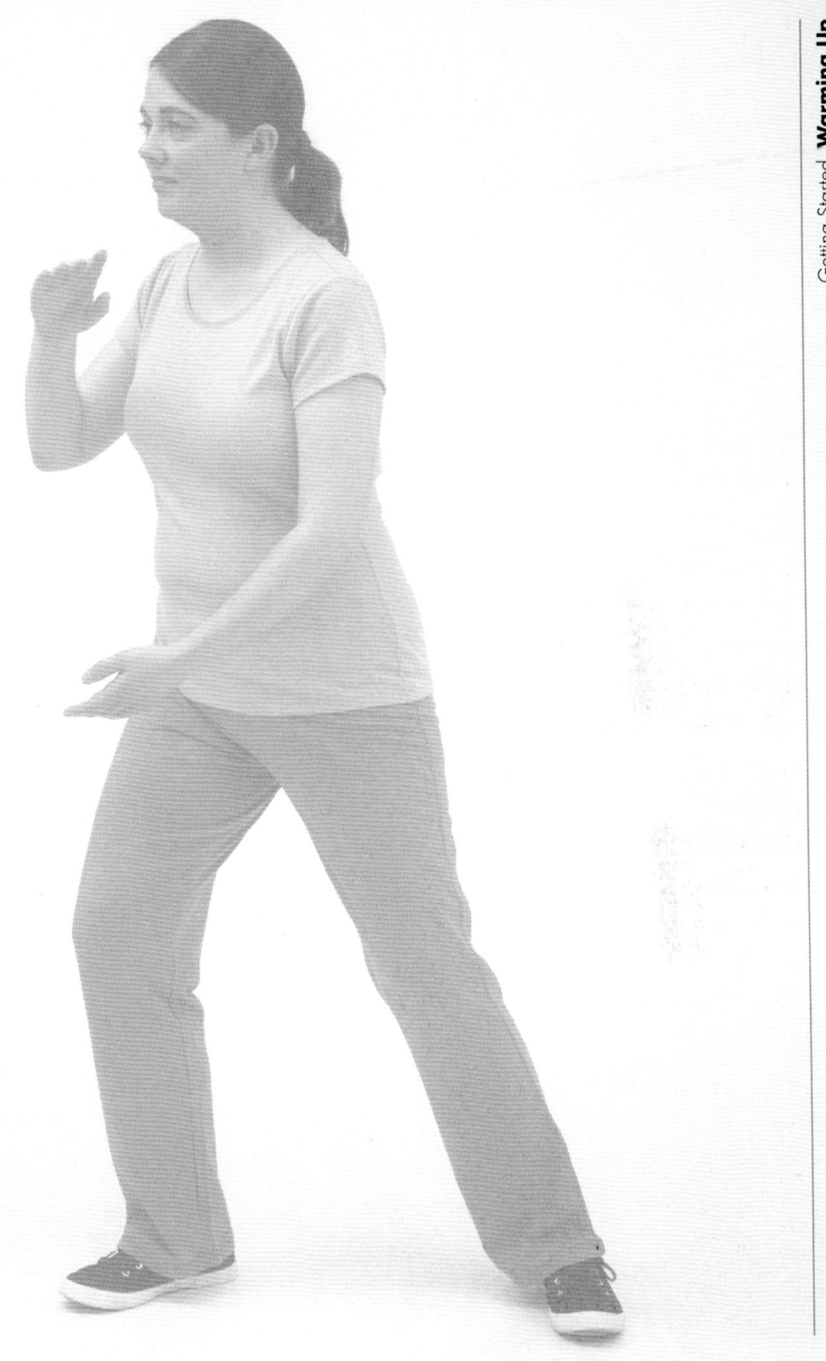

PREPARING FOR THE TAI CHI FORM

On the pages that follow are some simple movements that help to relax your muscles and open the joints. Before you start, go for a brisk five- or ten-minute walk, or try walking around your practice area

Relaxing the neck

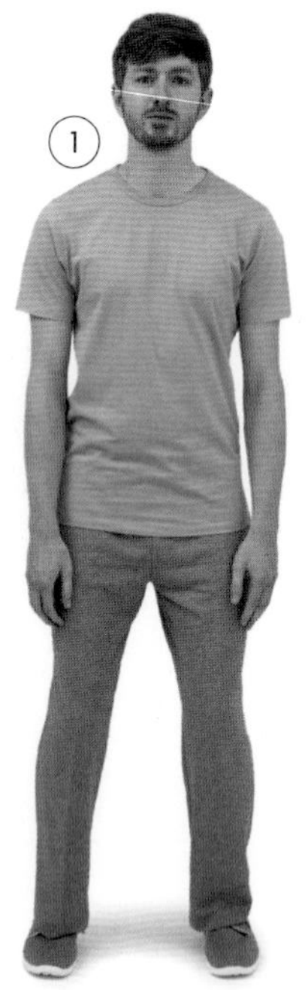

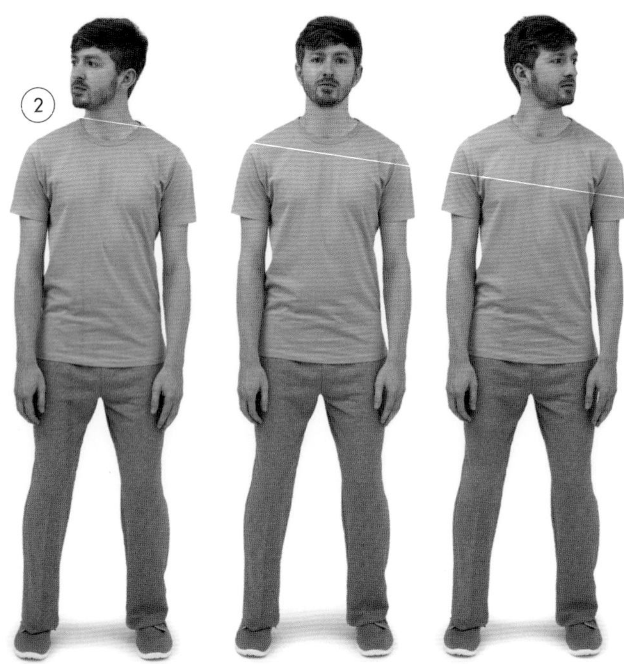

1 *Stand with your feet parallel and hip-width apart, knees bent, and check through the elements of tai chi posture (see page 28).*

2 *Turn your head to the right and then back to the center. Then turn it to the left and back to the center. Repeat eight times.*

in circles for a few minutes, gently shaking the arms and the legs as you go. Rub your hands together to warm them up, and then run them up and down your arms and shoulders, chest, lower back, legs, and feet until you feel warmer and energized.

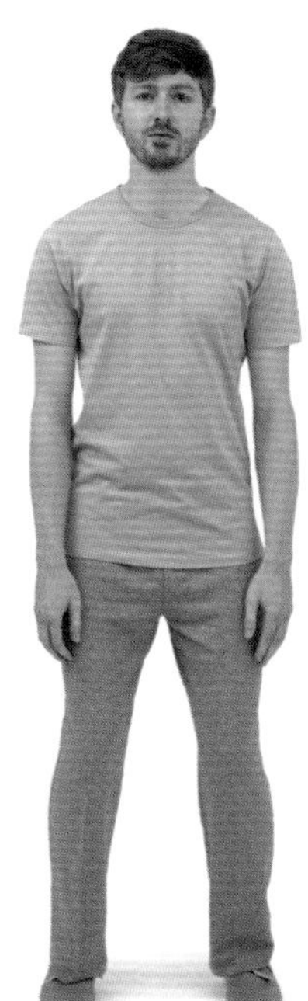

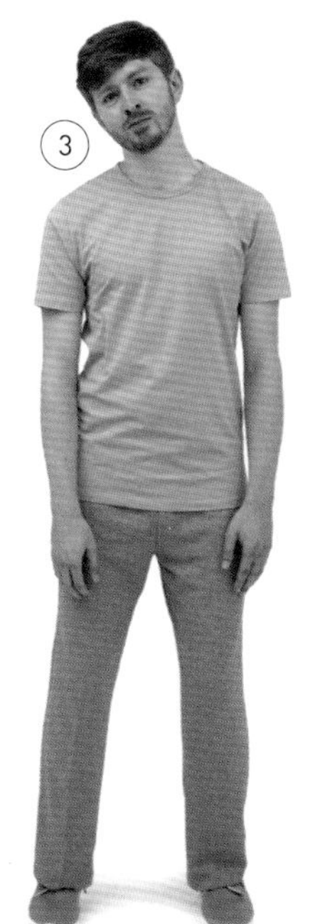

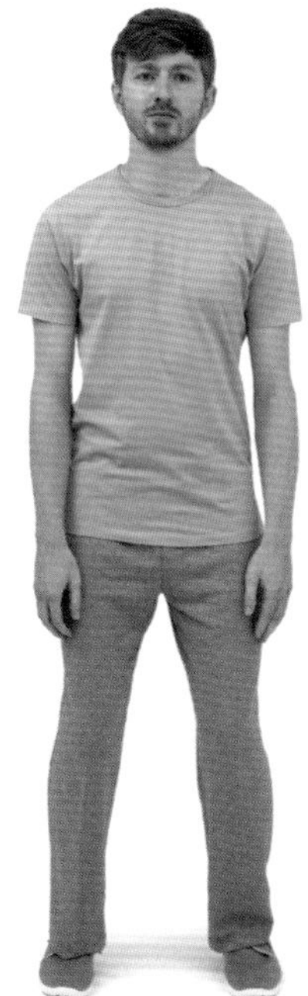

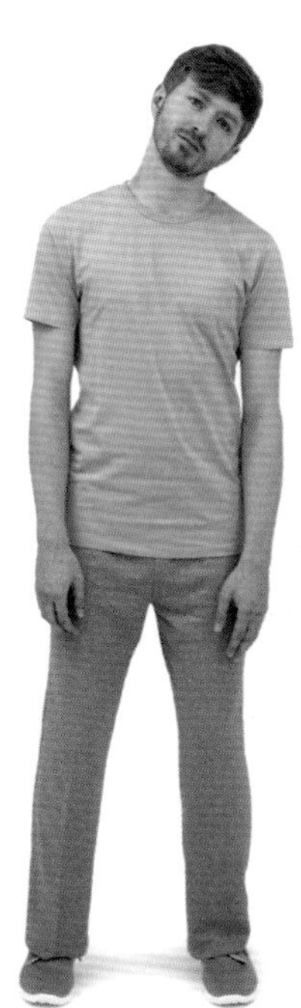

3 *Drop your head toward your right shoulder and then bring it back to the center. Then drop it toward your left shoulder and bring it back to the center. Repeat eight times.*

Continued overleaf

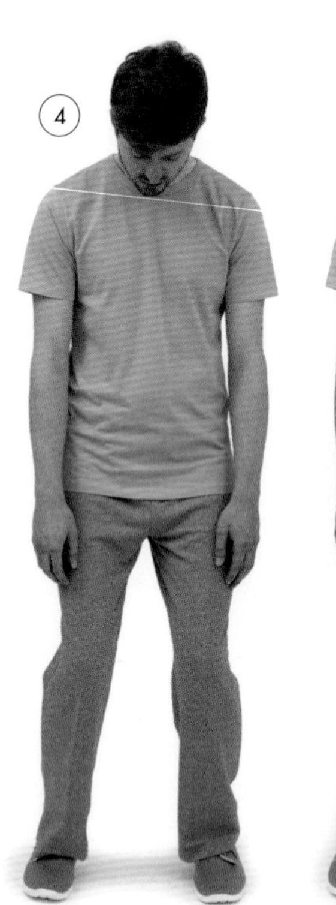

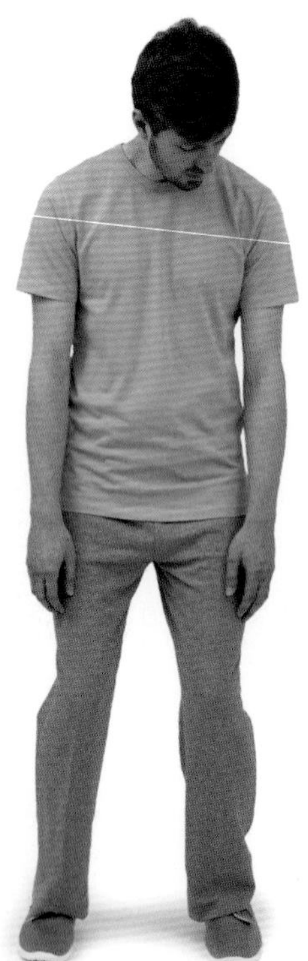

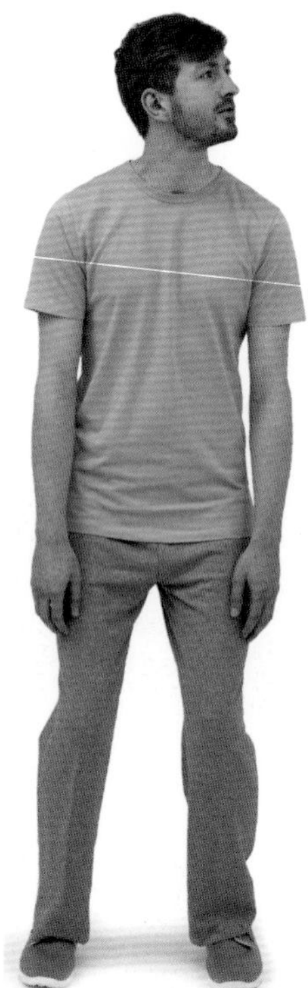

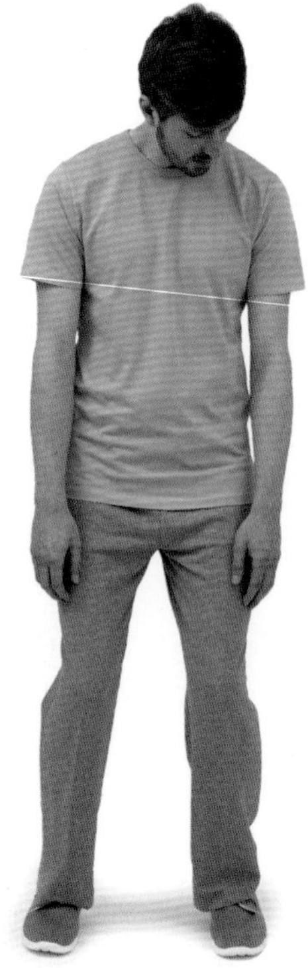

4 *Drop your head down toward your chest and then bring it back to the central point. Then, very slowly, raise it up and to the left, tilting it back just far enough so that you can see the ceiling. Do not drop the neck right back. Then do the same on your right side. Repeat eight times.*

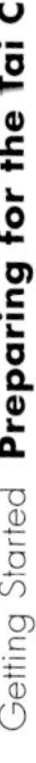

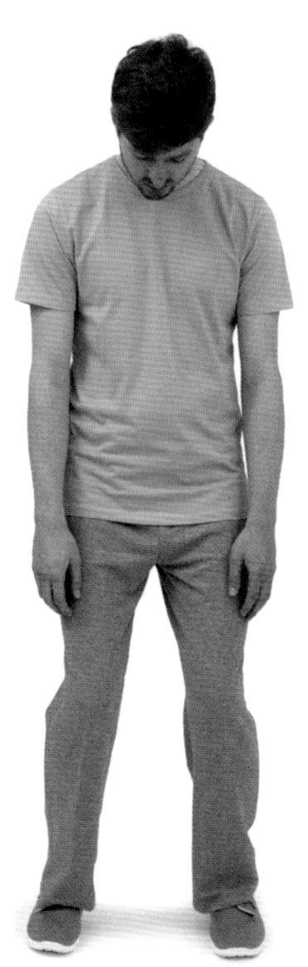

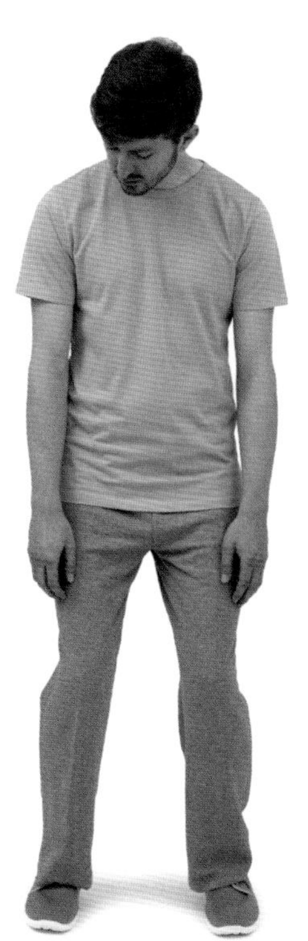

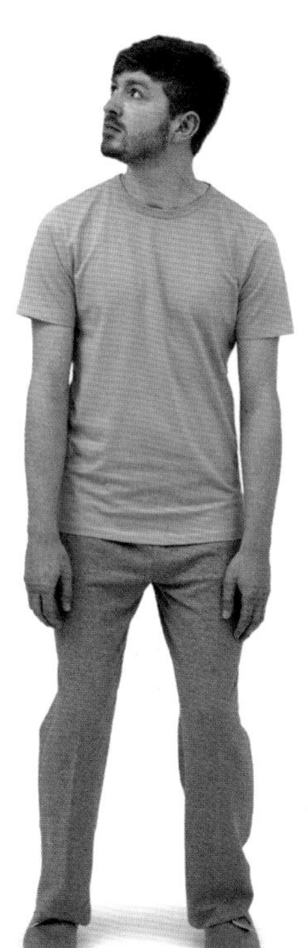

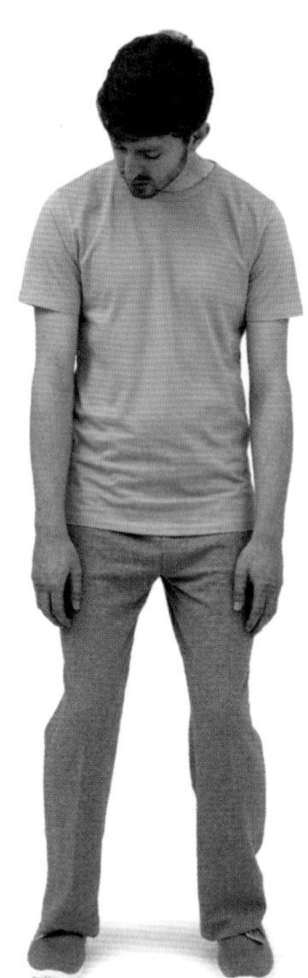

Safe Head Movement

Don't roll your head all the way around. That is, avoid tipping it back because this constricts the neck. It is much safer to move the head to one side, down to the chest, then to the other side, and back, like a pendulum.

Relaxing the shoulders

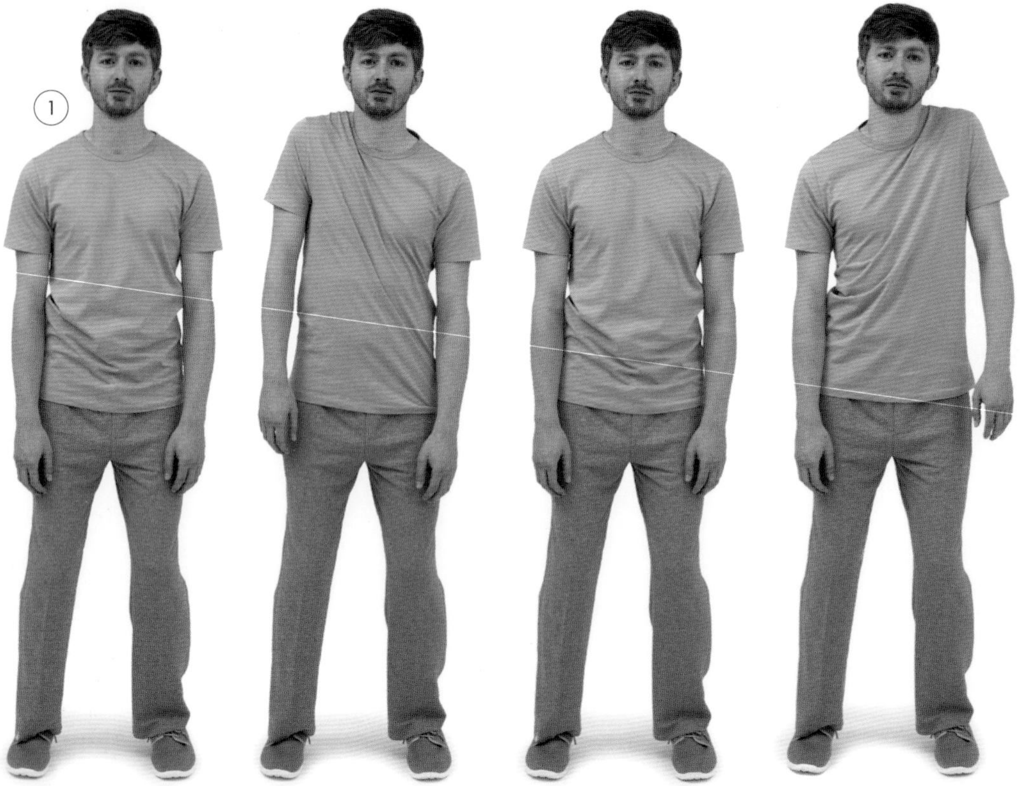

3 *Now make circles with both your shoulders. Bring them up toward the ears, then move them down and back before continuing the movement forward and up. Do eight circles this way, then reverse the action.*

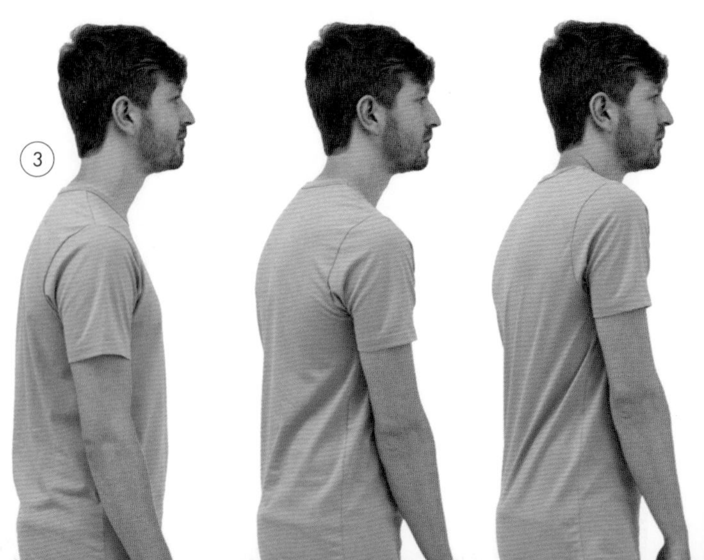

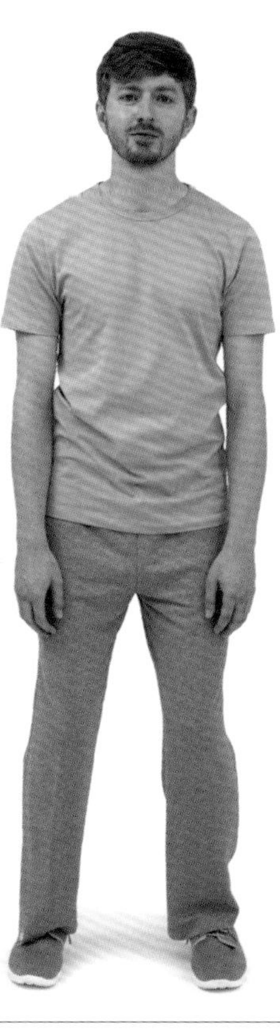

1 *Still standing with your arms by your sides, raise your right shoulder up toward your right ear, then let it drop down. Do the same with the left shoulder. Repeat eight times.*

2 *Raise both shoulders at once, then drop them back down together. Repeat eight times.*

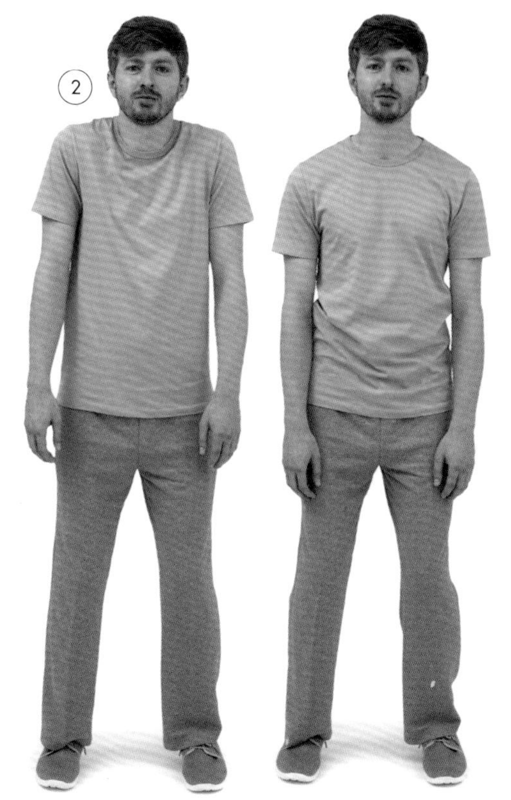

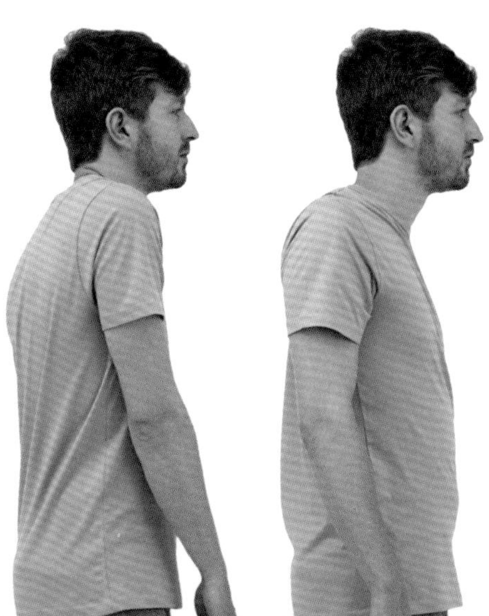

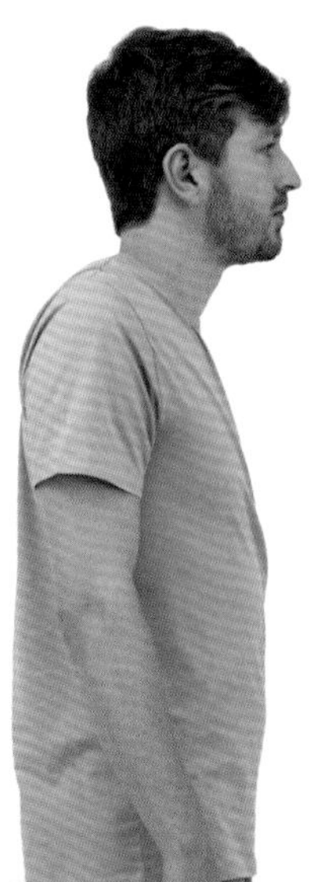

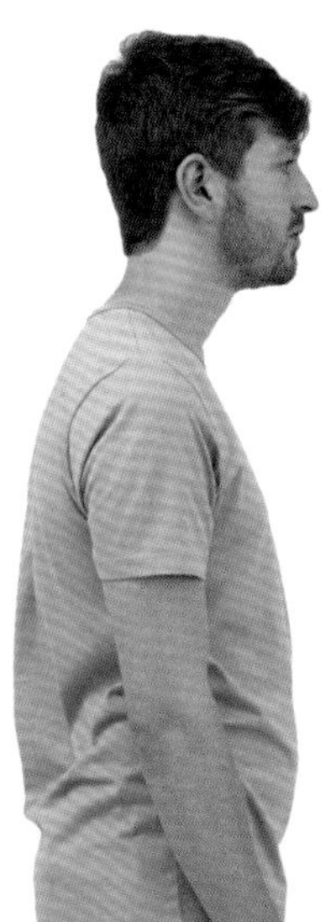

Energize the arms

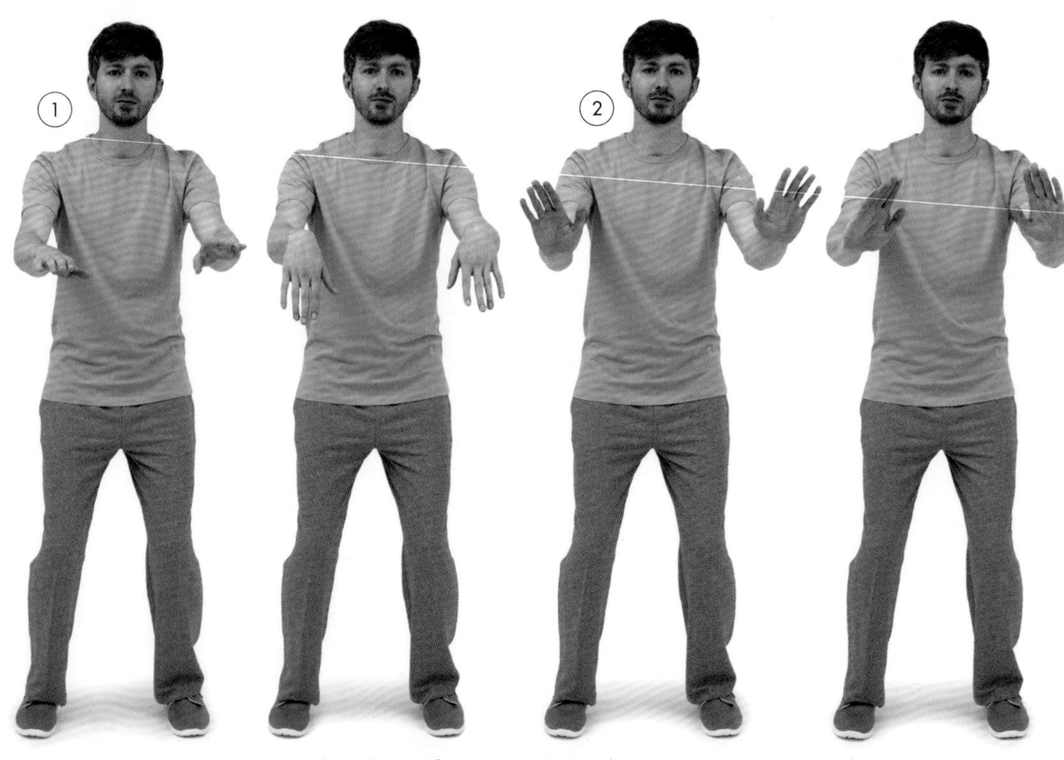

1 *Stand straight with your feet parallel and hip-width apart, knees bent. Raise your arms in front of you, no farther than chest height and with the elbows dropped. Drop and the raise your hands from the wrist eight to ten times.*

2 *Gently rotate your wrists inward for a few circles, then rotate them outward.*

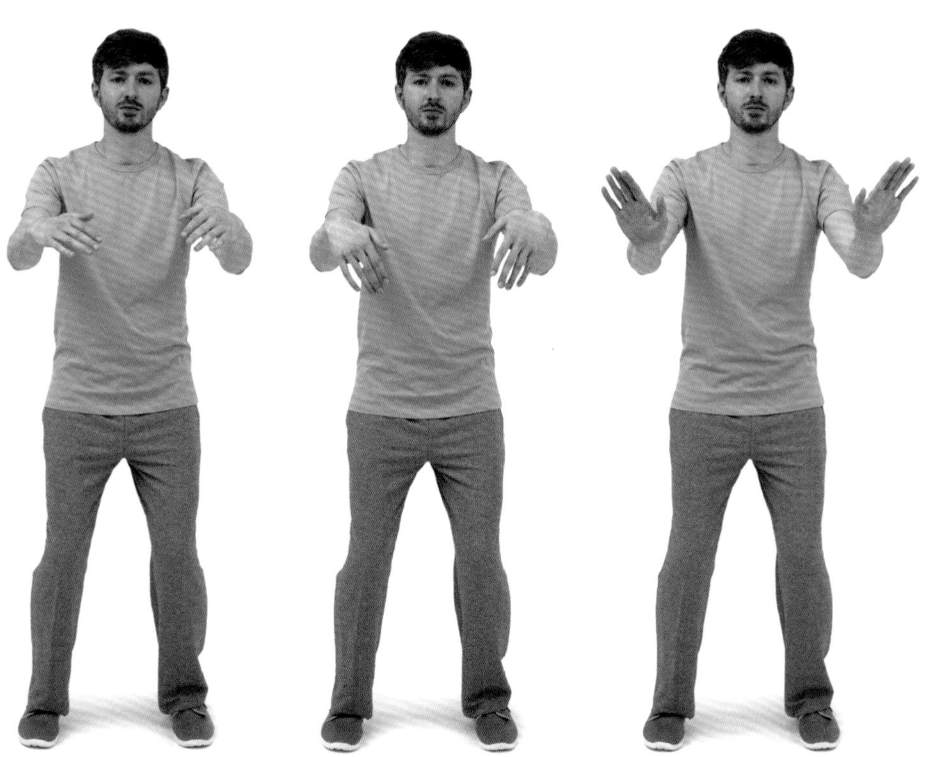

Continued overleaf

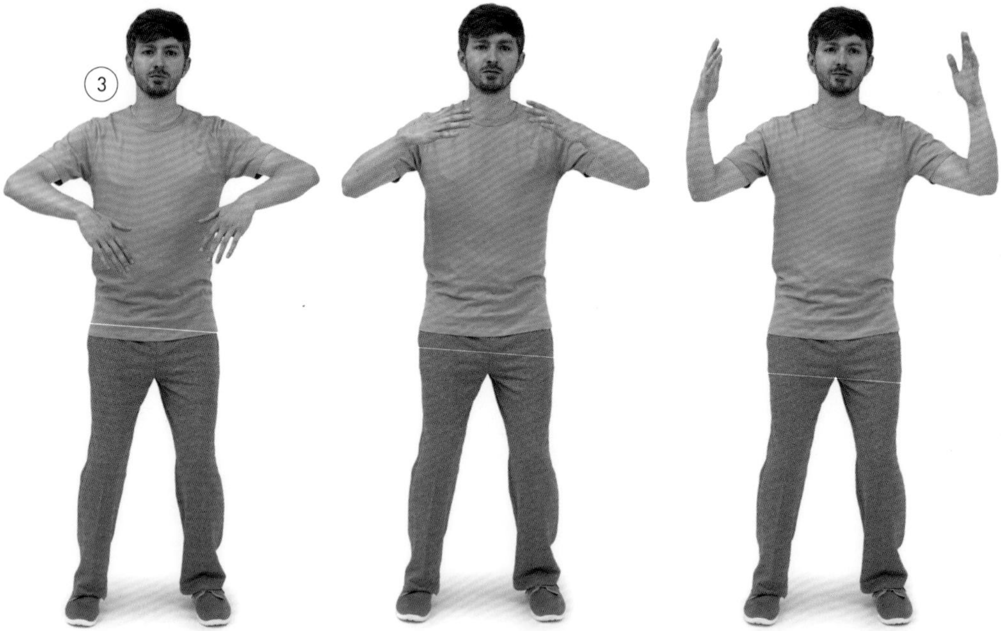

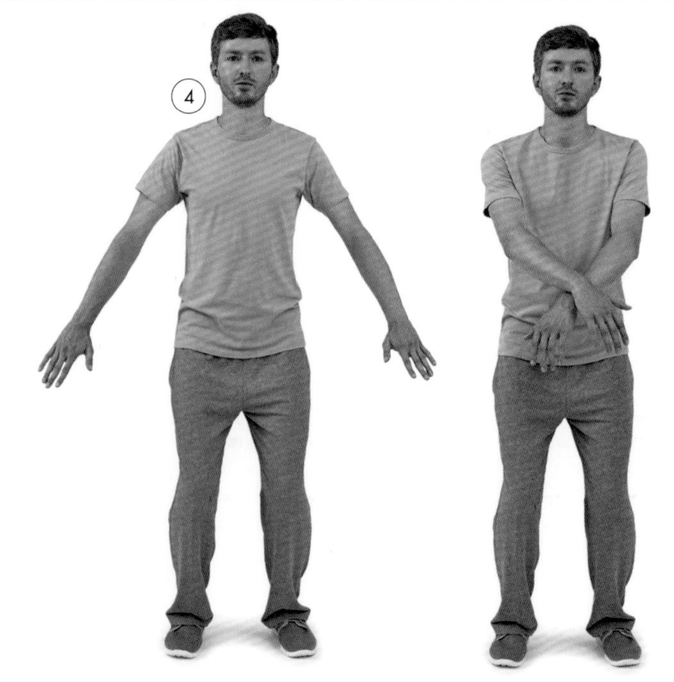

3 *Bring the movement to your elbows, circling them in one direction and then the other so that the forearms are moving but the upper arms stay relatively still. Bring the arms farther out to the sides to give yourself space to do this.*

4 *Then involve the whole arm in the movement, circling them out and then crossing one over the other in front of you to complete the circle. Do a few circles in one direction, then in the reverse direction. Take care that your spine remains erect, with your tailbone tucked in.*

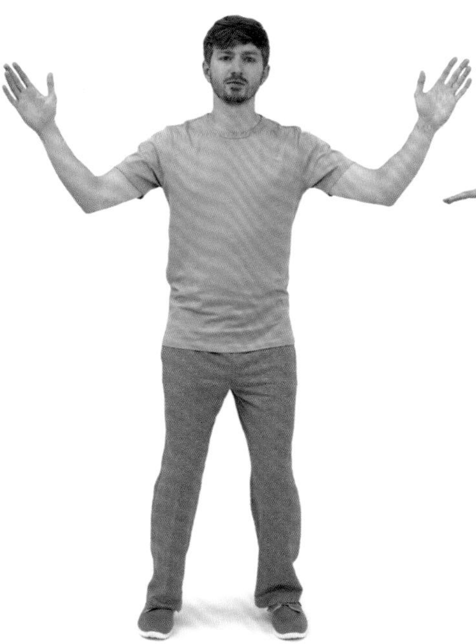

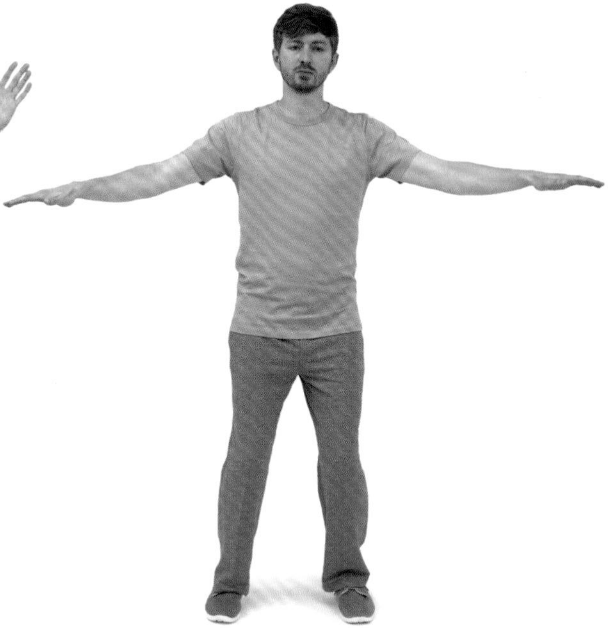

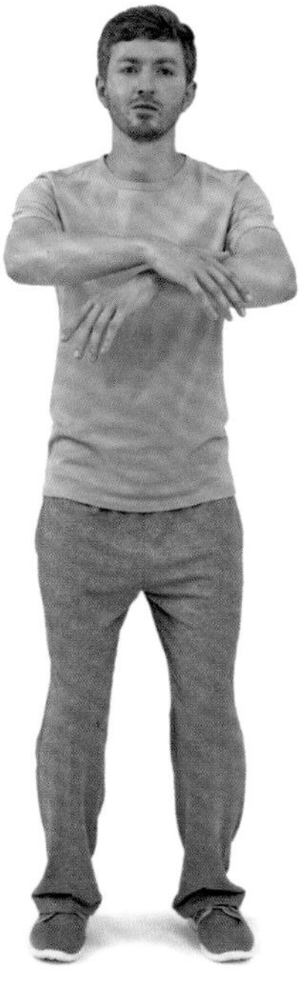

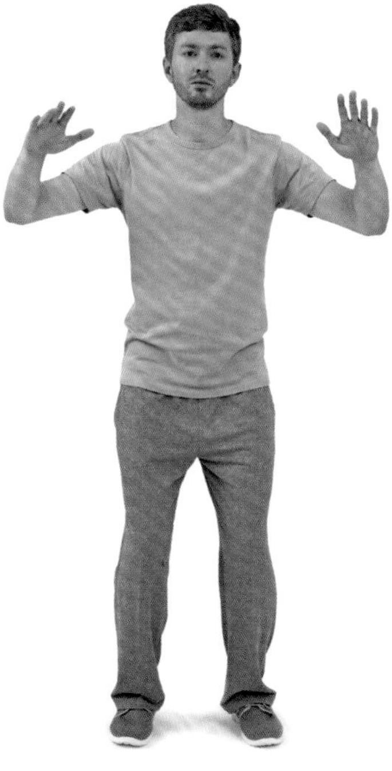

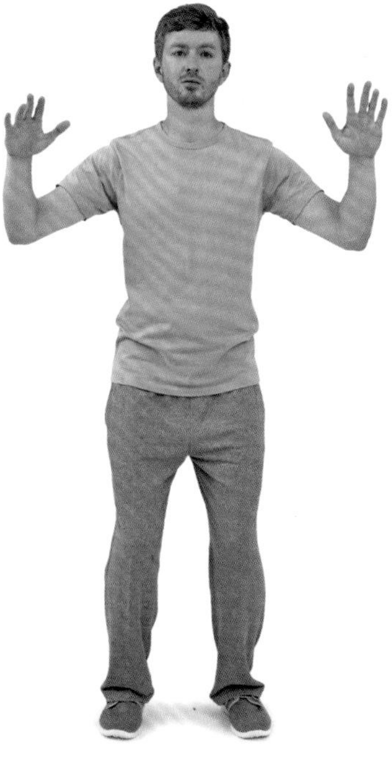

Waist turns

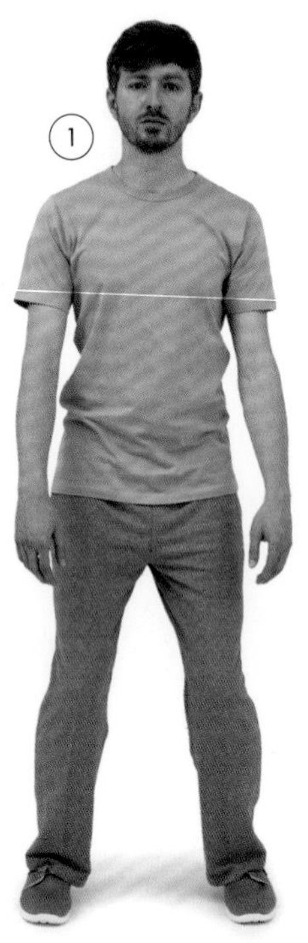

1 *Stand with your feet shoulder-width apart, arms by your sides with a small space in the armpits. Take a moment to run through the elements of tai chi posture. Your head should feel suspended above your body, as if by a cord, in line with a relaxed spine. Bend your knees and root your feet into the ground.*

2 *Use your abdominal muscles to turn your upper body and your ribs a little to the left. The arms should be loose and follow the movement of the upper body.*

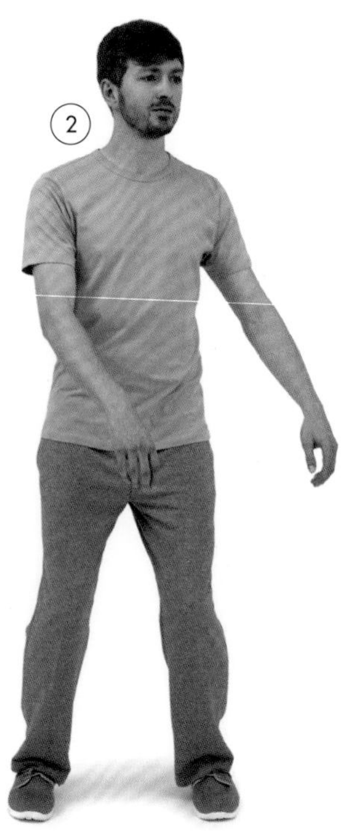

4 *Rotate in the same way to the right.*

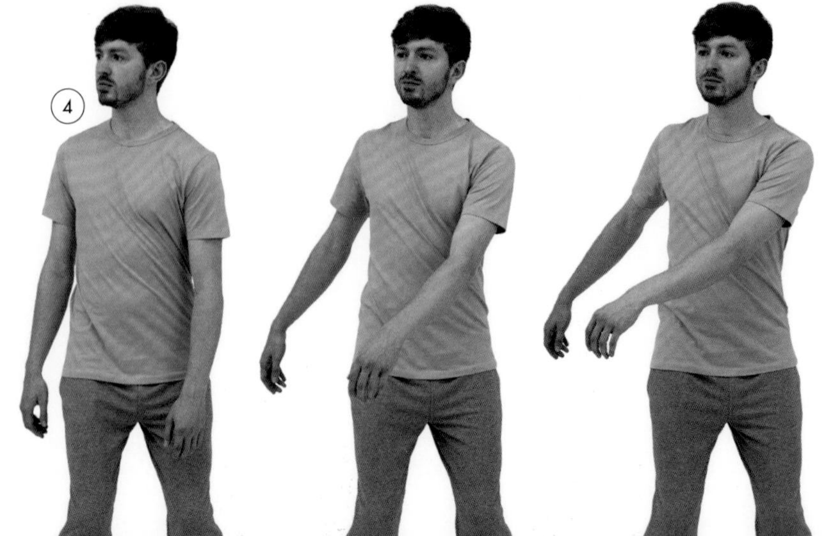

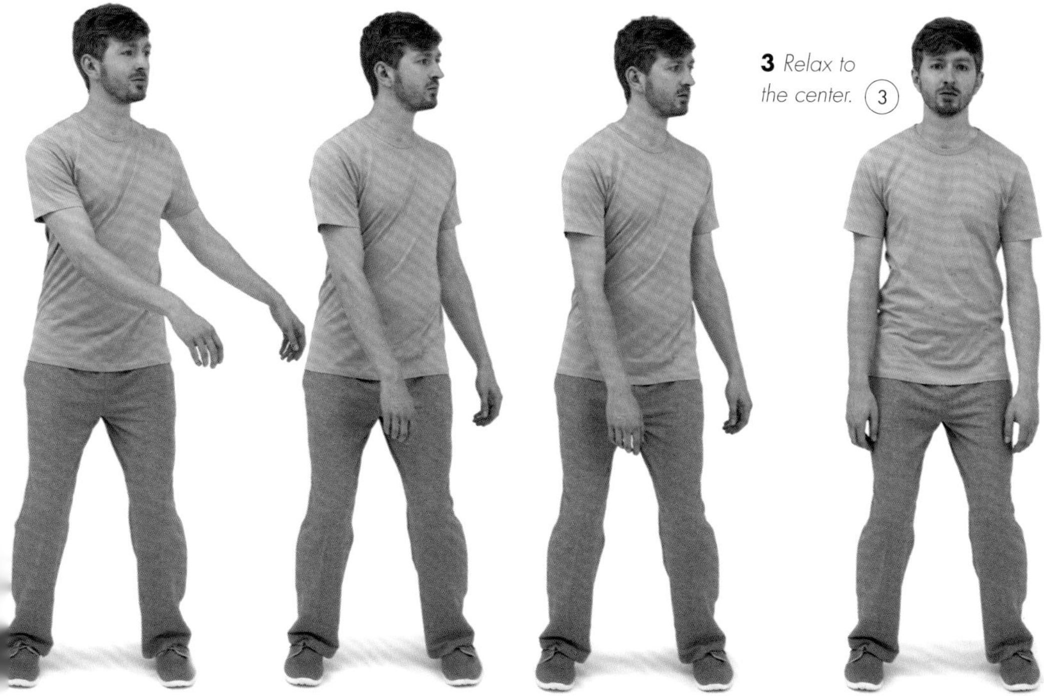

3 *Relax to the center.* (3)

5 *Relax to the center.*

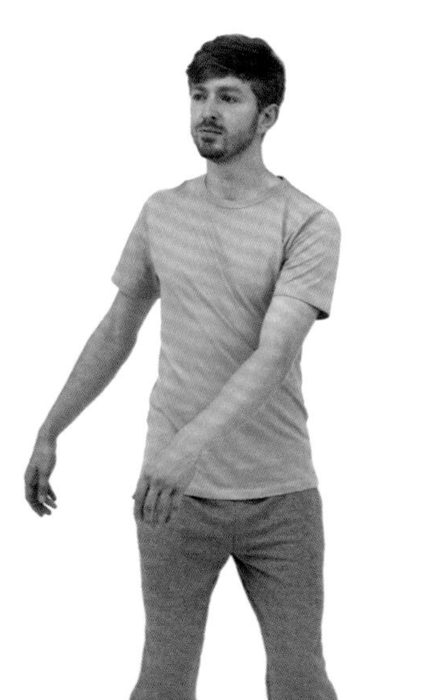

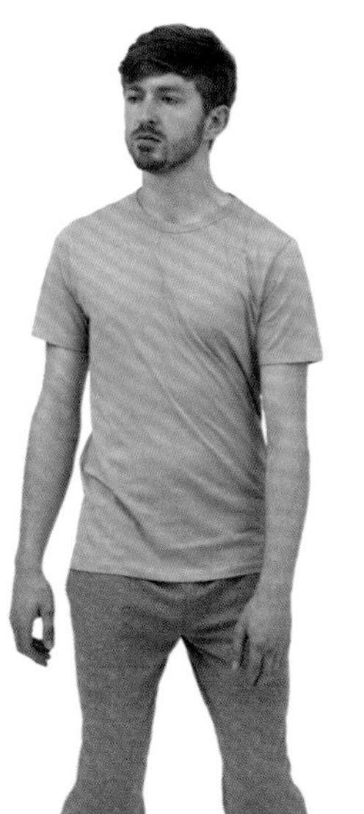

(5)

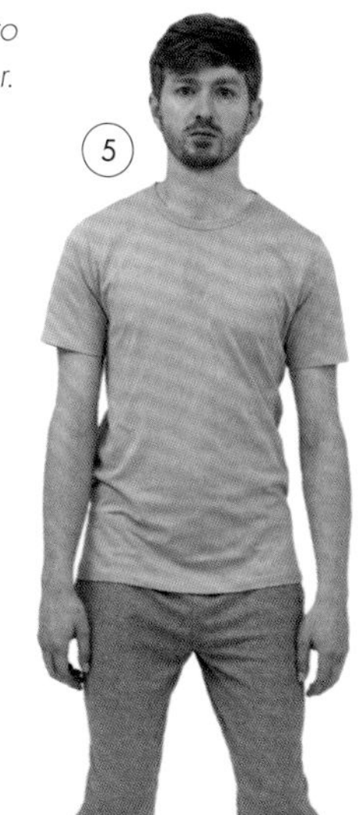

Swing the legs and arms

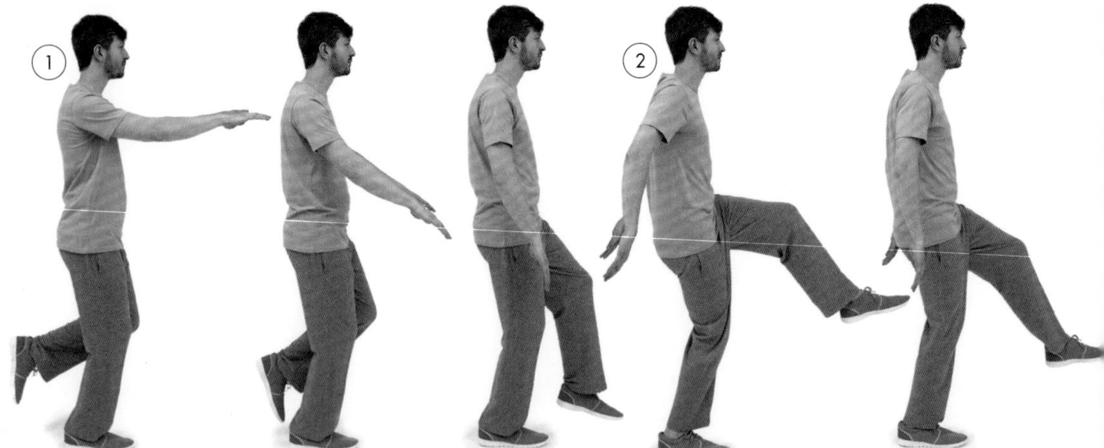

1 *Shift all your weight onto your right leg. Raise your left heel and then bring the whole foot off the ground, bending your knee, gently swinging your arms forward.*

2 *Swing your left leg slowly forward, keeping your right leg slightly bent, and let your arms drop and swing behind a little. Keep your shoulders relaxed.*

Ankle circles

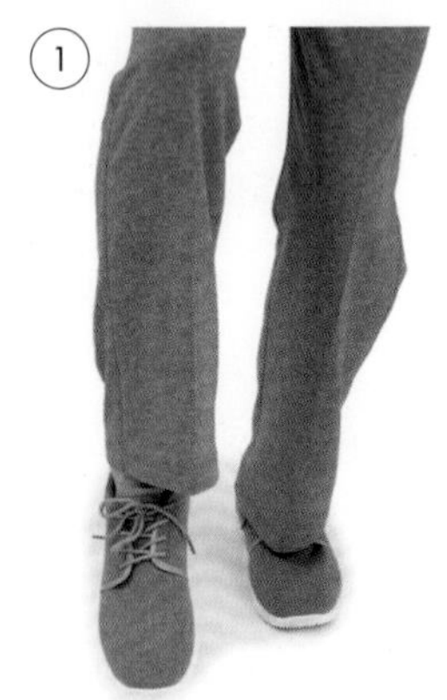

1 *Shift all your weight onto your left leg. Raise your right heel and then bring the whole foot off the ground, bending the knee.*

2 *Rotate your right ankle, as if you are drawing circles in the air with your toes. Do four circles in one direction and four in the other. Then repeat on the other side.*

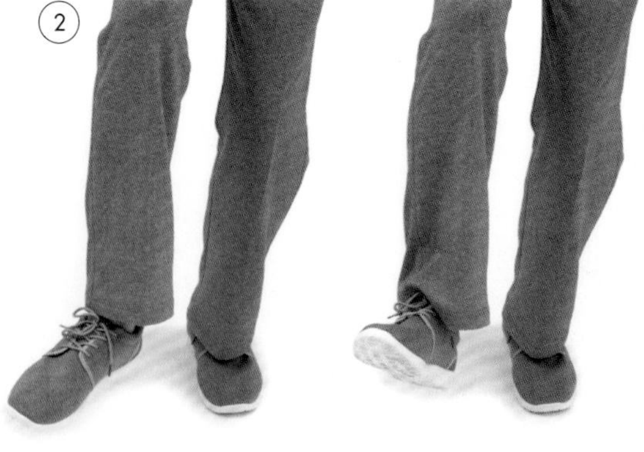

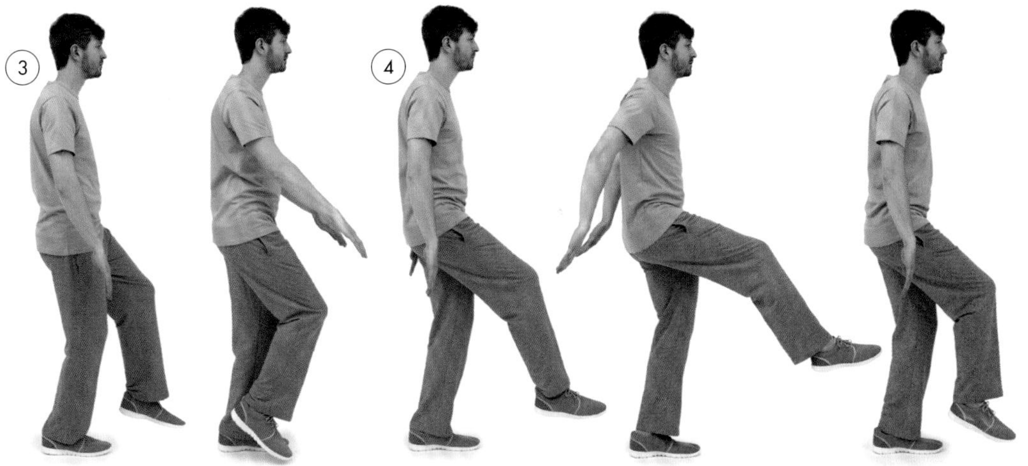

3 *Let your left leg return to the ground and your arms hang down.*

4 *Repeat steps 1 to 3, this time with your weight on your left leg and raising and swinging your right leg.*

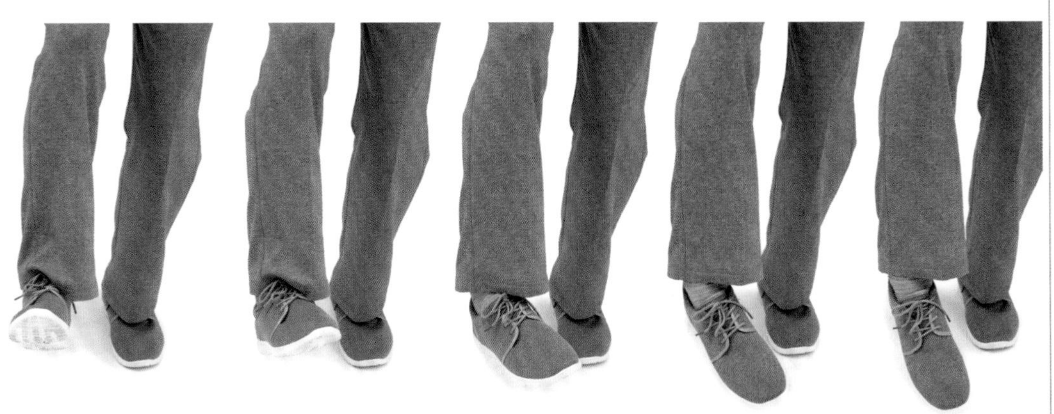

HOLDING THE BALL

This exercise introduces you to working with energy. You can practice it as a one-off exercise or as part of your warm-up. In the tai chi form, the hands often form a position known as Hold the Ball. The ball is a sphere of energy and experienced practitioners can sense it between the palms of their hands.

Finding the ball

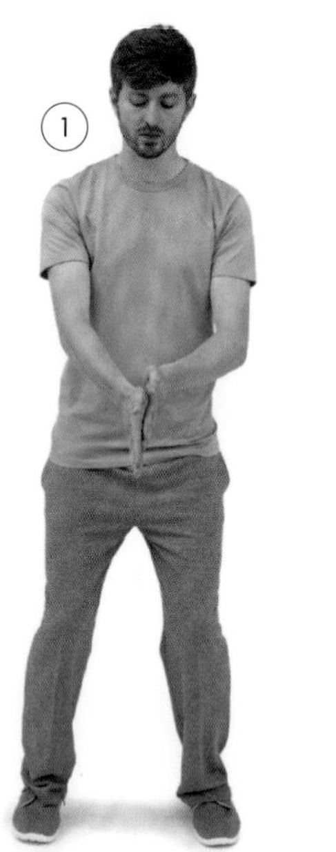

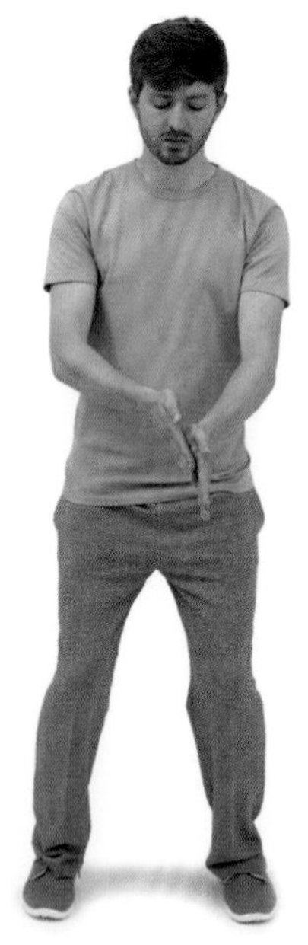

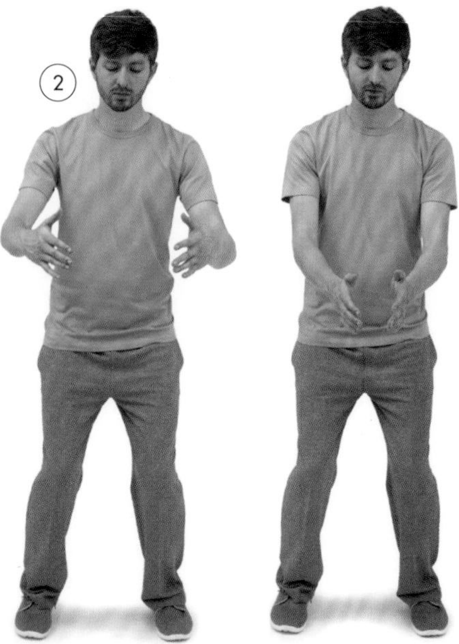

1 *Stand with your feet parallel and hip-width apart, and run through the fundamentals of tai chi posture (see page 28). Rub your hands together as if warming them. Keep your attention fully on your hands as they move and your shoulders relaxed.*

2 *Very slowly move your hands apart, letting them curve naturally so that the space formed between them is a sphere. Notice the warmth and energetic connection you feel here, and focus on the feeling until it starts to fade, then bring your palms close together without touching.*

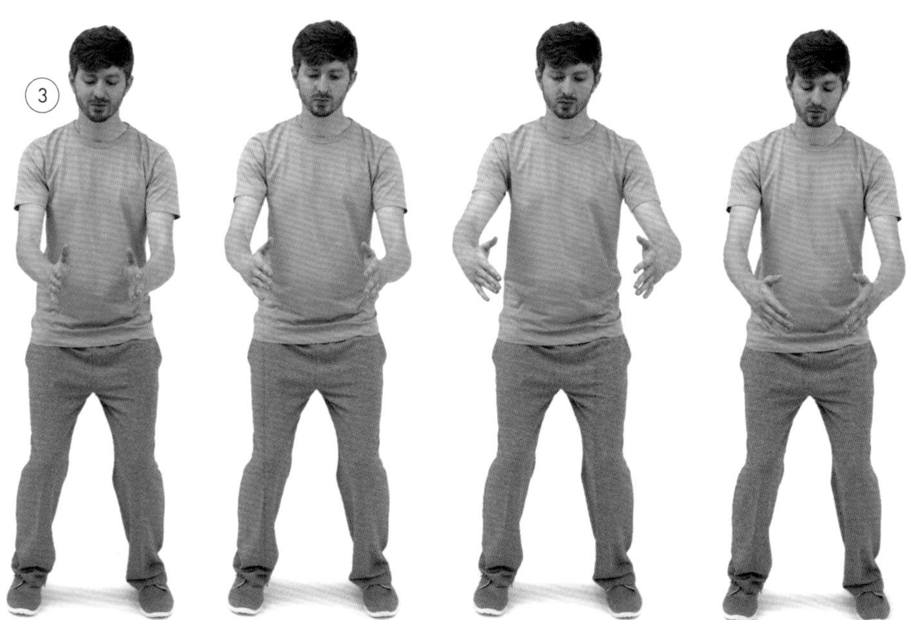

3 *Play with this movement, bringing the hands apart and together again, being aware of any resulting sensation. Do not worry if you do not feel anything—this may come in time. The important thing is to maintain a sense of focus and an openness to experiencing a change in sensation. At the end of the exercise, bring your arms to your sides again.*

Turning the ball

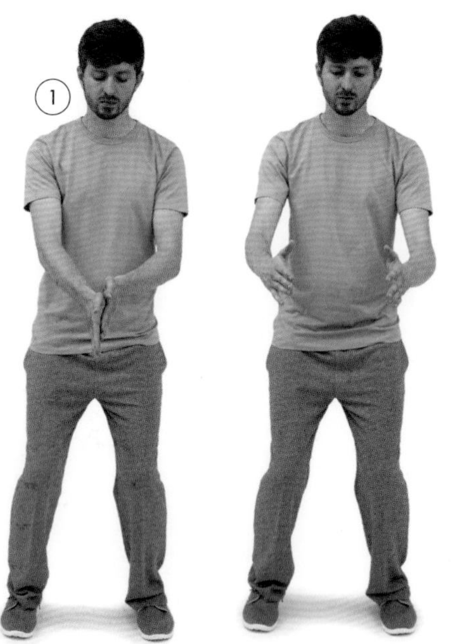

1 *Rub your hands together again and then move them apart as before. Keep your palms at dantien height.*

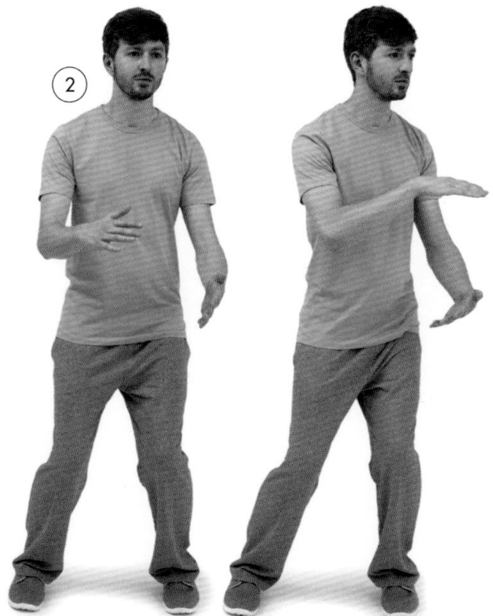

2 *Shift your weight onto your left leg, keeping your whole body soft as if suspended, and turn your hands so that the right hand is above the left, with your right palm facing down and your left palm facing up so that the space between them is still a sphere. Focus on any sensation between them. Return to the center with your palms at dantien height.*

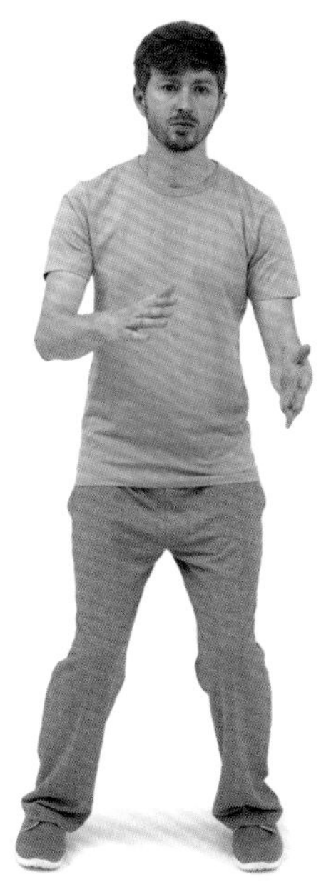

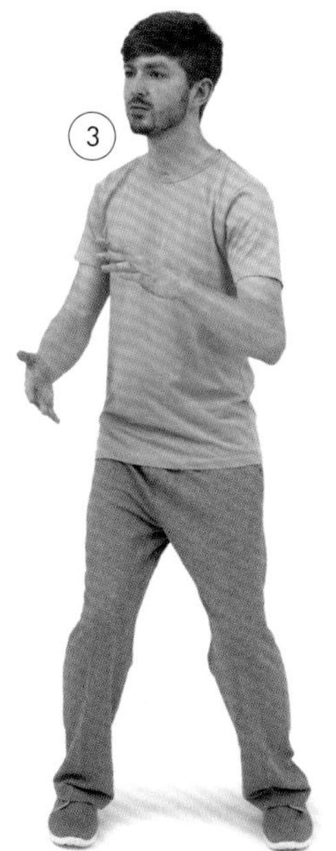

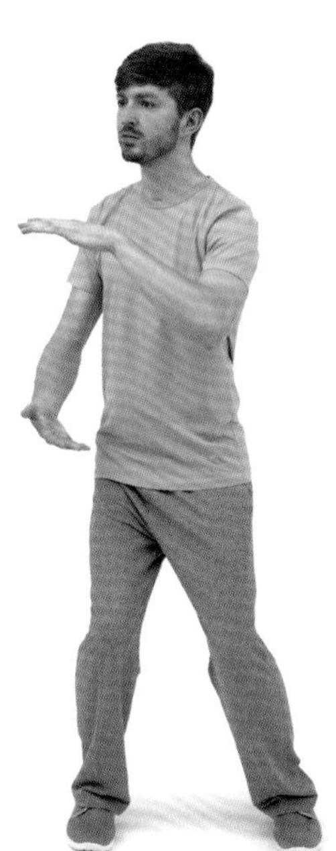

3 *Play with this action, reversing the leg that your weight is on and the position of the hands, but always keeping the spherical space between them, as if turning a ball around and around. Keep your movements smooth and regular. Return to the center with your hands at your sides to finish.*

Common Tai Chi Stances

The position of the feet is important in tai chi, and the same foot stances are returned to again and again. It is worth practicing these as a separate exercise so that you can assume the correct pose whenever it comes up and concentrate on other elements of the movement. You may like to do some foot stance practice after warming up and before starting the form. The foot stances are also useful standalone exercises for building strength in the legs and improving balance.

Horse stance

This stance is used at the beginning and the end of the Yang Short Form, and is the only time that your weight is evenly balanced between your two legs (though some practitioners also adopt this stance in the movement called Cross Hands—see page 118). It is an opportunity to bring the body into the correct tai chi posture, ensuring that your head and spine form a vertical axis, the weight is sunk, and the joints are relaxed (see page 28). Horse Stance is a very calming stance, and you can use it to practice conscious abdominal breathing as a form of meditation (see page 20).

Bow stance

This stance takes its name from the position an archer assumes when shooting an arrow. The majority of your weight—70 percent—is on your front leg, enabling you to deliver a punch or a push. Bow Stance crops up frequently in the form, together with its counterbalance, called Sit Stance, in which the foot position is the same but the distribution of weight is reversed, with 70 percent on the back leg and 30 percent on the front leg.

Empty stances

There are two empty stances: Toe Stance and Heel Stance. In both, the supporting foot carries the majority of your weight, known as "full," while the other is considered to be "empty." In Toe Stance, the toes of the empty foot rest on the ground, whereas in Heel Stance, the heel of the empty foot rests on the ground with the toes slightly raised.

Empty stances are transitional, designed for use between movements or before a kick. The feet are closer together than in Bow Stance. Some teachers advise bringing 10 percent or more of your weight onto the empty leg, to help with balance.

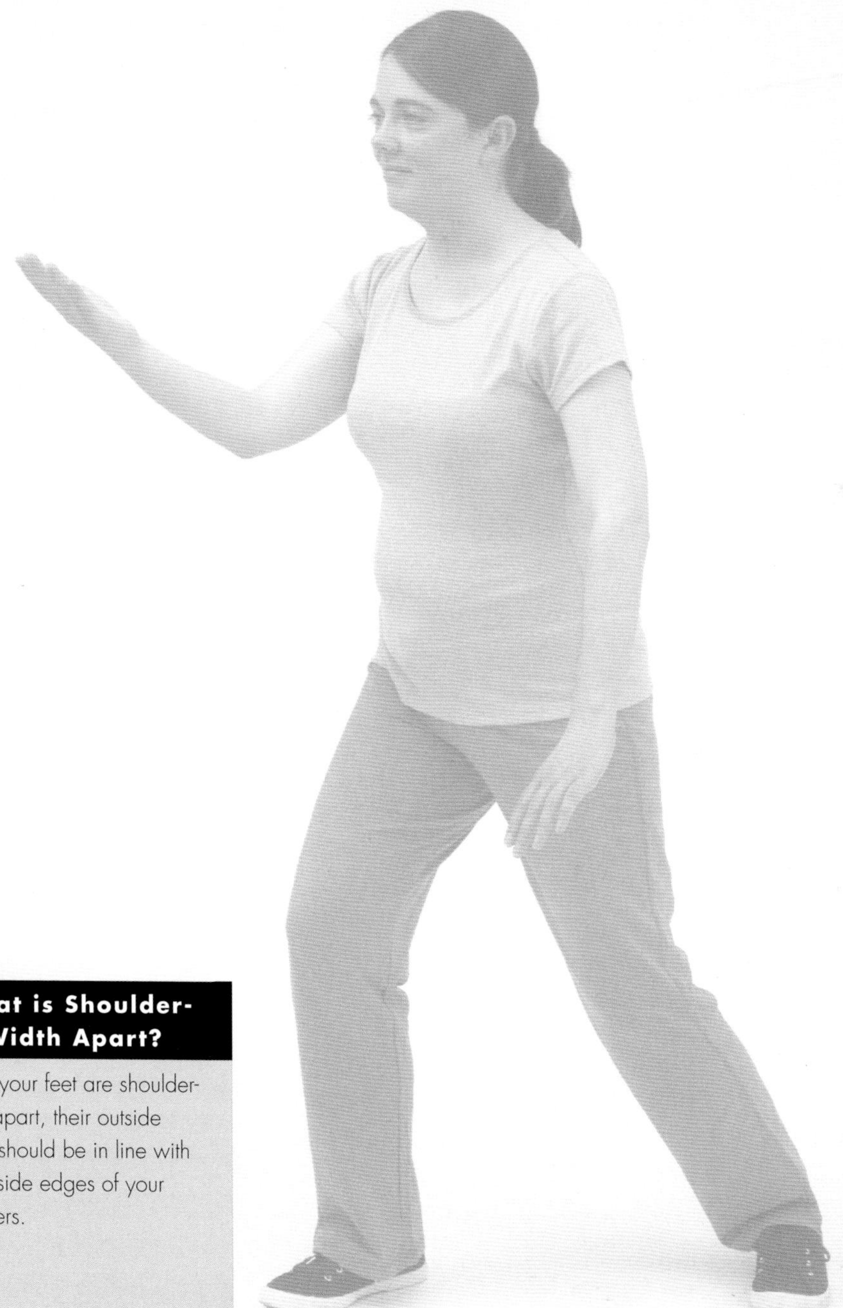

What is Shoulder-Width Apart?

When your feet are shoulder-width apart, their outside edges should be in line with the outside edges of your shoulders.

THE BASIC STANCES

All stances apart from Horse Stance involve weighting the body toward one leg or the other. Where percentage splits of total body weight between the two legs are given—70/30 in the case of Bow Stance—they are

Horse stance

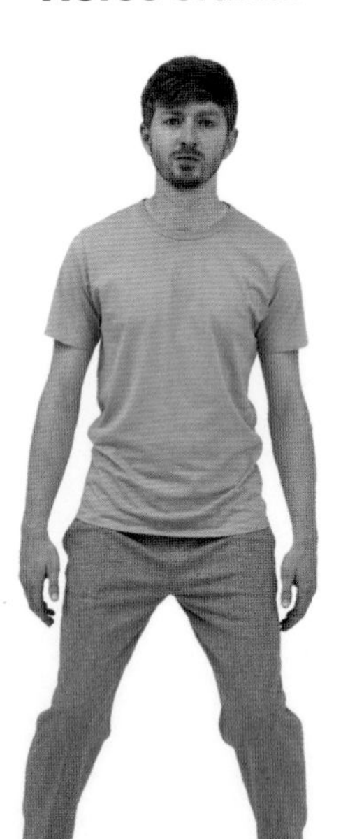

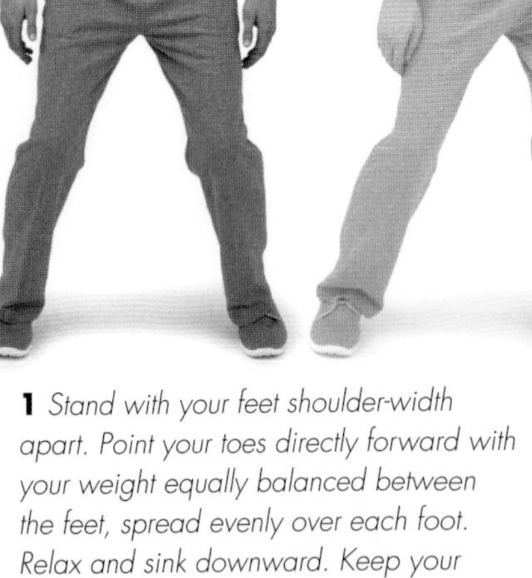

1 *Stand with your feet shoulder-width apart. Point your toes directly forward with your weight equally balanced between the feet, spread evenly over each foot. Relax and sink downward. Keep your head straight. Relax and breathe naturally.*

Bow stance

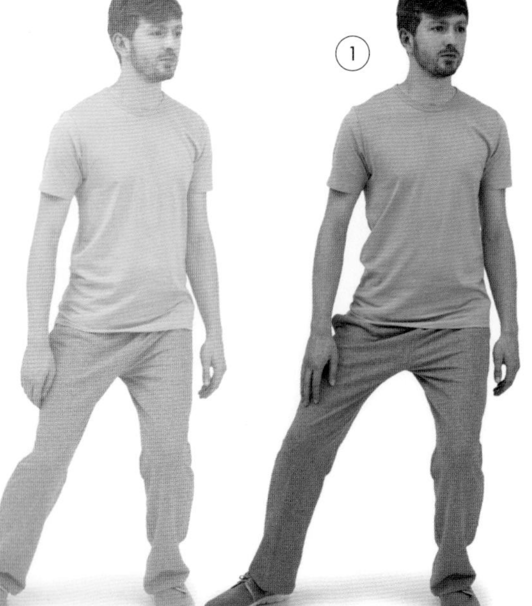

1 *From Horse Stance, bring your weight onto your left leg, raise the toes of your right foot and pivot on your right heel to turn them 45 degrees, then roll the foot down.*

meant as guidelines, and it is important not to get hung up on precisely what, say, 70 percent of your weight feels like, as this can distract you from other elements of the practice. In any case, some teachers recommend slightly different percentage splits.

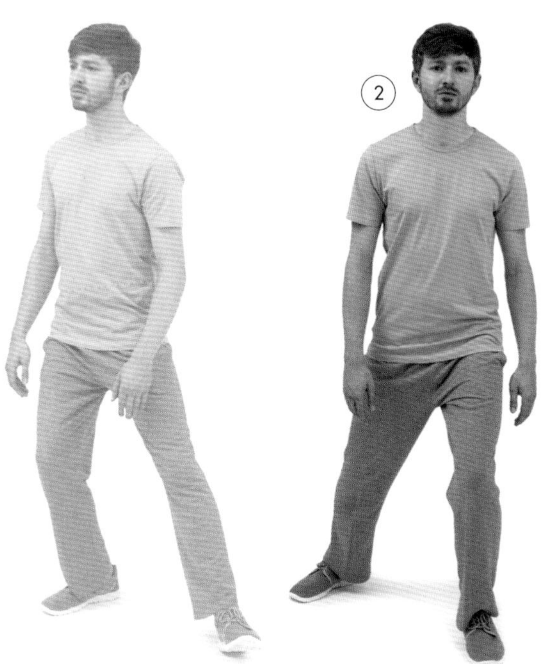

2 *Now bring your weight fully onto your right leg and step your left foot forward. Softly place your left heel down and then roll the foot down; your heels should be shoulder-width apart. Shift 70 percent of your weight onto your left foot, letting your left knee bend and your back (right) leg straighten while maintaining a soft knee. Bring your waist and hips to face the same direction as your front leg.*

Sit stance

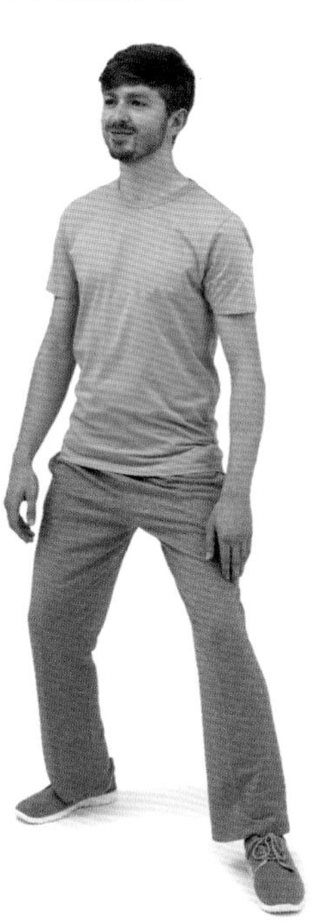

1 *To move into Sit Stance, keep your feet where they are, but then shift 70 percent of your weight onto your back leg. As you shift your weight, bend your back leg and straighten your front leg.*

2 *Now practice with your feet in the opposite position. Take a moment to settle into the stance, checking that your spine is vertical and that your knees do not protrude over the toes.*

Toe stance

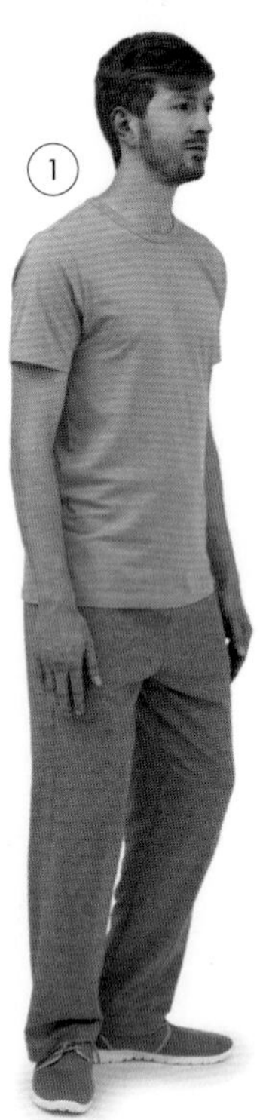

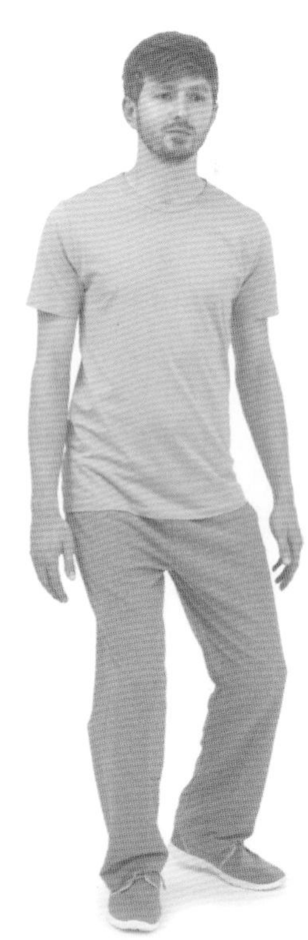

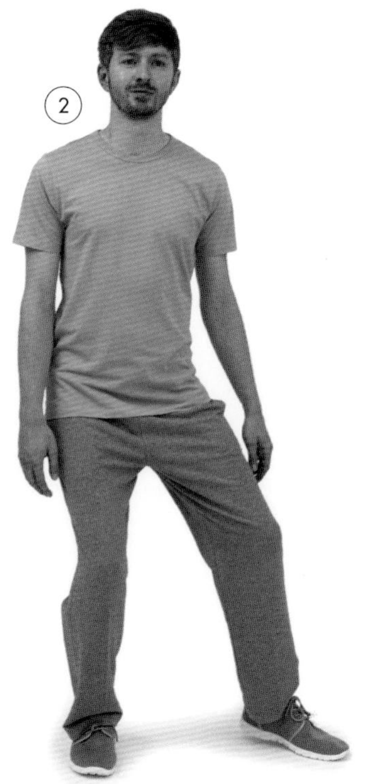

1 *Stand with your heels together and your toes pointing outward at a 45-degree angle so that your feet are at right angles to each other.*

2 *Bring all your weight onto your right leg, bending the knee to facilitate this, then step your left foot forward, bringing the toes down but leaving the heel slightly raised. Keep your weight on your back (right) leg. Settle into the stance and hold. Then step your foot back and repeat on the other side.*

Heel stance

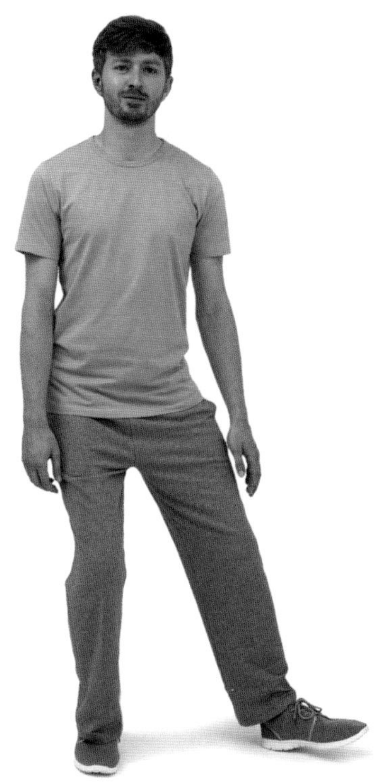

1 *Stand with your heels together and your toes pointing outward at a 45-degree angle so that your feet are at right angles to each other. Bring all your weight onto your right leg, bending the knee to facilitate this, then step your left foot forward, bringing the heel down but leaving the toes slightly raised. Your heels should be aligned. Keep your weight on your back (right) leg.*

2 *Settle into the stance and hold. Then step your foot back and repeat on the other side.*

One-Legged Stance

The form includes a movement called Golden Rooster Stands on One Leg where you move from Toe Stance to a position in which, as the name suggests, you are standing on one leg. This requires good balance and takes practice. From Toe Stance, bend your front knee and raise it to hip level or as close as feels comfortable (if you are wobbling, you have gone too far), keeping the toes relaxed, pointing downward. Breathe naturally and hold this position for a short period, then touch your toes back to the ground. Repeat on the other side.

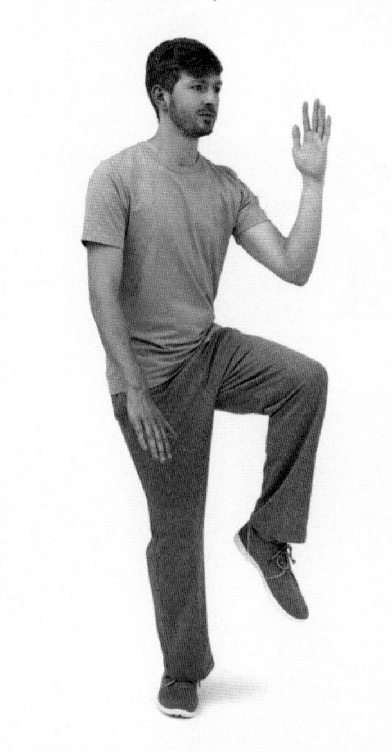

THE YANG SHORT FORM PART 1

This chapter introduces the first part of Yang Short Form, as devised by Cheng Man Ching (see page 15). This opening section of the form contains around half the total number of postures, if you discount the sequences that are repeated. It is sometimes known as the Short Half for this reason. The Short Half begins and ends in the same position, so it can be practiced as a discrete set of movements.

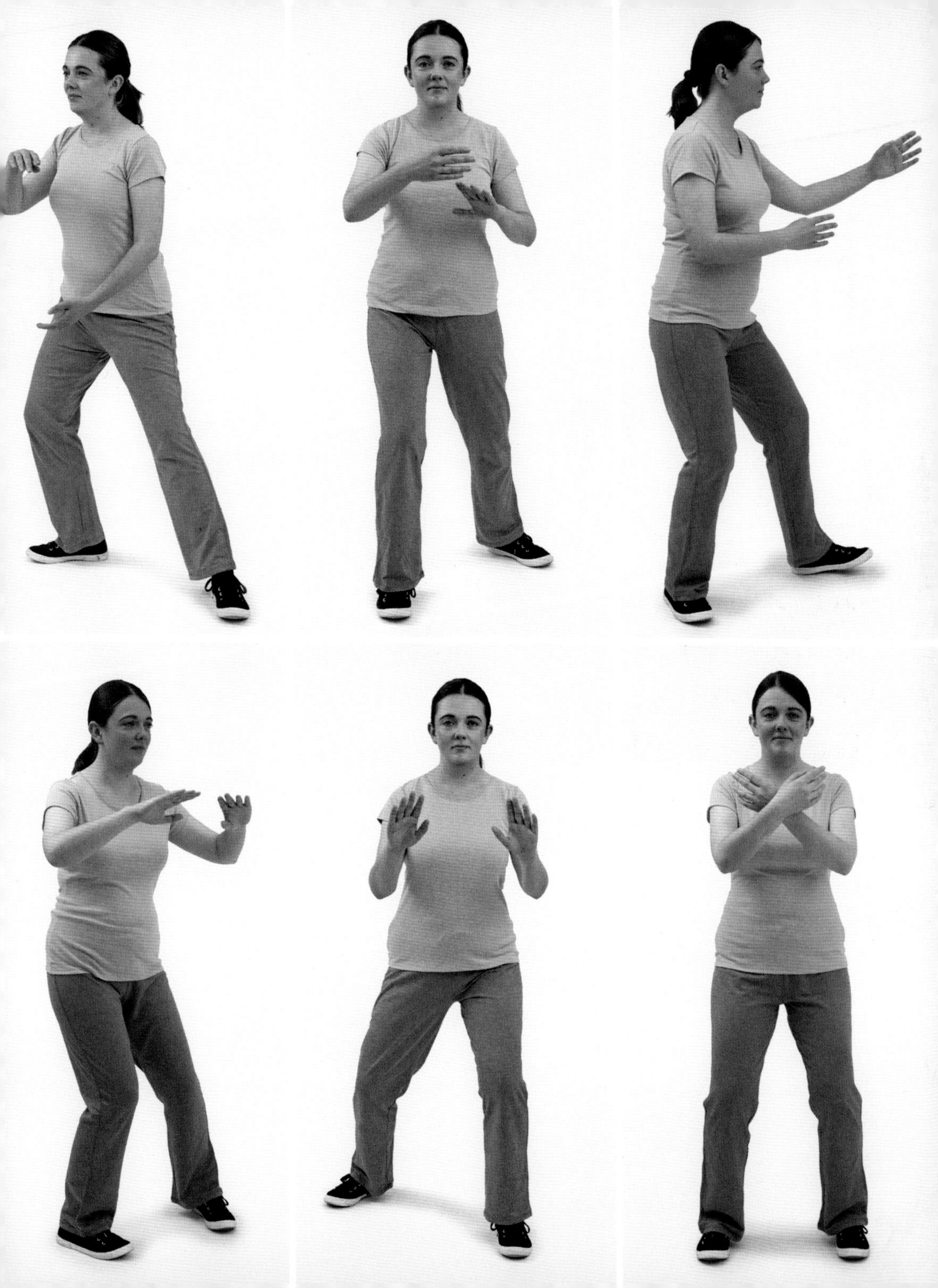

The Yang Short Form

The Yang Short Form came into being because the master teacher Cheng Man Ching wanted to make Yang-style tai chi more accessible and easier to learn. He reduced the traditional form, consisting of 108 postures, to a mere 37, mainly by omitting many of the repeated sequences. His short form is much quicker to perform, taking seven to ten minutes rather than the thirty or so required for the long form. However, it retains the essence of the original practice as well as its health benefits.

Getting started

It takes time to learn the form, and it can take a decade or more to perfect it. Try to integrate the fundamental principles of tai chi right from the beginning while you are learning the placement of the feet and the arms and other aspects of the physical movement. Focus on maintaining a relaxed yet straight posture and making your movements smooth and slow.
The more relaxed you are, the easier it is for energy to flow. All your attention should be on your movements, but your mind should be relaxed rather than overly focused.

As you become familiar with the movements, you can begin to refine your internal awareness of the principles, feeling how to shift your weight in the most fluid way and how to place your feet for greater stability. The more you practice, the more you will begin to realize how multilayered the form is—the external movements are actually a very small aspect of it. Tai chi is not about making perfect shapes with your body, and once you have learned the basic choreography of the sequences, there is much to refine and deepen.

It is best to concentrate on one posture at a time, only moving to the next when you have committed the movements to memory and are feeling a sense of flow and relaxation as you perform them.

Relaxation is key, not only in your body but in your mind. The form begins with Preparation (see page 82), which you can use as a transitional exercise to take you from the busyness of the day into the flow of the tai chi form. At the start of Preparation, take a few moments to mentally run through the eight points of tai chi posture (see page 28), standing tall yet relaxed.

Points of the Compass

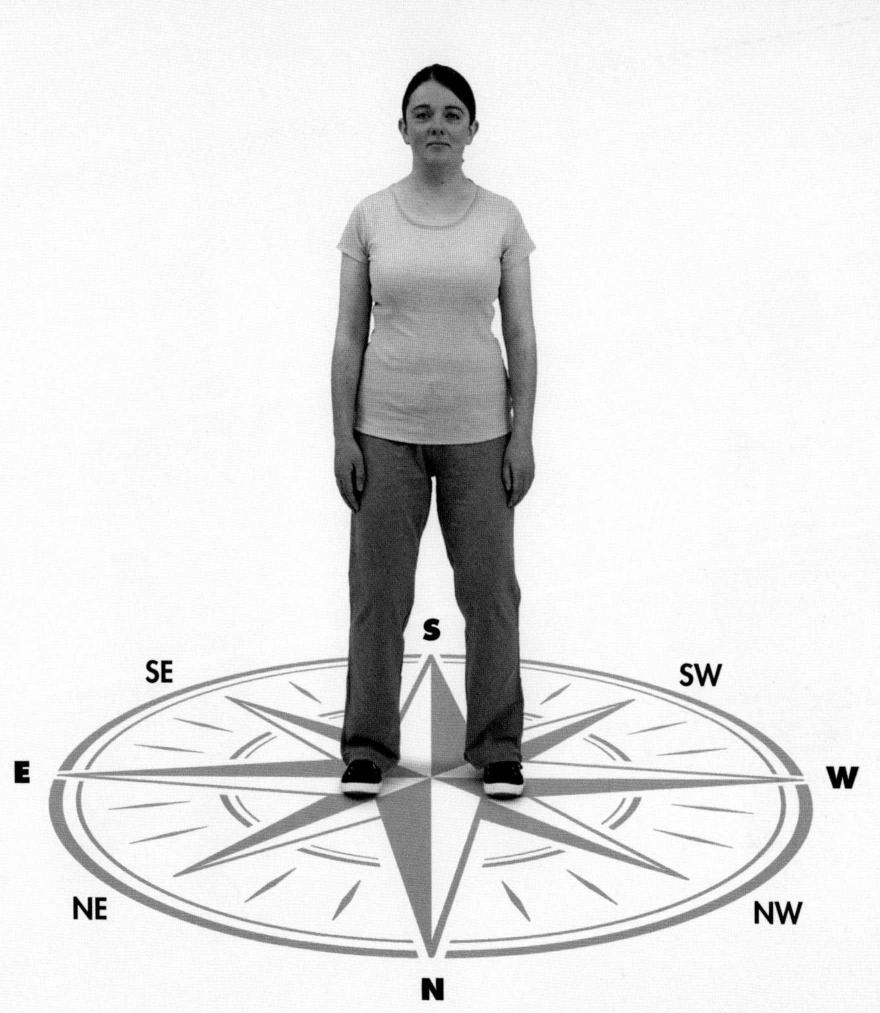

In tai chi, it is customary to orient yourself using the points of the compass. The way you are facing at the start is taken as north, east is directly to the right of you, northwest is diagonally ahead to the left, and so on. Of course, the compass points you use in your tai chi practice do not have to correlate with those of an actual compass—it is just a useful shorthand way of reminding yourself which way to turn at any given stage in the form.

PREPARATION

Preparation is an opportunity for you to come into the moment and steady your mind before beginning the form. It can be a perfect reminder of the need to let go of one activity before continuing with the next. Take three long, slow,

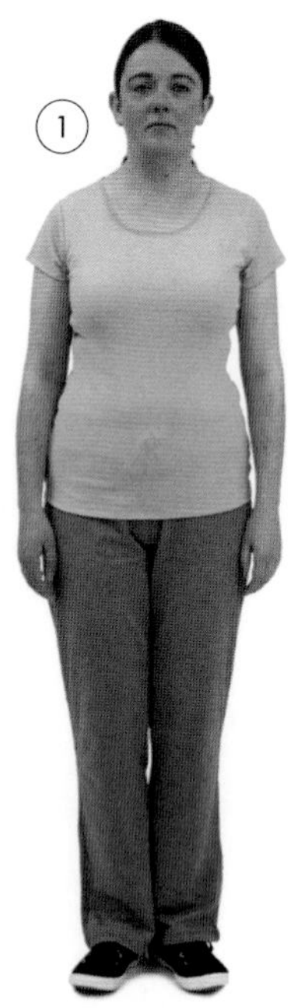

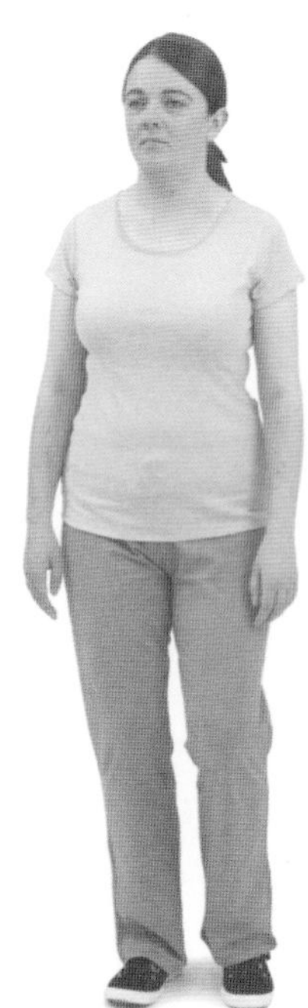

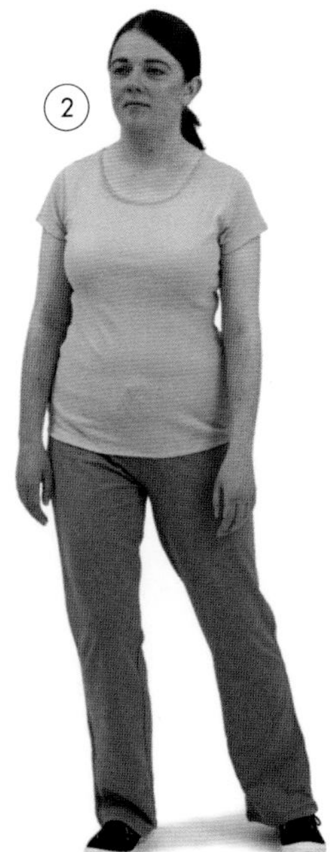

1 *Facing forward (north), stand with your heels touching and your feet pointing outward. Let your arms hang comfortably by your sides, shoulders relaxed, and breathe naturally. Your weight should be equally balanced between your feet.*

2 *Bend your right knee as you pour your weight into your right leg, letting your weight sink downward, and bring your arms slightly forward and away from your body. Then raise your left foot from the ground and step it to the left so that it is a shoulder-width distance from your right foot. Bring your heel to the ground first, placing the toes so that they face directly forward.*

deep breaths from the belly, imagining your breath traveling into the dantien (see page 24) and then out of it, before you begin shifting your weight.

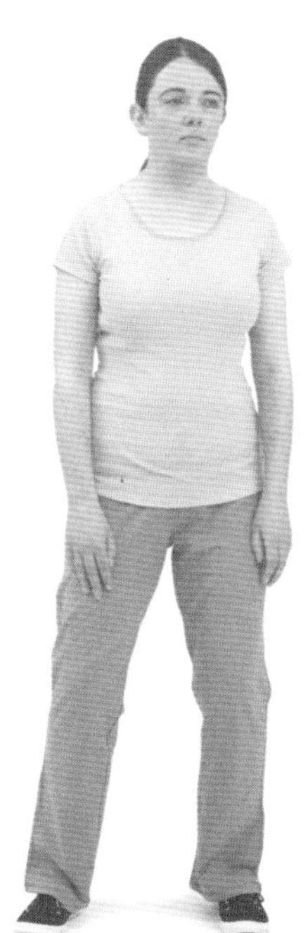

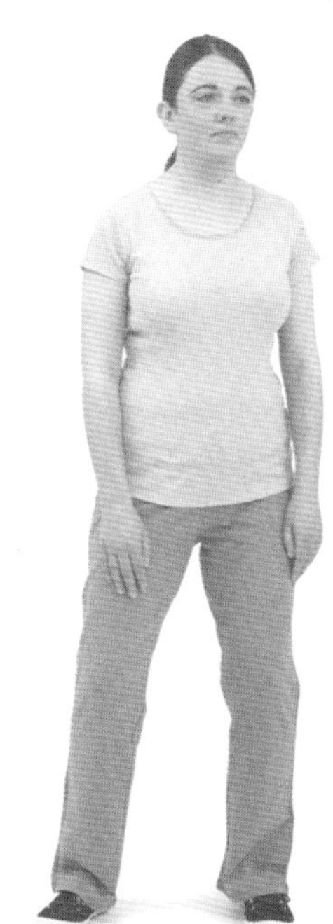

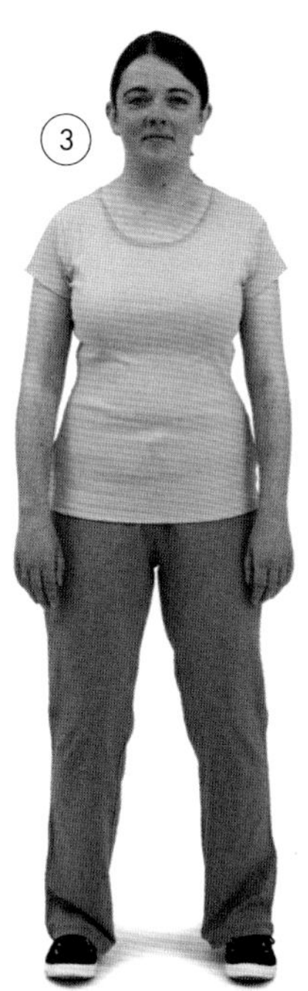

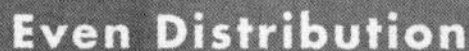

Even Distribution

Acknowledge your connection with the earth beneath your feet. Check that the soles of your feet make even contact with the ground—your weight should be evenly distributed across the sole of each foot, from inside to outside, toes to heel.

3 *Sink more of your weight into your left leg (about 70 percent) and slowly pivot your right foot so that it, too, faces directly forward. Center your weight, keeping your knees bent. You should now be facing forward with both feet parallel, ready to begin the form, weight evenly distributed.*

BEGINNING In this movement, also known as Commencement, only the arms move while the feet remain still with your weight centered evenly between them. The knees are slightly bent and the weight sunk downward. The movement of the arms is

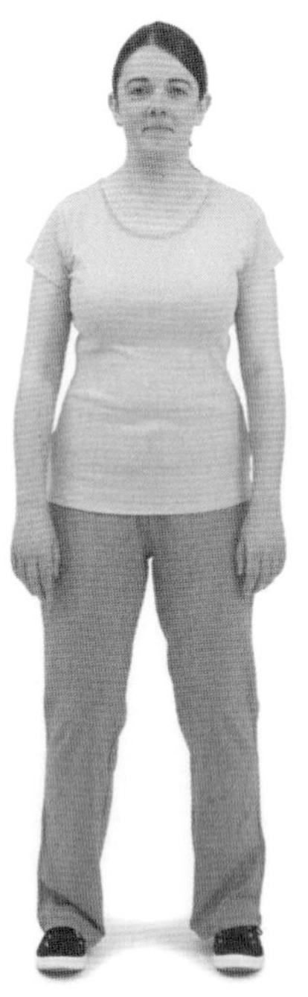

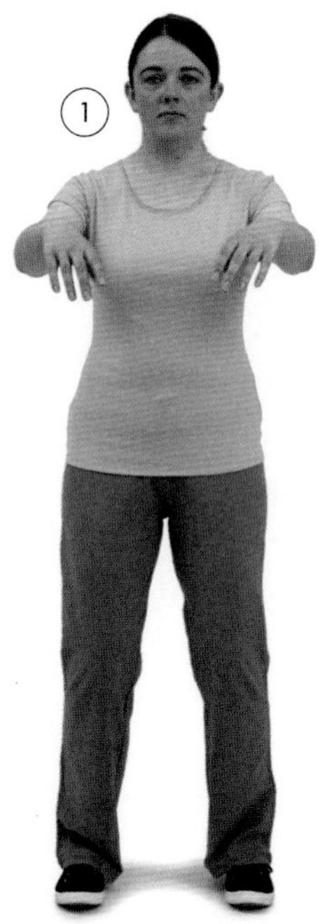

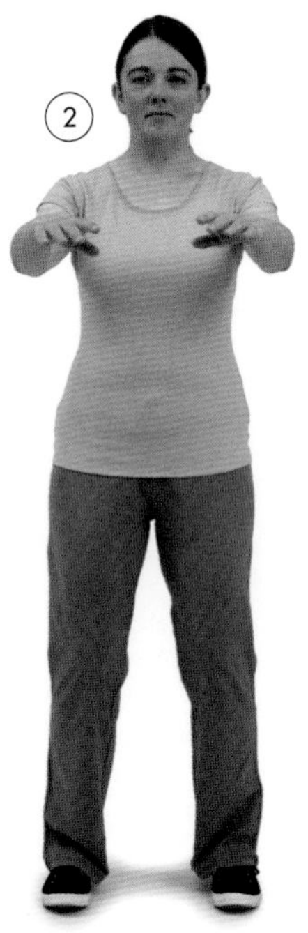

1 *Float your arms gently upward until they are parallel with the ground, roughly at shoulder height, with your hands shoulder-width apart. Keep your wrists and hands relaxed, palms facing down and fingers pointing toward the ground.*

2 *At the point when your hands reach shoulder height, draw your fingers upward so that they straighten a little and are in line with your arms and shoulders. Maintain the softness in your wrists and hands, and keep your shoulders relaxed.*

slow, controlled, and relaxed, as if the arms are rising through water. Make sure that the arms mirror each other in their movements, with the shoulders staying relaxed and elbows remaining below shoulder level throughout.

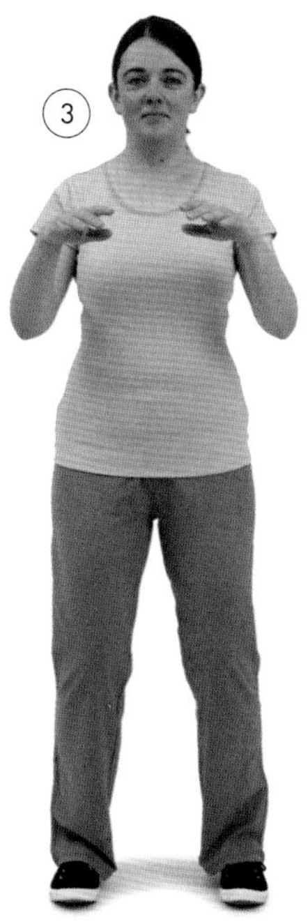

3 *Release your shoulders more, then bend your elbows and draw them down toward your body, letting the hands follow the movement and draw back toward the shoulders, palms facing downward.*

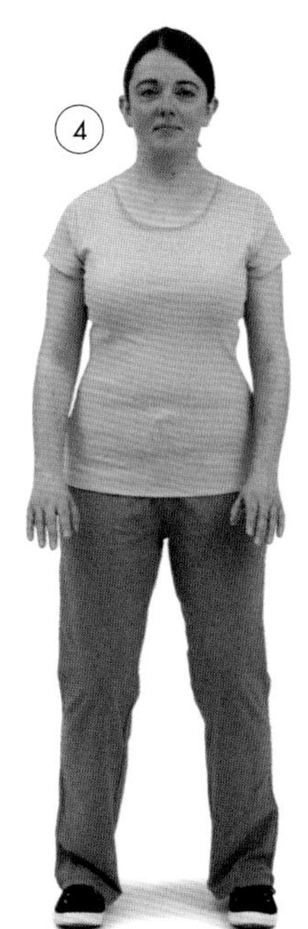

4 *Continue the movement by letting your hands float slowly downward so that they end by your thighs with your palms facing backward. As you do so, soften your whole body as if supported by a cord from above and sink into the posture.*

Holding an Egg

Maintain a space in the armpits so that your arms are held slightly away from your body. Some tai chi teachers suggest imagining that you are holding an egg under each armpit.

Focus on Grasp the Sparrow's Tail

The form begins with a group of sequences known collectively as Grasp the Sparrow's Tail. Like many of the movements, it draws on the natural movement of an animal for its inspiration.

The agile sparrow

Given that tai chi is based on a martial art, it may seem odd that this sequence is named for a small and practically defenseless bird, whereas other tai chi nature movements are inspired by creatures with obvious fighting prowess, such as the white crane or the rooster. One theory is that this sequence encapsulates the tai chi way of absorbing and moving away from an opponent's attack, leaving him or her grappling with nothing—or grasping at a tiny bird's tail that flutters away before you can get a hold of it. Cheng Man Ching recommended Grasp the Sparrow's Tail for two-person training sequences (called Push Hands), a very gentle form of slowed-down sparring that can help make the martial application of the movements much clearer.

Four moves, four times

This sequence includes the four fundamental techniques of tai chi, which are Ward Off, Rollback, Press, and Push. These postures incorporate the main ways in which energy manifests in the body—upward energy (Ward Off), backward energy (Rollback), forward energy (Press), and downward energy (Push). The sequence moves between expansive outward energy and yielding absorbing energy in beautifully flowing movements.

Grasp the Sparrow's Tail is repeated four times in total in the form, which is an indication of how important it is; only Single Whip, which follows it, features more frequently. It is also often recommended as a self-contained exercise, practiced first on one side and then repeated on the other.

Hold the Ball

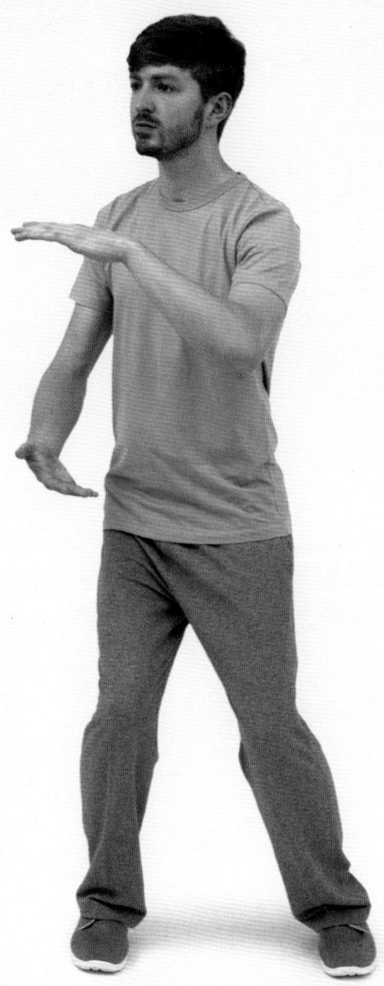

Grasp the Sparrow's Tail also incorporates the Hold the Ball hand movement in which one hand is held in front of the chest, palm facing downward, the other in front of the *dantien* (see page 24) palm facing upward. This occurs frequently, and is a useful movement to practice. Visualizing a sphere of energy between your hands will help you to get them into the right position.

WARD OFF LEFT This is the first part Grasp the Sparrow's Tail. In the final move, the left arm comes up, bringing energy upward and outward to deflect an

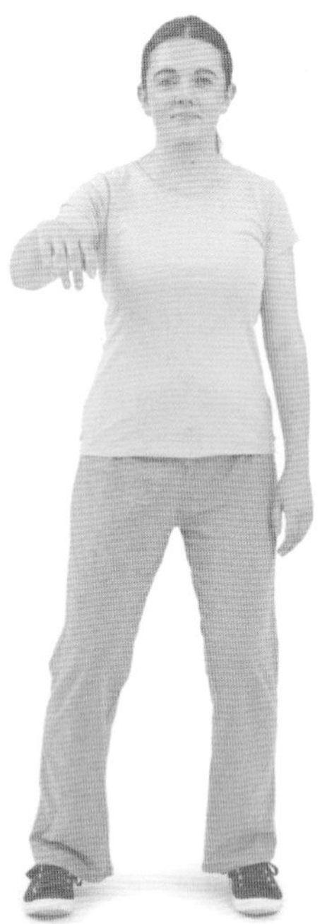

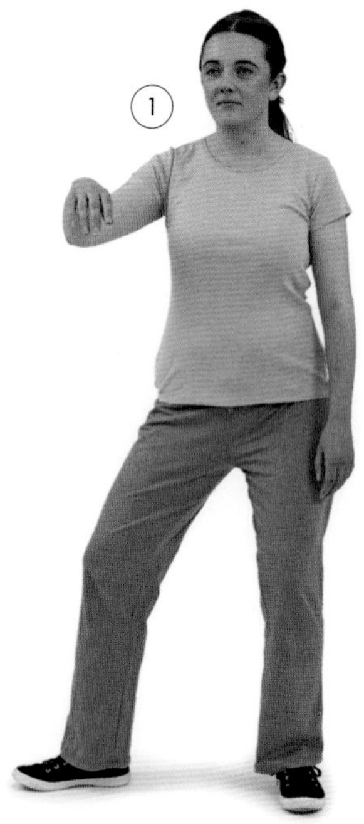

1 *Shift all your weight onto your left leg, relaxing your left hip as you bring your right hand up to chest height, palm facing down, and then turn to the right (east), letting your right foot pivot on the heel 90 degrees to the right.*

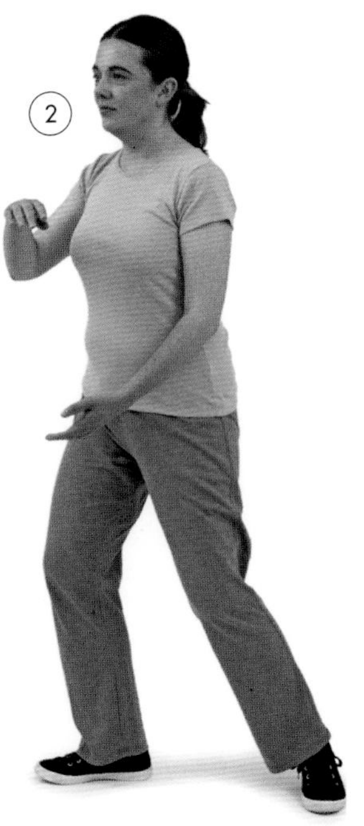

2 *Bring the toes of your right foot down so that they face right. Then shift all your weight onto your right foot, letting your left heel rise from the ground, and bring your left hand in front of the dantien, palm facing upward, to assume the Hold the Ball position (see page 87).*

attack from an imaginary opponent. When you reach the Ward Off position, check that your tailbone is dropping down and your head is gently upright.

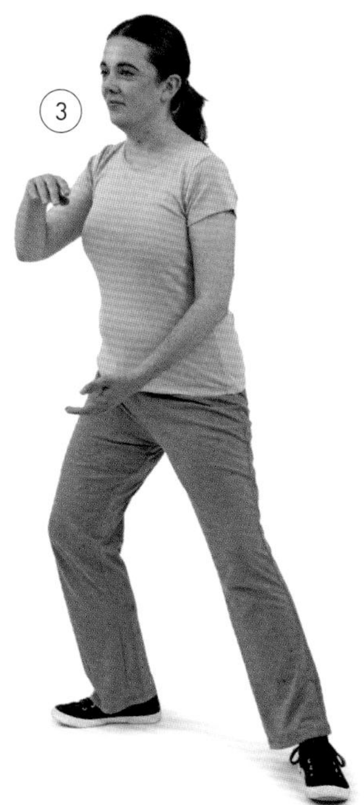

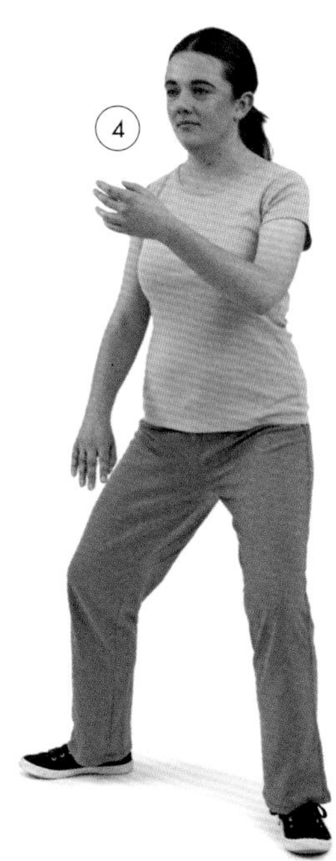

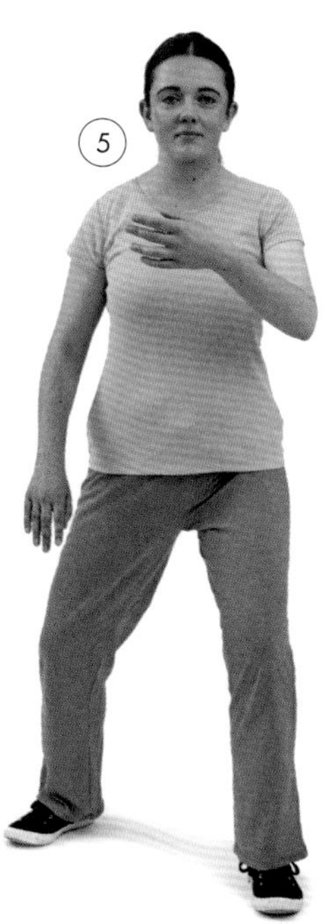

3 *Take a step forward with your left foot, placing first the heel and then the toes down so that they face forward (north). Your feet should form an L shape and the distance between them should be shoulder width.*

4 *Start shifting your weight onto your left foot, floating your left hand up to chest height with the palm facing in, and letting your right hand float down, palm facing behind you.*

5 *When the weight is roughly equal between your feet, turn your body to face forward and bring the toes of your right foot in by 45 degrees. Continue shifting your weight as you do so, ending with it about 70 percent on your left leg (Bow Stance—see page 74). This is Ward Off Left.*

WARD OFF RIGHT

Remember that tai chi is a continuous sequence of movements that flows like a river, so you progress smoothly from Ward Off Left to Ward Off Right. This is not simply a reverse of the previous sequence—notice that the arms

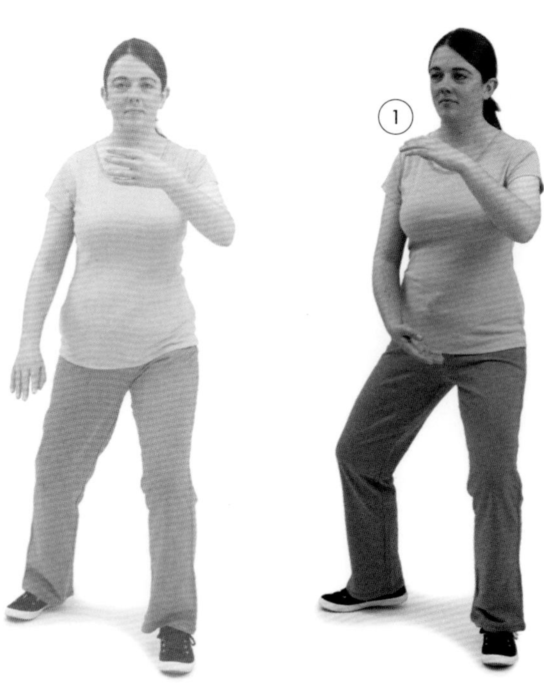

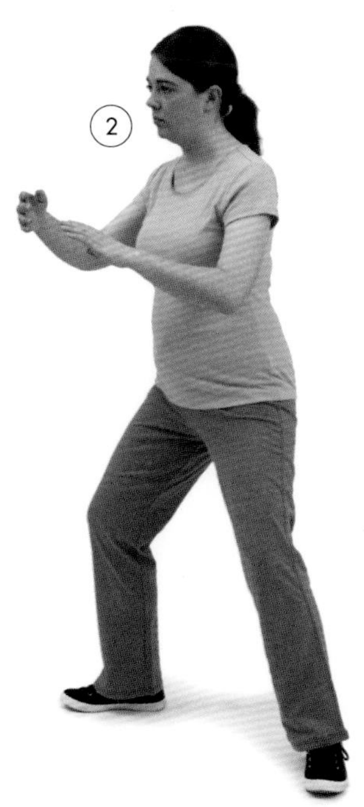

1 *Transfer all your weight onto your left leg, letting your right heel rise up from the ground. Turn your body to the right, as you pivot on the ball of your right foot through 45 degrees, to face northeast. At the same time, bring your hands into the Hold the Ball position (see page 87), this time with your left hand at chest height, palm facing downward, and your right hand underneath, palm facing upward. Imagine there is a ball of energy between your hands.*

2 *Step your right foot out to the right, placing the heel down first, so that your foot points to the right (east). Your feet should be at right angles to each other, with a shoulder-width distance between your heels. Continue turning to the right, with your arms following your body and your right hand beginning to rise with the fingers facing left, while the fingers of your left hand point toward the palm of your right hand.*

are in a different position at the end. Keep your knees in line with your toes at all times, and do not let them drift farther out than the beginning of the toes. Maintain softness and fluidity in your movements, enabling them to emanate from the center.

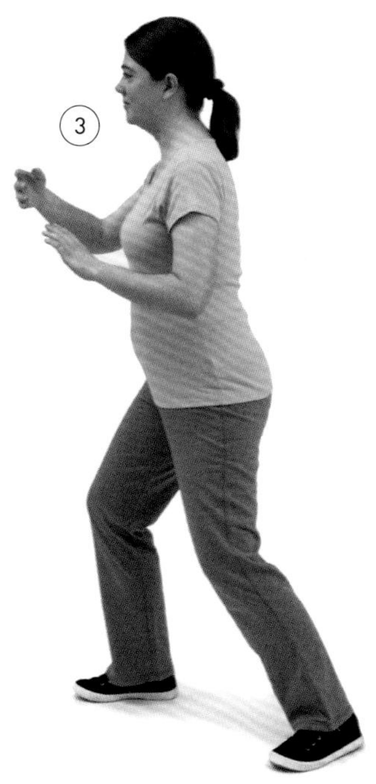

3 *Transfer about 70 percent of your weight onto your right leg. Turn your body to the right so that it is facing the same direction as your right foot, and bring the toes of your left foot in by 45 degrees (Bow Stance—see page 74). This is Ward Off Right.*

Correct Positioning

In Bow Stance (see page 74), your hips should be square and your heels should be placed so that if you moved the front one backward they would be shoulder-width apart.

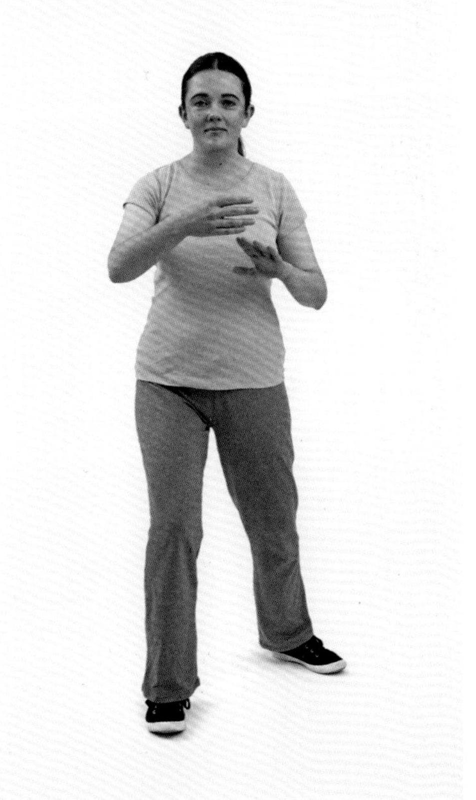

ROLLBACK After Ward Off Right comes the soft yielding posture of Rollback. In martial art terms, this is a defensive move that enables you to absorb the force of an attack from an opponent, which has the effect of throwing him or her off balance.

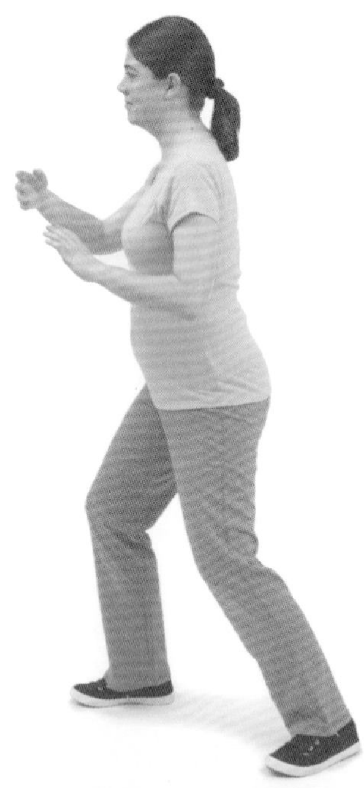

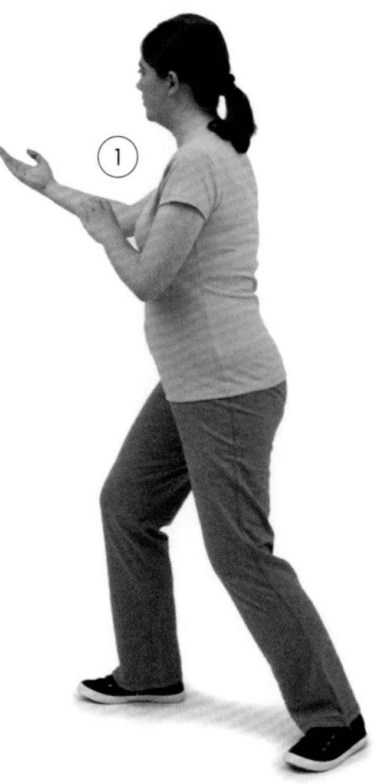

1 *Turn a little to the right, bringing more of your weight onto your right leg. As you do so, turn your right palm upward, with the fingers of your left hand pointing toward your right wrist.*

Moving from the Waist

Remember to move from the waist area—which means the lower abdominal area, encompassing the hips and the spine—while keeping the feet rooted into the ground. To help you move from the waist, try to imagine yourself sitting as you stand.

You then glide into the outward power of Press and Push. Notice that the feet remain in the same stance throughout—be sure to maintain their stable connection with the ground as you shift your weight from one leg to the other and back again.

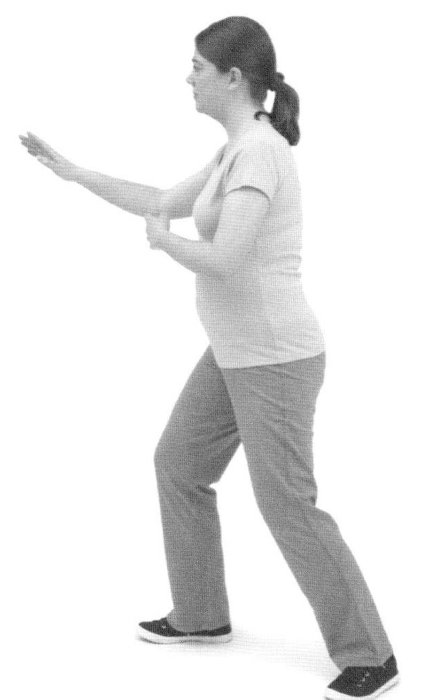

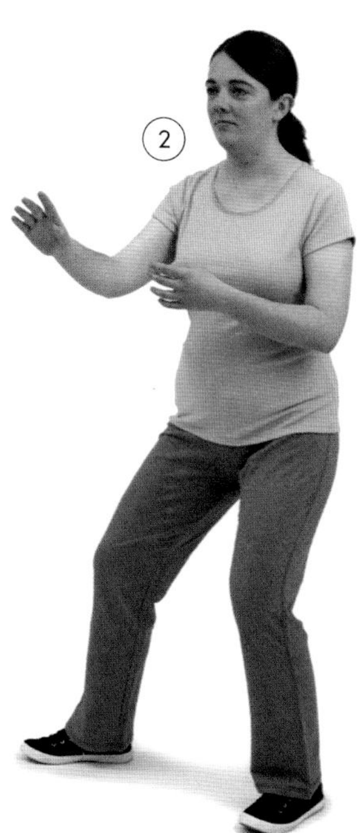

2 *Transfer your weight onto your left leg, turning your right palm to face forward while your left palm continues to face your body. As you transfer your weight, turn your hips to the left (northeast), keeping your shoulders and elbows relaxed, with your arms being carried by your body's movement. This is Rollback.*

PRESS & PUSH

The last phase of the Grasp the Sparrow's Tail sequence consists of the movements Press and Push, which send energy forward and then

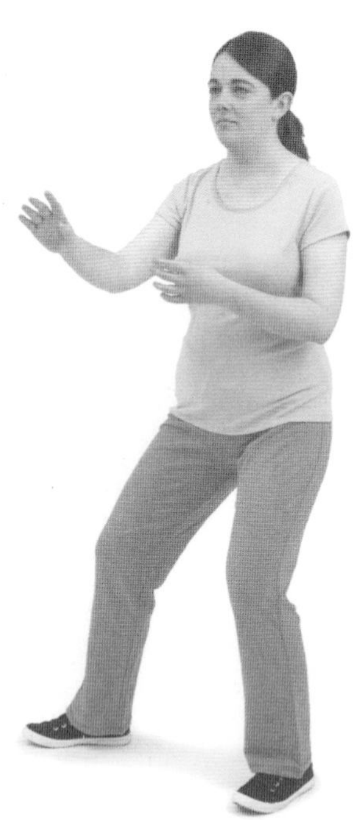

Press

1 *Bring your right arm slightly toward you, turning your right palm to face your chest, while you raise your left arm slightly with your left palm facing outward and bring it across so that the bases of your hands touch.*

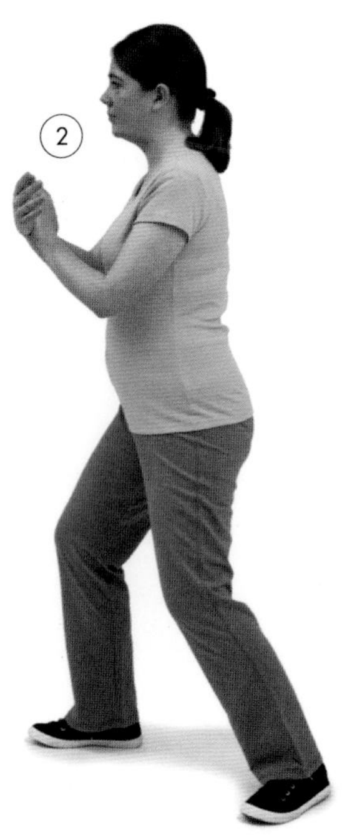

2 *As you do this, return your weight mostly to your front (right) leg so that you are facing the same direction as your right foot. This is Press.*

upward after the receptive gathering that occurs in Rollback. Keep the hands soft and curved rather than straightening them as you push.

Push

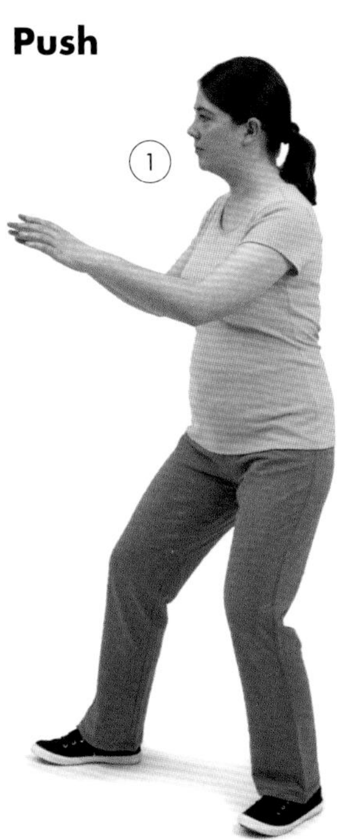

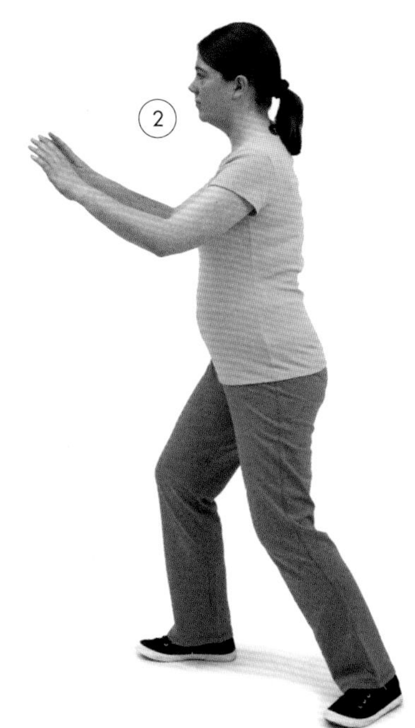

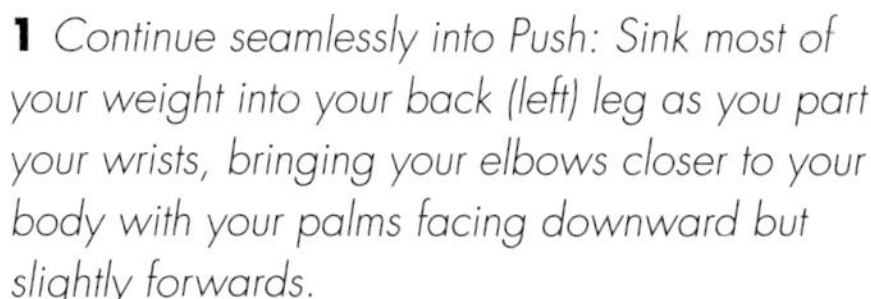

1 *Continue seamlessly into Push: Sink most of your weight into your back (left) leg as you part your wrists, bringing your elbows closer to your body with your palms facing downward but slightly forwards.*

2 *Then shift your weight back onto your front (right) leg as you push forward, raising your hands so that they are at chest height and chest-width apart in the Beautiful Hands position (see page 27). At the end of the movement, 70 percent of your weight should be on your front (right) leg and 30 percent on your back (left) leg. This is Push.*

Focus On Single Whip

This movement encapsulates tai chi's grace and beauty, and is probably the most well-known posture—it is often depicted in old photographs of tai chi masters demonstrating their prowess. Single Whip appears 5 times in the 37-movement form, and features with slight variations in all tai chi styles.

The posture

In Single Whip, the feet are in Bow Stance (see page 74), while your body may be slightly angled. One hand extends forward in a Push position, as if blocking or pushing an imaginary opponent, while the other forms a relaxed hook (beak) to the side, ready to deliver a jab or to grab the opponent's wrist once the initial attack has been deflected.

It's quite difficult to bring the hands into these two very different positions, in the same way that we struggle to rub our belly and pat our head simultaneously. It is worth practicing the Single Whip on its own to get the hang of it so that you can perform it without breaking the flow of the form, and it is also a useful posture for building strength and balance.

You may also like to spend time practicing how to form the beak, where the fingers and thumb are connected at a single point. Try imagining that a pea is placed on the inner tips of your fingers, or that a strand of fine silk is passing through them.

Making a beak

Hold your arm out to the side so that the arm is at or just below shoulder height and the elbow is dropped. Bend your wrist so that your fingertips are pointing toward the ground. Then bring the tip of your little finger to rest on the pad of the thumb followed by your ring finger, middle finger, and index finger—the pressure should be soft. Keep the wrist bent and relaxed, and make sure that the forearm and shoulder remain relaxed, too. Release the fingers slowly and in reverse order, and then repeat. This is a good exercise for the muscles of the fingers, hand, and wrist.

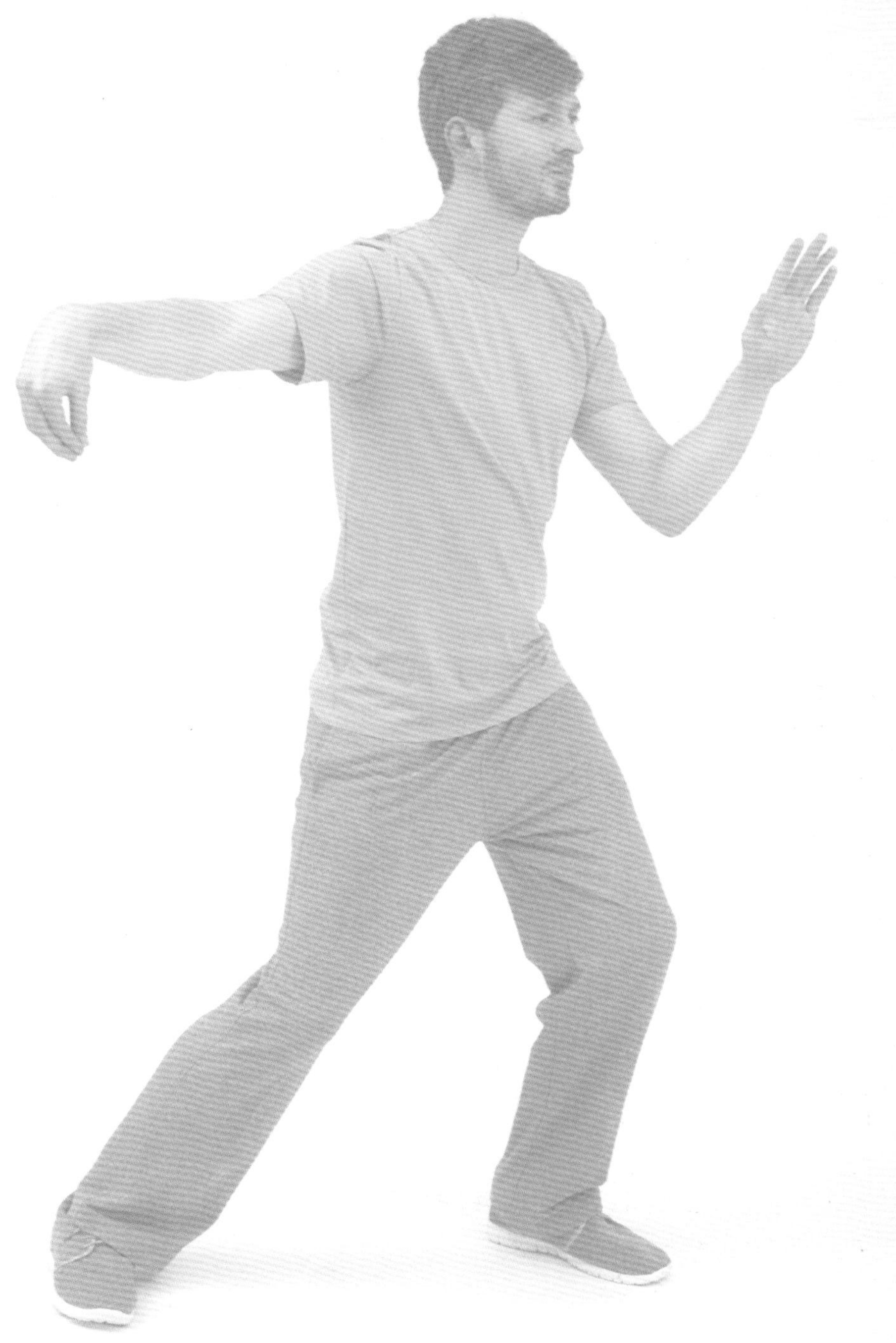

SINGLE WHIP

Single Whip is a complex and beautiful movement that encourages the flow of energy around the body. Try to keep the arms and shoulders relaxed throughout, and do not permit the hooked hand to rise above shoulder level.

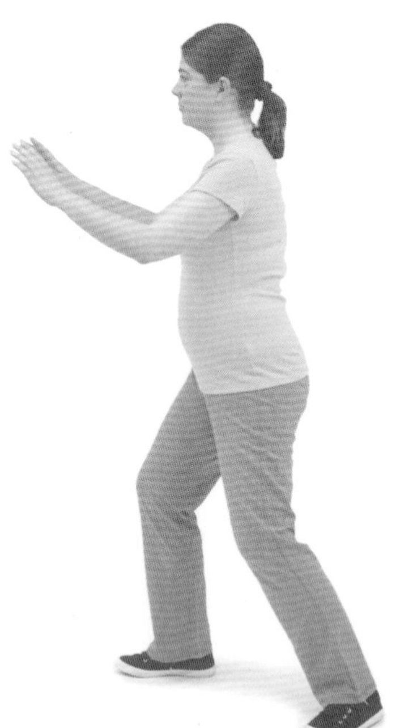

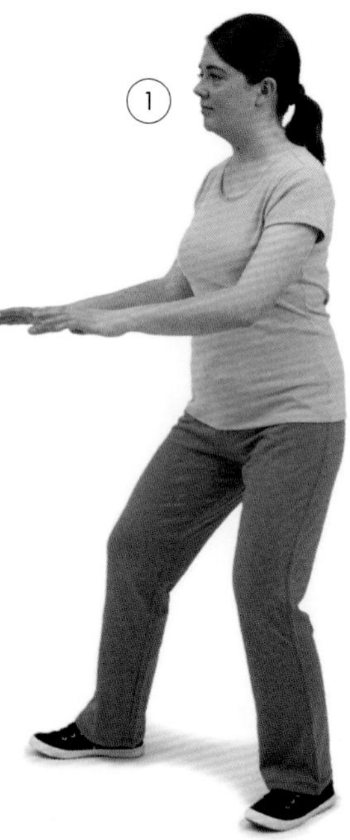

1 *Start transferring your weight back onto your left leg, lowering your forearms with a slight downward pressure so that they are parallel to the ground with the palms facing downward.*

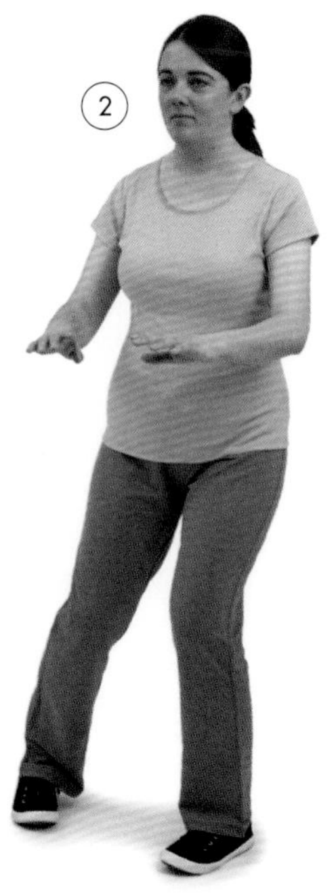

2 *Continue shifting almost all your weight onto your left leg as you turn to the left as far as you can comfortably go by pivoting your right foot on the heel to face forward (between north and northeast), leaving your left foot in the same position. Follow the movement of your body with your arms.*

It is useful to practice Single Whip as an individual sequence, holding the final posture to build balance and strength—this will also help you to master the various tricky hand positions.

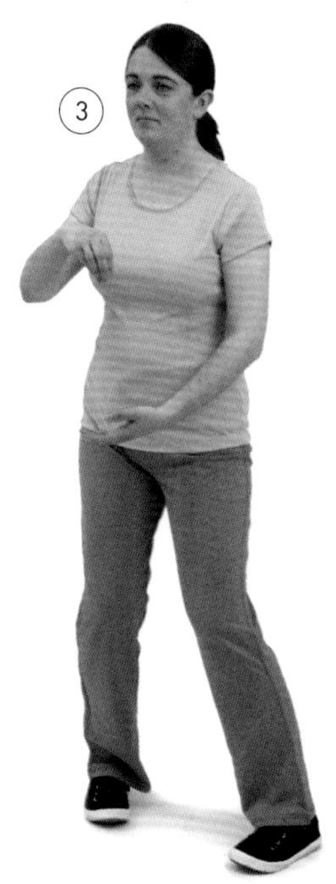

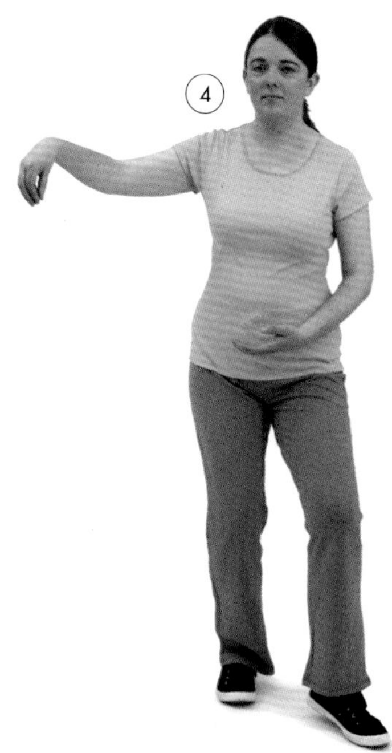

3 *Now transfer all your weight onto your right leg. As you do so, drop your left hand, turning the palm upward as in the Hold the Ball position (see page 87). Move your right arm in front of your chest, bending the elbow and forming a beak with your fingers (see page 96).*

4 *Turn to the left on the ball of your left foot so that the toes are facing northwest while your body faces north. Extend your right arm out to the right, keeping your hand in the beak position and your elbow relaxed.*

Continued overleaf

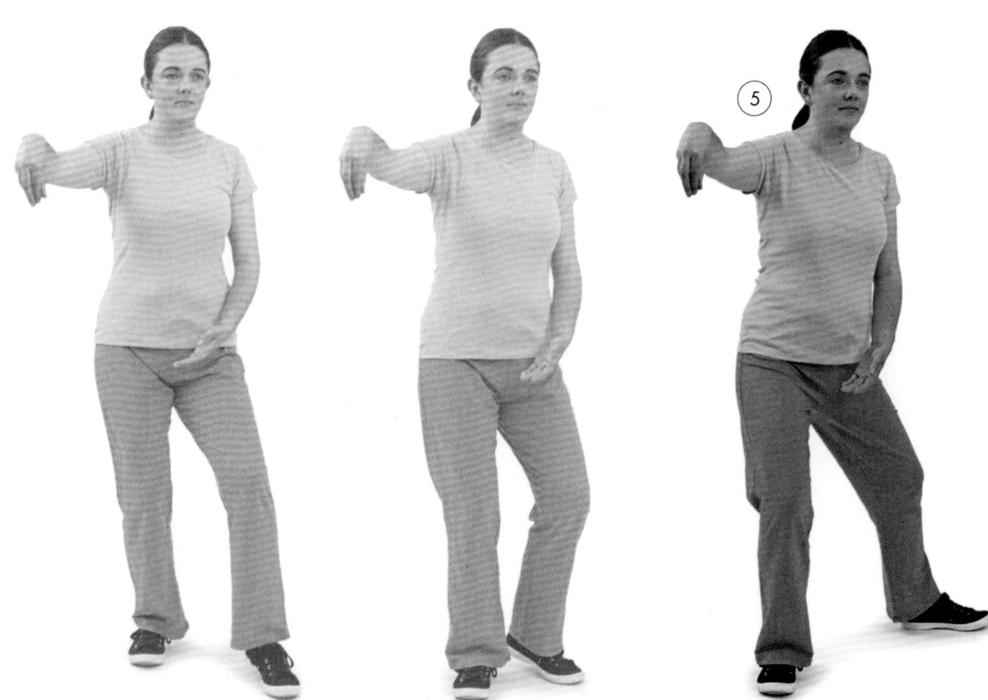

5 *Step out with your left foot so that the toes are facing west, turning to the northwest as you do so, placing the heel down first and keeping the weight on your right foot (you may wish to step back briefly first to help you balance). Your heels should form an L shape with a shoulder-width distance between them.*

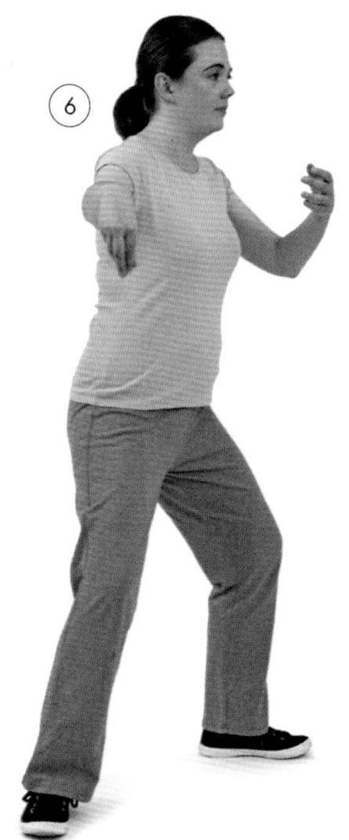

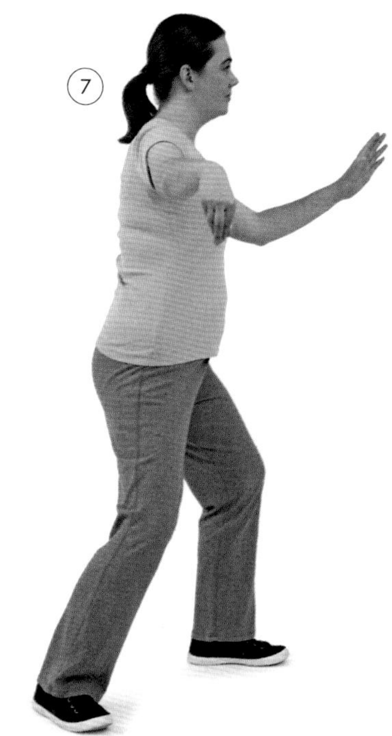

6 *Now pour about 70 percent of your weight into your left leg and bring your left hand up so that the palm is facing your chest.*

7 *Pivot on your right heel so that the toes are pointing northwest and turn your body to the left to face west in Bow Stance again (see page 74). As you end the movement, turn your left palm to face outward in the Beautiful Hands position (see page 27). This is Single Whip.*

LIFTING HANDS, SHOULDER STROKE

The form continues with these two short movements. Try to feel the energy between your palms in the

Lifting hands

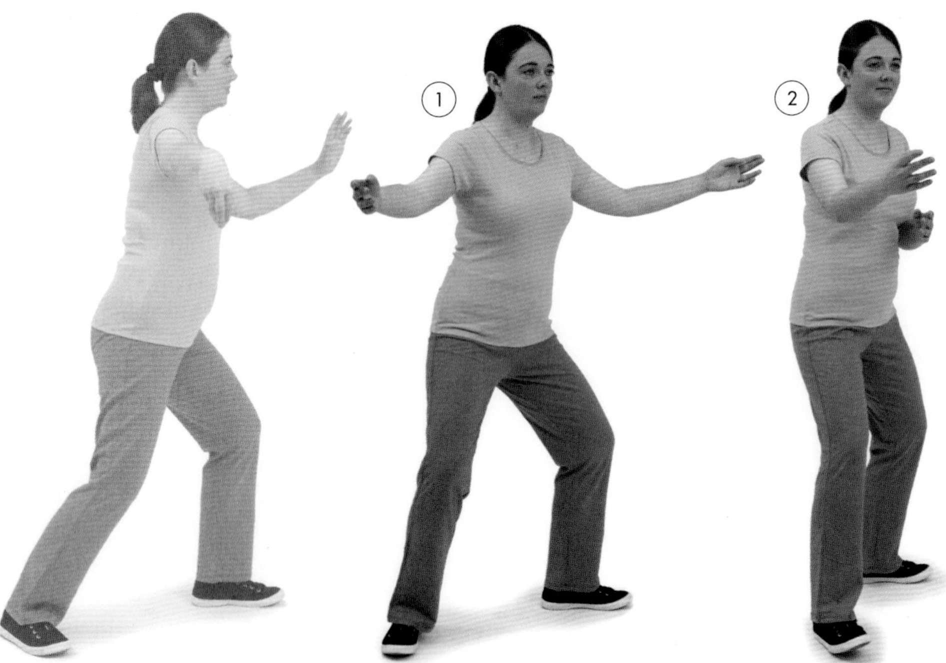

1 *Sink all your weight into your left leg. Raise your right heel and pivot on the ball of your right foot, turning your body to the right so that it is facing northwest. As you do this, release your right hand from its beak and turn both palms inward, keeping the arms wide.*

2 *Step your right foot to the left, placing only your heel down in front of your left heel. Keep most of your weight on your left leg. This is Heel Stance. At the same time, bring your arms closer together with your right hand at shoulder height and your left palm facing your right elbow. Turn your head to face in the same direction as the toes of the right foot. This is Lifting Hands.*

final position of Lifting Hands; the same hand position crops up in reverse in Strum the Lute (see page 110).

Shoulder stroke

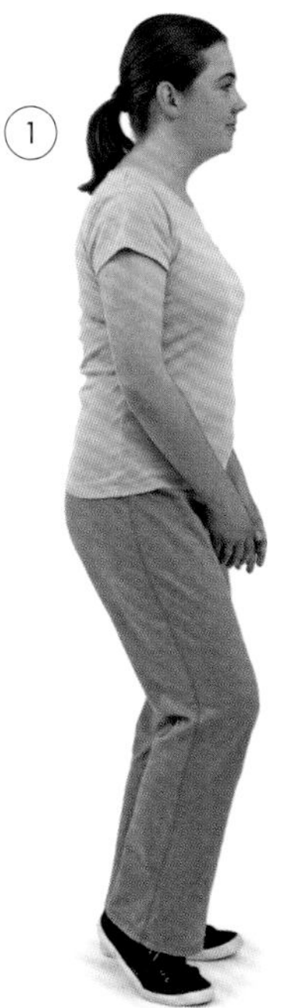

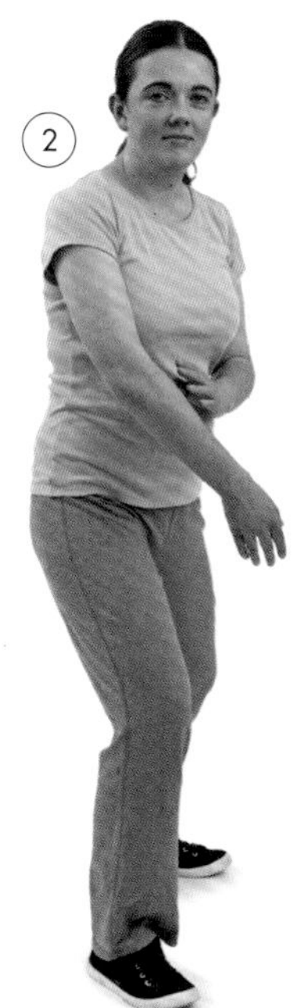

1 *Bring your right foot back toward your left heel, keeping your right heel raised. Bring your arms down so that your right hand is in front of your left thigh, palm facing in, and your left arm is by your left side, and turn to the left so that your right shoulder faces forward (north).*

2 *Step your right heel forward, then roll the rest of the foot down. Sink 70 percent of your weight into your right foot and turn slightly to the right to face northwest. As you transfer your weight, raise your left hand to bring the palm opposite your inside right elbow and curve your right arm slightly, bringing your right hand in front of your groin. Look over your right shoulder. This is Shoulder Stroke.*

Focus On White Crane Spreads Its Wings

The white crane is the most important bird in Chinese mythology, representing longevity or immortality. It also symbolizes patience because of its habit of standing on one leg and remaining perfectly still, waiting for the perfect opportunity to strike. The fighting abilities of the white crane are said to be the inspiration for tai chi, and the bird also lends its name to a form of kung fu.

You can regard the white crane as the perfect expression of the forces of yin and yang in harmony—its beauty and patience on the one hand, and its power and resilience on the other. In tai chi, it is seen as representing integrated movement, its wings blocking an attack while the beak stabs at the opponent.

Balancing opposites

In the final posture, the body forms a channel between sky and earth. The right hand arcs upward, while the left hand moves down, palm angled toward the earth. The lightness in the right hand is mirrored by the lack of weight in the left leg, and the downward action of the left hand is reflected in the weight and rootedness of the right leg. There is a clear energetic connection with both heaven and earth, and you can play with this idea in your practice if you like, imagining chi raining down from the heavens and bubbling up from the earth.

Toe stance

This posture introduces the Toe Stance to the form (see page 76). Almost all your weight is on the back leg, with 10 percent on the front to help stabilize you. Some teachers recommend that you place your entire weight on the back leg so that the front leg is free to move swiftly for a kick—its martial-art application.

This is a good position to practice separately from the form, especially if you want to improve your balance. Try holding it for a short period each day and you will notice that you can progressively maintain it for longer. Always practice on both sides. You can try asking someone to press gently on your arms to test your balance—when the posture is held correctly, you will stand firm.

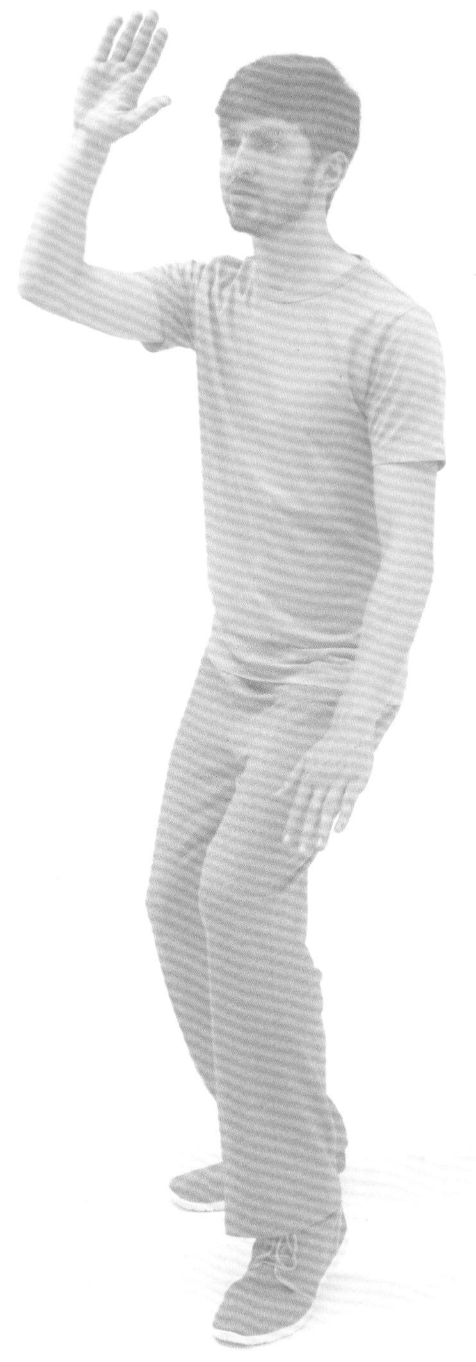

WHITE CRANE SPREADS ITS WINGS This pose is based on a bird opening its wings and standing on one leg, as the white crane does when it

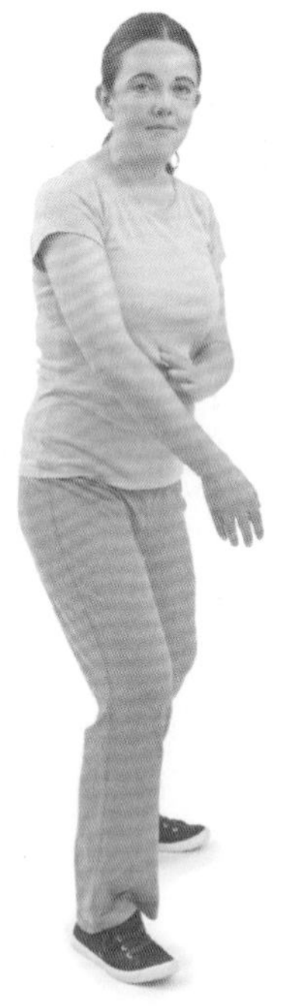

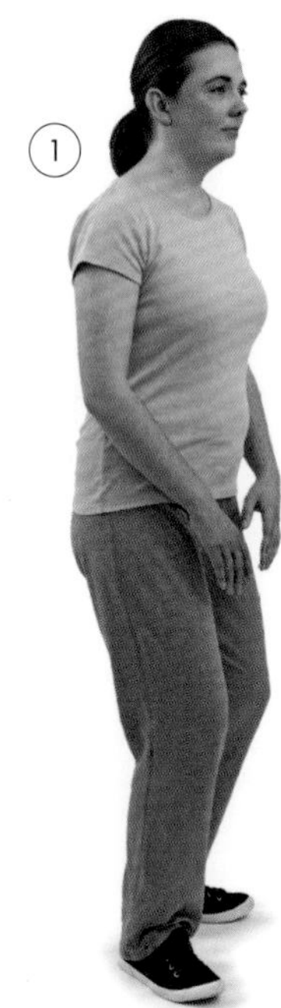

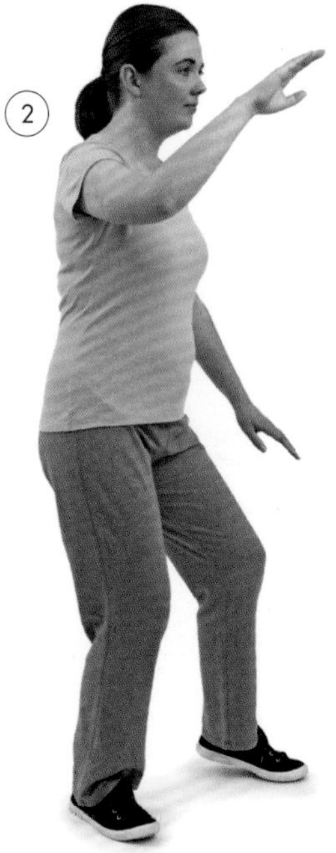

1 *Relax the neck, transfer all your weight onto your right (front) leg, brush the left hand down the right arm so that it is in front of the stomach as you start turning your body to the left (west), and draw in your left foot.*

2 *Step your left foot forward, toward the west, resting on the ball of the foot and keeping the heel off the ground. Your heels should be hip-width apart. Transfer 10 percent of your weight from your right leg to your left leg. This is Toe Stance. As you are turning and positioning your feet, bring your right hand upward and your left one downward.*

is poised to strike. Try to keep the shoulder relaxed in the final movement, raising the right arm only as far as feels comfortable and keeping the elbow soft.

Opposing Pairs

In the posture, notice how the body balances opposites, with the limbs working in opposing pairs. The left arm and right leg are weighted and rooted downward toward the earth, while the right arm and left leg are unweighted and expansive, with the right hand pointing to the sky. Try to maintain a feeling of openness and lightness in the front of the body, while simultaneously sinking downward.

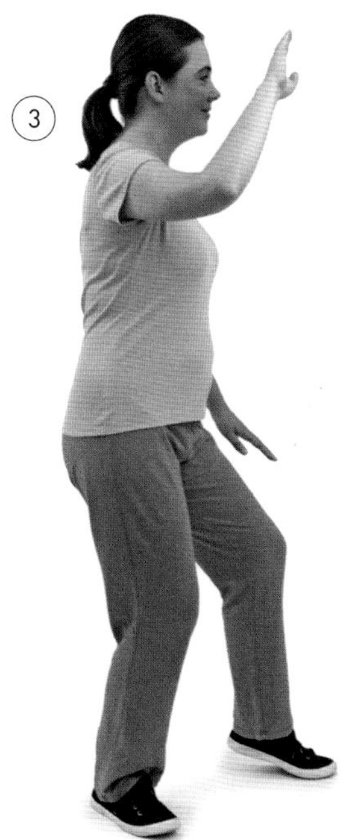

3 *As you complete the turn to the left so that you face west, finish the upward movement of the right arm when it reaches above your head and then turn the palm to face forward, while bringing the left hand to rest outside your left thigh, palm turned slightly backward. Maintain the weight distribution of 90/10 between your right and left legs.*

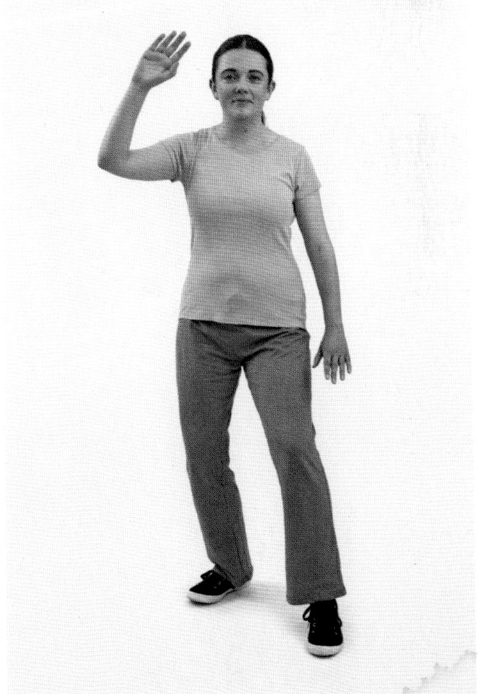

BRUSH LEFT KNEE & PUSH

This sequence appears for the first time here and is then repeated after the following movement of Strum the Lute. As in White Crane Spreads Its Wings sequence, the left arm is paired with the right leg,

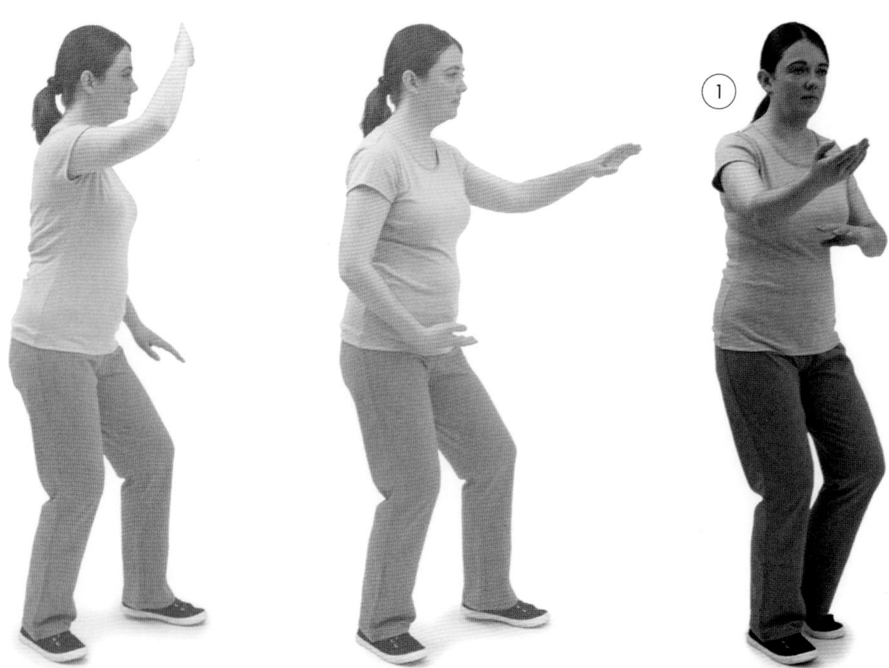

1 *Transfer all your weight back onto your right leg as you turn to the right. Meanwhile, lower your right arm in front of you, palm facing upward, then circle it up to shoulder height, palm facing you; bring the left arm up and then fold in at chest height.*

and the right arm with the left leg, so it is important to harmonize their movements. When you turn to the right, take the turn only as far as feels comfortable. If your spine and head are pulled out of alignment, you are going too far.

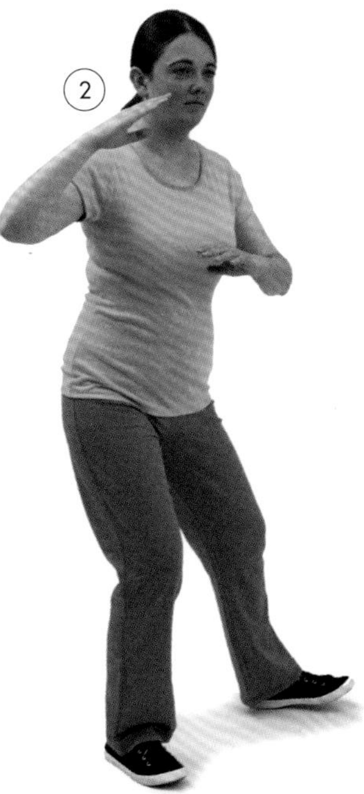

2 *Step your left foot to the west, heel down first, and as you do so, bend your right elbow and bring your right arm in near the shoulder with the palm facing to the front and down.*

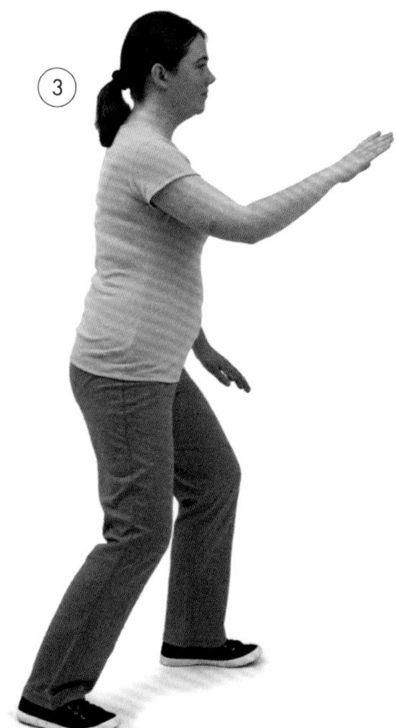

3 *Transfer 70 percent of your weight to your front (left) leg, bringing your right foot inward slightly and turning your body to face west, while brushing your left hand over the top of your left knee (without touching) and bringing your right hand up and forward into the Push position* *(see page 95).*

Smooth Movement

In the final movement, the fingertips are brought forward by the turn of the body. Keep your hand in line with your right shoulder, as well as with your back leg. The movement should be smooth and continuous throughout.

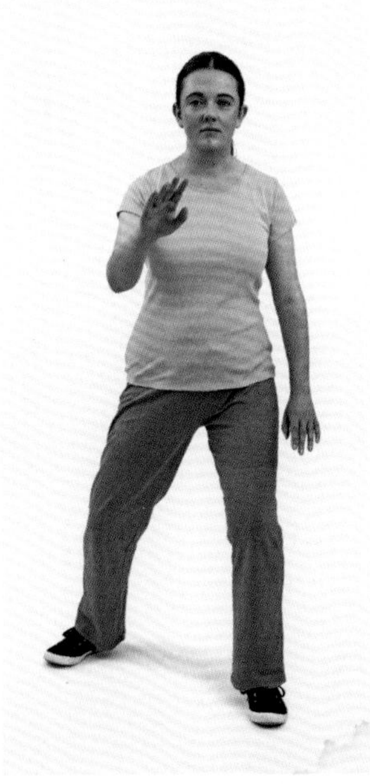

STRUM THE LUTE, BRUSH LEFT KNEE & PUSH

This movement is also known as Play the Guitar or Play the Pipa, named for the placement of the hands, which appear poised to strum a musical instrument. It can be helpful to

Strum the lute

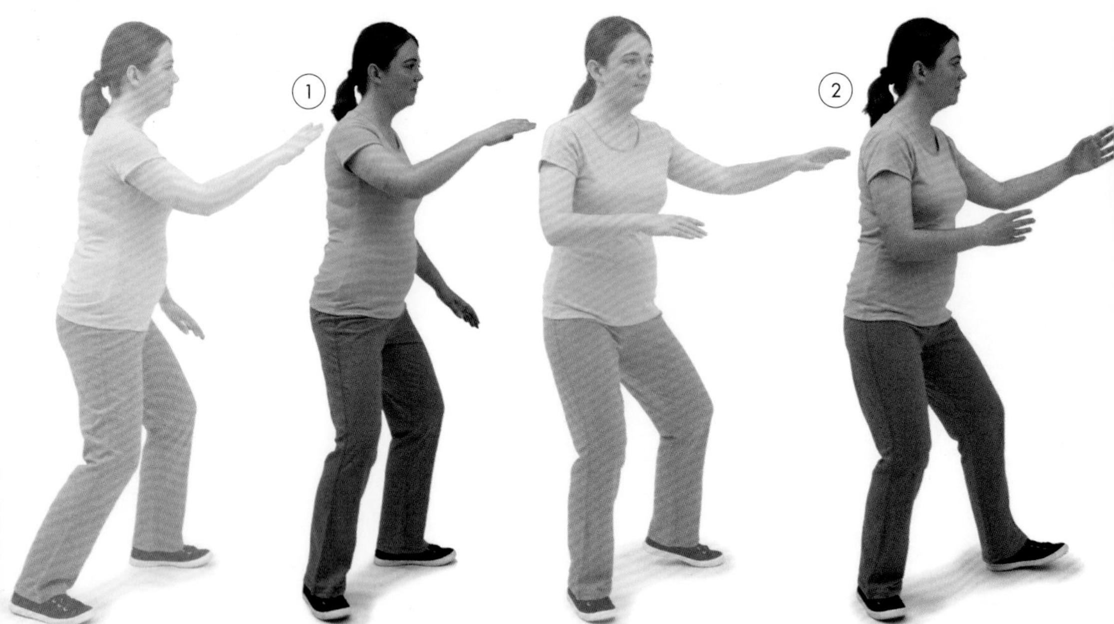

1 *Bring your weight fully onto your left leg, raise your right heel and then take a half-step with your right foot to bring it closer to your left (about half a shoulder-width apart), placing the ball of the foot down first facing between north and northwest.*

2 *Now sit back onto your right leg, letting your left arm come up and forward while lowering your right arm a little. Lift your left heel from the ground and step the heel forward and inward as you turn your palms inward. This is Strum the Lute.*

visualize the instrument in the empty space between your hands to check that they are in the right position. Strum the Lute is followed by a repetition of Brush Left Knee and Push.

Brush left knee & push

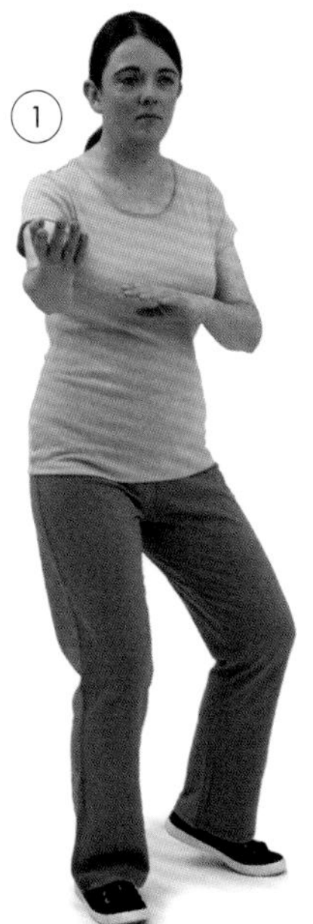

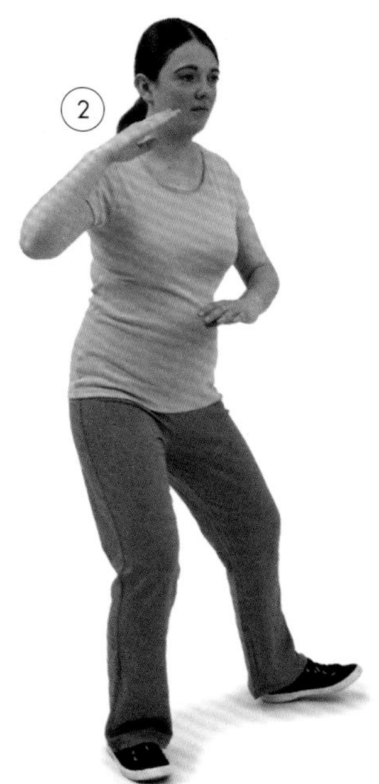

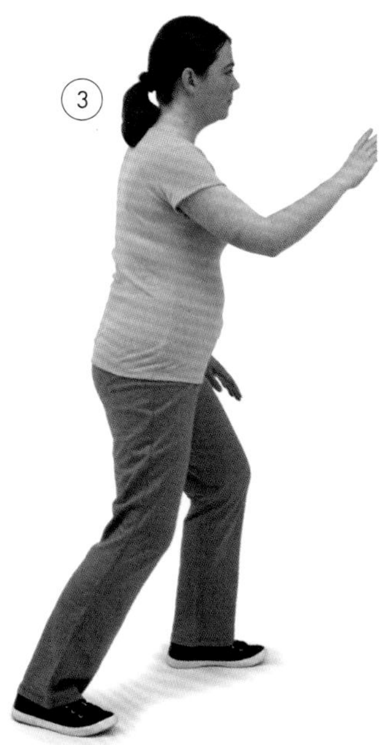

1 *Transfer all your weight back onto your right leg as you turn to the right, taking a short step back with the left foot to help you balance. Meanwhile, lower your right arm in front of you, palm facing upward, then circle it up to shoulder height, palm facing you; fold the left arm in at chest height.*

2 *Step your left foot to the west, heel down first, and as you do so, bend your right elbow and bring your right arm in near the shoulder with the palm facing forward.*

3 *Transfer 70 percent of your weight to your front (left) leg, turning the toes of the right foot inward slightly and turning your body to face west, while brushing your left hand over the top of your left knee (without touching) and bringing your right hand up and forward into the Push position (see page 95).*

STEP FORWARD, DEFLECT DOWNWARD, INTERCEPT & PUNCH

This is the first part of a series of movements that continues with Intercept and Punch overleaf. It introduces the Tai Chi Fist into the form

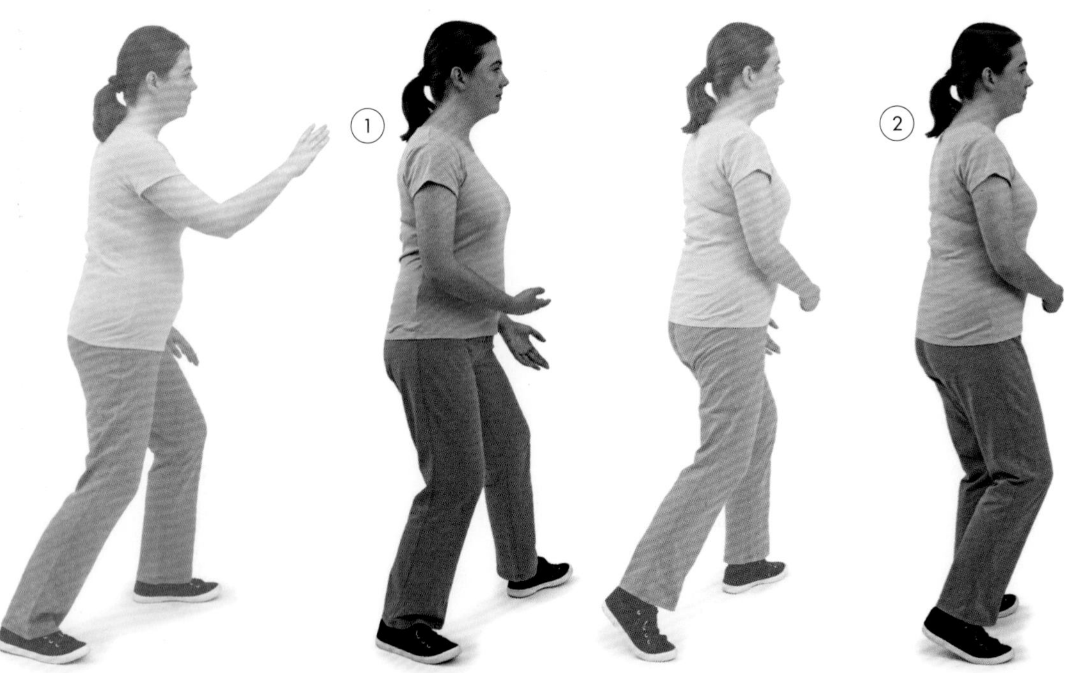

1 *Bring all your weight back onto your right leg while opening your left hip so that the toes of your left foot face southwest, then relax your left foot onto the ground. At the same time, lower your right arm to below the navel, palm facing upward, while turning your left palm to face forward.*

2 *Sink all your weight into your left leg, and with this forward shift of weight, let the right heel lift off the ground. Form a soft Tai Chi Fist with your right hand (see page 115), then draw the toes of your right foot in to your left ankle.*

for the first time. Remember that the movements of the hands and arms are directed by the turning of the body, and that they draw power from the rootedness of the legs and feet. Try to keep your waist area relaxed throughout.

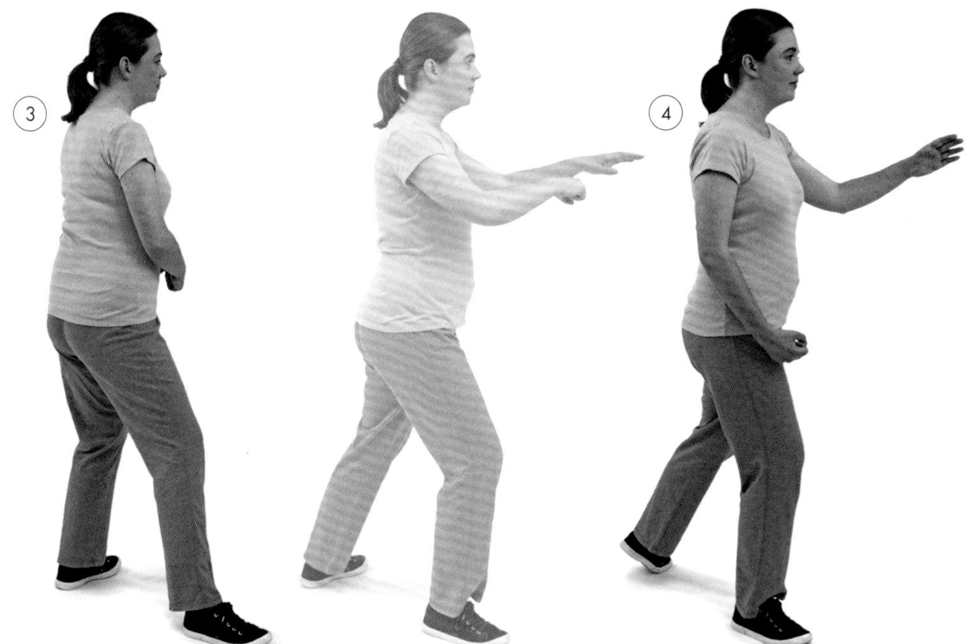

3 *Step forward with your right foot, placing it heel first and with the toes pointing comfortably toward the northwest.*

4 *Transfer your weight onto your right leg, bringing your arms up, then as you turn to the right, leave the left arm in place with the palm facing forward while dropping the right-hand fist to outside your right thigh.*

Continued overleaf

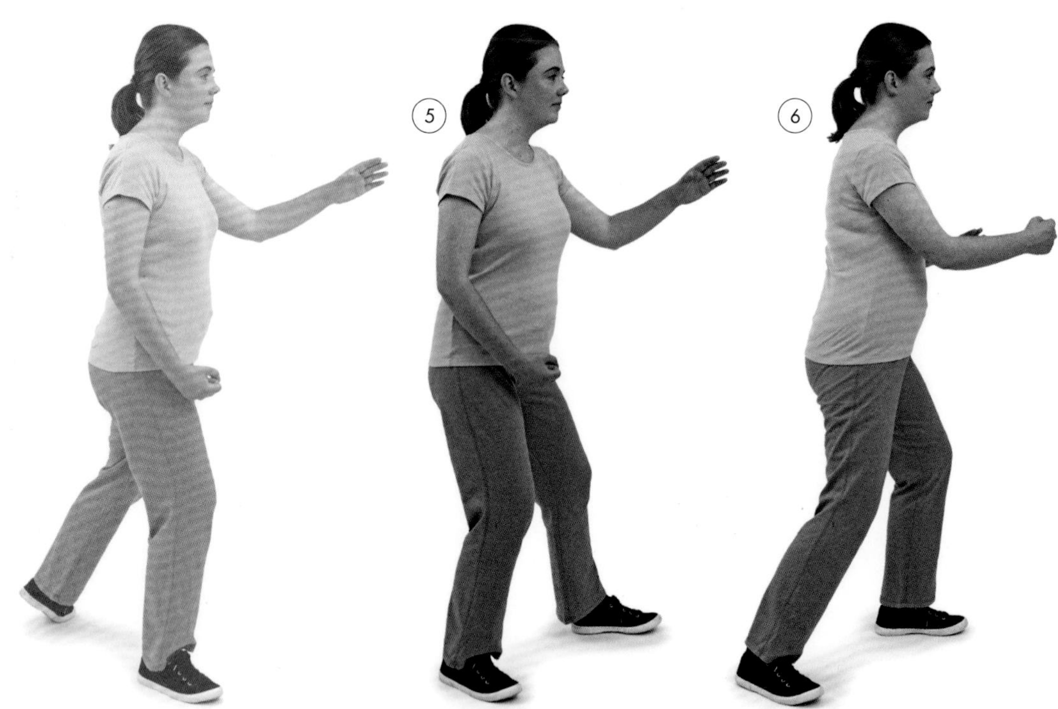

5 *Step forward with your left foot, toes facing west and keeping your body facing northwest.*

6 *Transfer 70 percent of your weight onto your left leg (Bow Stance—see page 74). At the same time, bring your right-hand fist up and forward, rotating it through a quarter turn to the left (counterclockwise) and then delivering the Punch. Keep your left hand in its protective position, palm facing your right forearm at the end of the movement.*

Stable Posture

In the final moments of this movement, check that your Bow Stance (see page 74) has the right distribution between your left and right legs and your body is correctly aligned.

Avoid leaning the body too far forward with the punch
Keep your spine correctly aligned with the neck and head
30 weight
70 weight

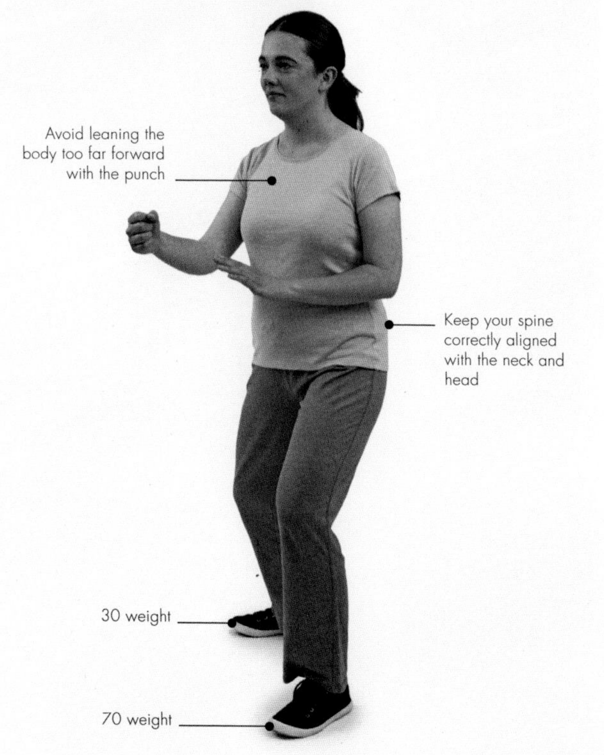

Making a Tai Chi Fist

The fist should be relaxed and light rather than clenched and hard. Bend your thumb and place it outside your fingers, over the first set of knuckles. Keep your wrist straight.

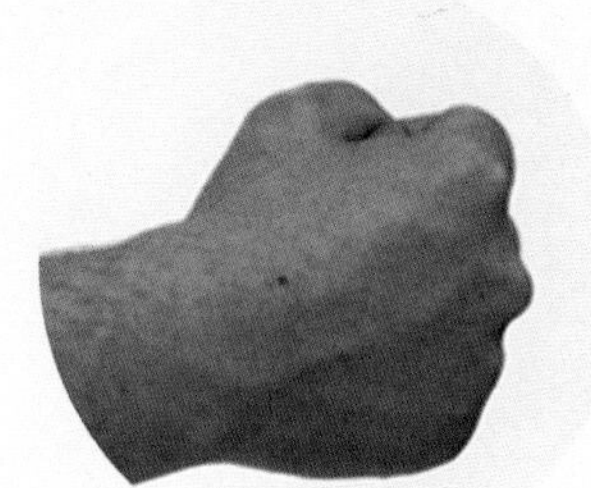

WITHDRAW & PUSH

After the outward energy of Punch, the form continues with the countermove of withdrawing and then gathering new energy and sending it outward once more in a Push that involves both hands. Use the shift in

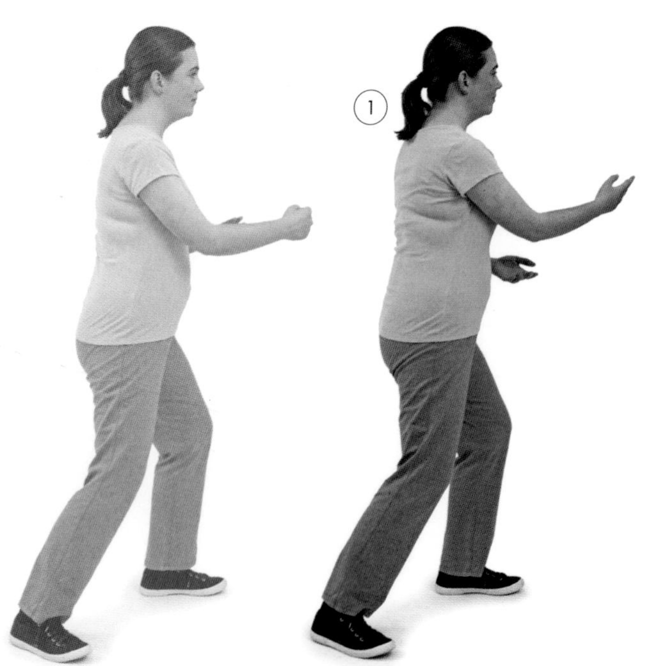

1 *Turn the upper body slightly to the left, maintaining the position of the feet and the 70/30 weight distribution between your left and right legs. Release your right hand from its fist as you drop your right elbow and your right hand rises. Lower your left hand and turn the palm upward, as if cupping your right elbow.*

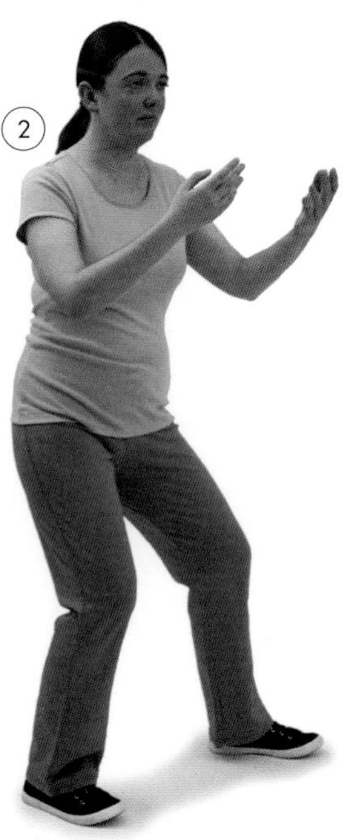

2 *Sink your weight into your right leg as you turn back to the right and face northwest, with both hands in front, palms upward.*

weight from the back leg to the front to propel your hands forward, imagining that they are moving against some invisible force as you do so.

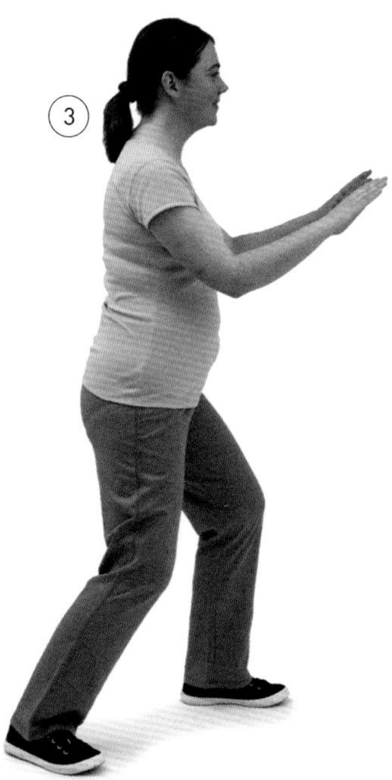

3 *Turn the palms outward as you transfer about 70 percent of your weight onto your left leg, turning back to the left to face west (Bow Stance again—see page 74). This is Push.*

And Breathe . . .

Keep your belly relaxed and your breathing even and natural. Some practitioners like to exhale when their hands are moving upward or outward, as in Push, and inhale when they are moving downward or inward. You may find that your breathing naturally coordinates with the movement in this way, but it is best not to try too hard to achieve this until you are very familiar with the form.

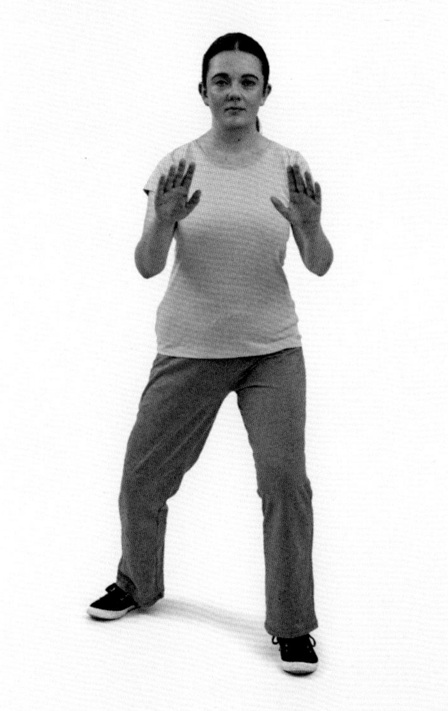

CROSS HANDS

This is the final sequence of the first section of Yang Short Form. It brings you back to face north again, with both feet facing forward.

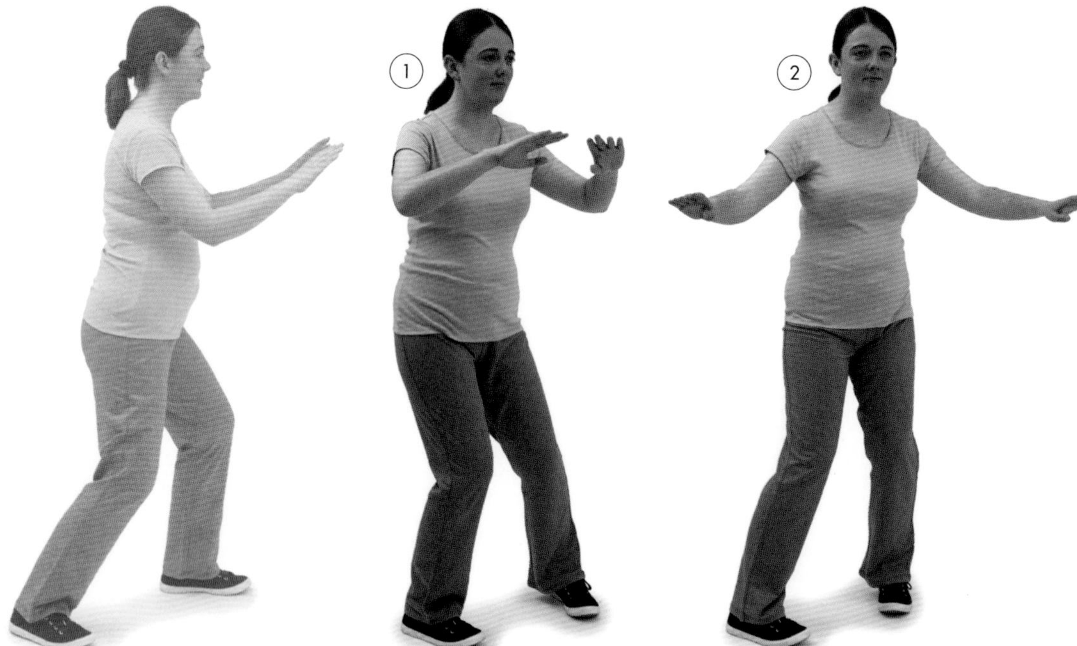

1 *Sink your weight back into your right leg, carrying your arms comfortably with you. Turn your left toes in as close to north as is comfortable.*

2 *Turn out your left heel slightly and transfer some weight to your left leg, moving your arms apart and outward at waist height.*

At the end of the posture your weight appears to be equally balanced between the right and left leg, but is in reality more strongly weighted on the left.

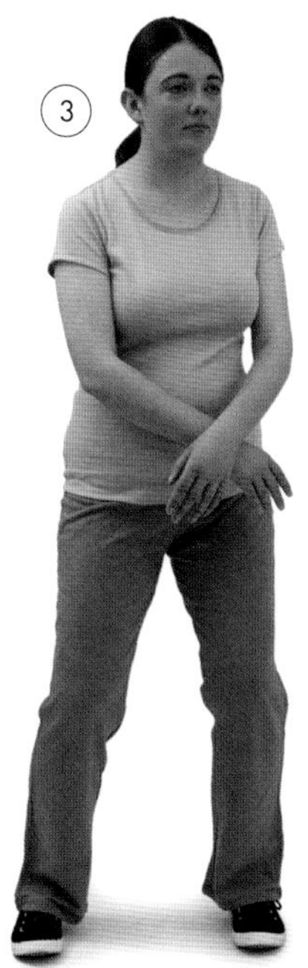

3 *Step your right foot back so that it is a shoulder-width distance from your left foot and parallel to it. Circle your hands in, crossing your left wrist over your right wrist in front of your navel, palms facing inward.*

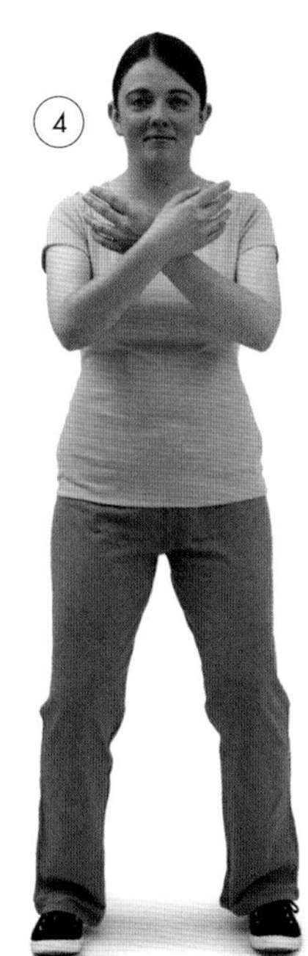

4 *Shift about 40 percent of your weight onto your right leg, leaving 60 percent on your left leg, while you float your hands up until they are in front of your chest, palms facing inward, so that the right hand is now on the outside.*

Early Closing

If you are learning the form in stages, you can balance your weight equally between the feet at the end of step 3 and use this as a closing movement. It is also a good position to practice on its own for building stamina and strength. Try to sink into it as if sitting down, and watch that the shoulders are relaxed, and the knees do not extend any farther forward than the toes.

THE YANG SHORT FORM PART 2

The second section of the Yang Short Form includes some already familiar postures, such as the Grasp the Sparrow's Tail sequence (see page 86), and introduces some more complex movements including backward and sideways stepping. There is also a directional shift—instead of just moving east to west, we now perform the movements on the diagonal (northwest to southeast). It is best to progress to this and subsequent sections only when you are fully comfortable with the first section.

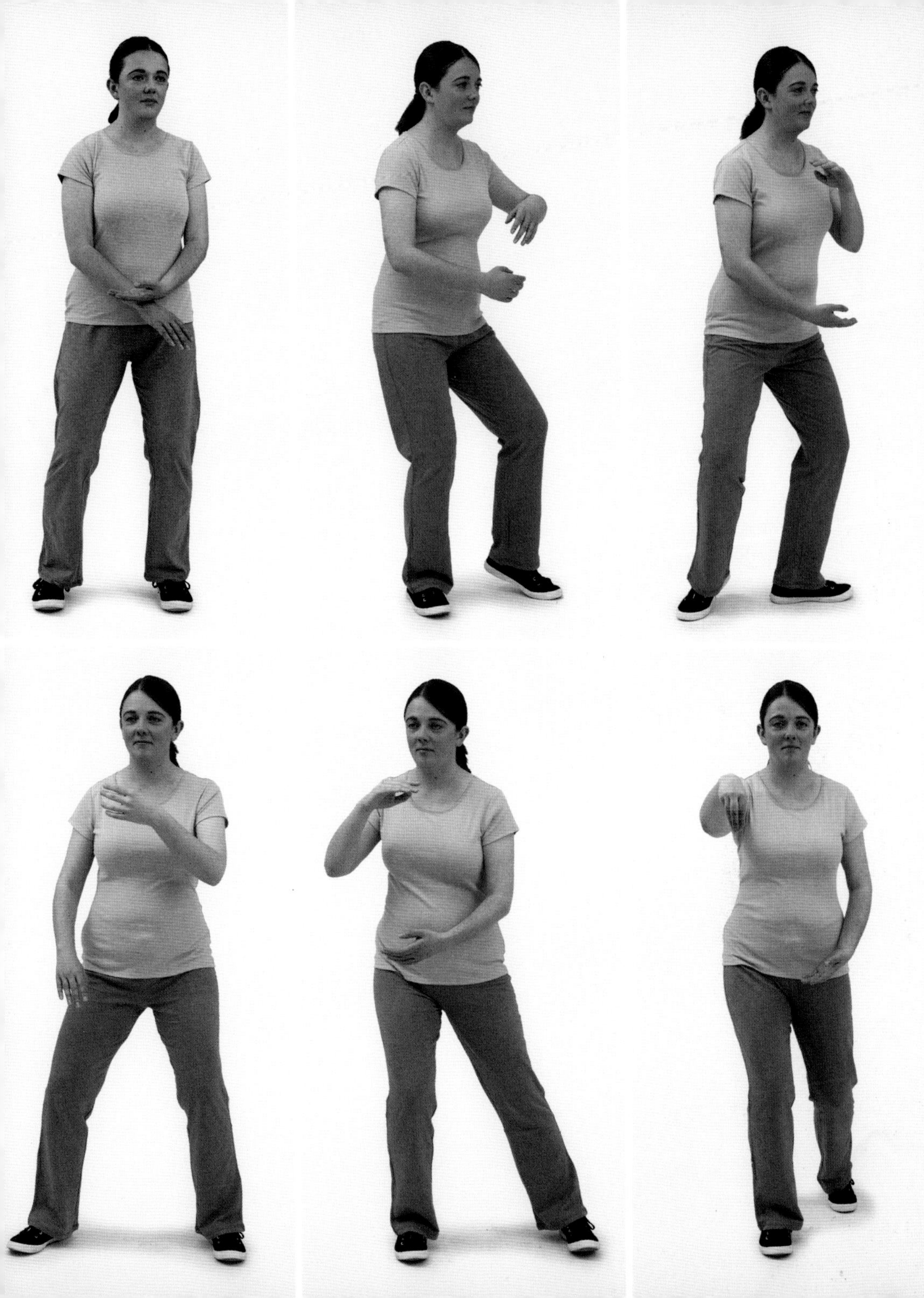

Continuing the Form

This section of the form begins with the posture Embrace Tiger, Return to Mountain. Many tai chi postures have beautifully colorful names. This nomenclature both helps practitioners to remember the moves and provides a visual element that can inform and inspire the practice.

The name of this posture is often said to refer to the position of the hands—lifting the tiger, which is a symbol of energy, and returning it to the mountain, a place of rest. However, students have long questioned this interpretation because the notion that anyone can lift an animal the size of a tiger (or would want to) and carry it up a mountainside is an impossibility. A more plausible theory about the name suggests that given that this posture is intended to thwart an attack from the rear, the "embrace" signifies turning to face the tiger (your attacker), while "return to mountain" is a reference to the stable posture you assume once the initial attack is deflected.

Stepping back & to the side

Backward stepping is brought into the form in the Punch Under Elbow and in the poetically named movement Step Back to Repulse Monkey. In martial art terms, being able to retreat while averting an attack is an essential skill. When stepping backward, you always place the toes and ball of the foot down first before rolling down the rest of the foot; conversely, when stepping forward, it is always heel first.

Backward walking is a useful general skill to develop, and will improve your balance. Its inclusion in the form is one reason why tai chi can be so beneficial for older people, since as we age we often lose the ability to maintain balance when changing direction. Cheng Man Ching emphasized the importance of this movement in relaxing the muscles and opening up the energy pathways of the lower body, enabling chi to circulate freely.

This section of the form also works on sidestepping in the soft, meditative movement of Cloud Hands, which promotes a sense of general wellbeing as well as building strength in the back and torso (see page 142).

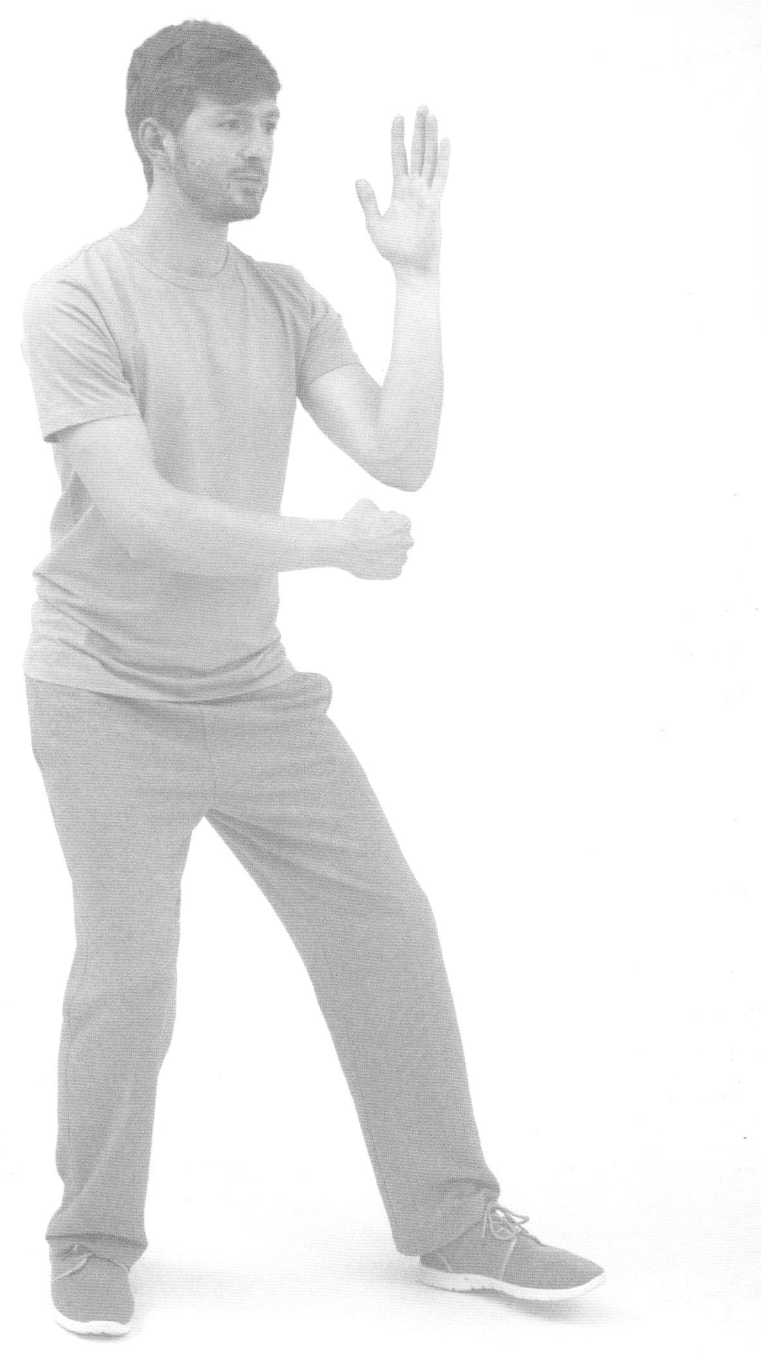

EMBRACE TIGER, RETURN TO MOUNTAIN

In this movement, you change direction to deal with an imaginary attacker who comes from behind your right side. Your right hand moves outward as if to block a kick from your

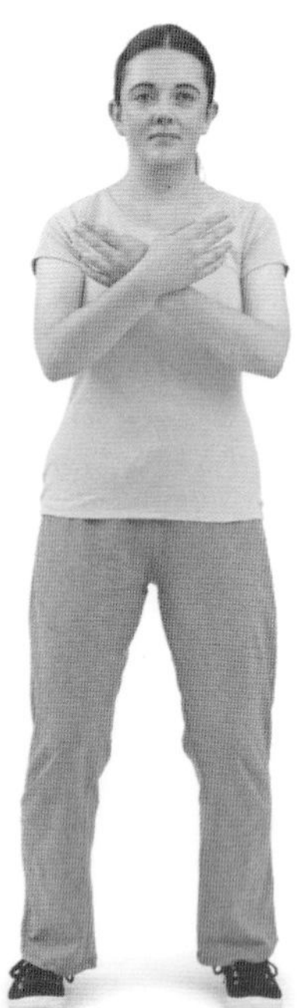

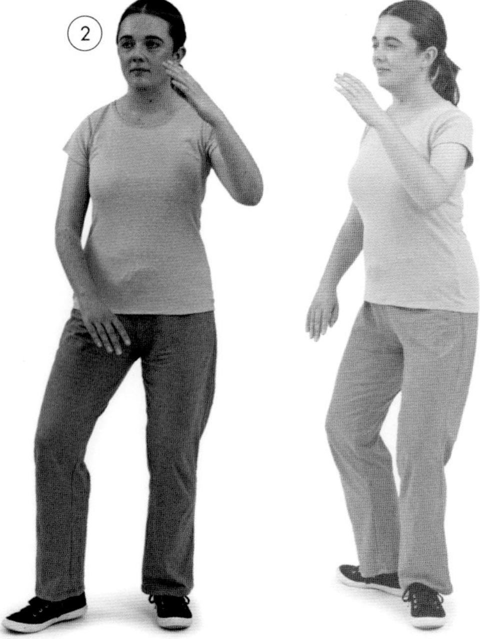

1 *Pour most of your weight into your left leg as you bring your arms down with the right palm facing down and the left palm facing up. Turn slightly to the left as you do this.*

2 *Keep your weight on your left leg as you pivot on the ball of your right foot to pivot the heel inward. When you turn, float your left hand up to relax near the shoulder, while your right arm hangs down, protecting your groin.*

opponent, while the left hand is used as if to push him or her off balance. Be sure to integrate the turns of the waist with the movements of the arms, since this is what gives them their power.

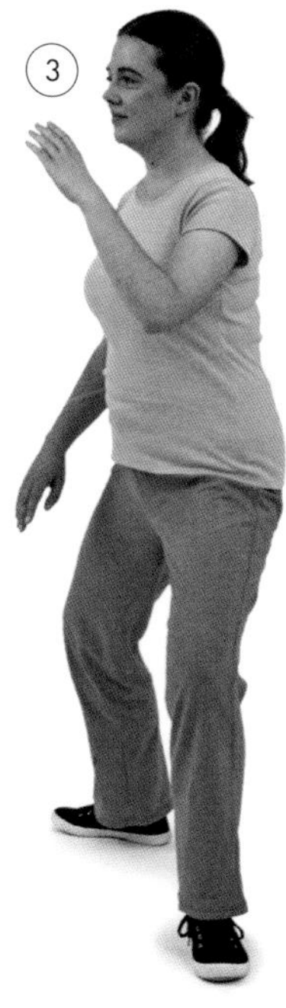

3 *Bring the toes of your right foot behind your left heel, then step back to the south with your right heel, placing the heel down first and with your toes facing southeast. This is quite a big step, so make sure that you are firmly rooted on your left leg before you take it to avoid twisting your knee.*

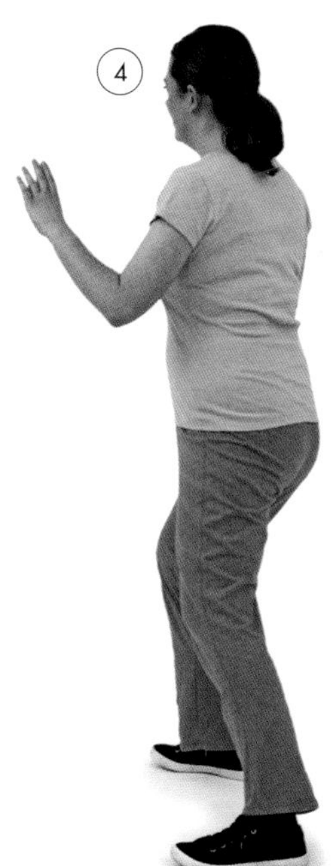

4 *Pour 70 percent of your weight into your right foot as you turn to the right so that your body faces the same southeast direction as your right foot, brushing over your thigh with your right hand. Lift the toes of your left foot and pivot the heel inward (Bow Stance—see page 74). Turn the right palm forwards and up, and turn the left palm forward just outside the shoulder. Both shoulders should be level and relaxed.*

Reverse View

In step 4 the right hand brushes the thigh, seen here from the other side.

ROLLBACK The form continues with the pleasing movement of rollback, but this time you move on the diagonal rather than from side to side. Remember that your feet do not change position in Rollback, or in the postures that follow. They maintain a firm connection with the ground while your weight shifts from one foot to the other.

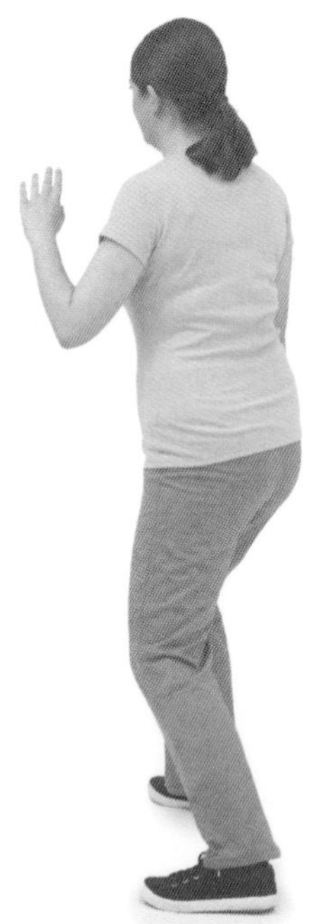

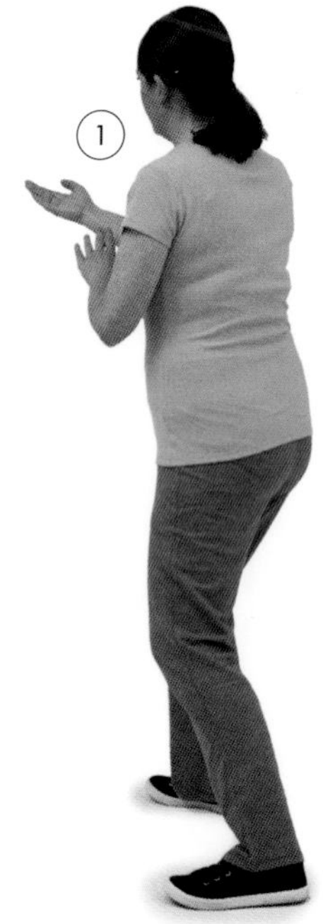

1 *Turn a little to the right, sinking your weight into your right leg. As you do so, float your right arm up so that your upward-facing palm is close to shoulder height, and start to lower your left arm, fingers pointing toward your right wrist.*

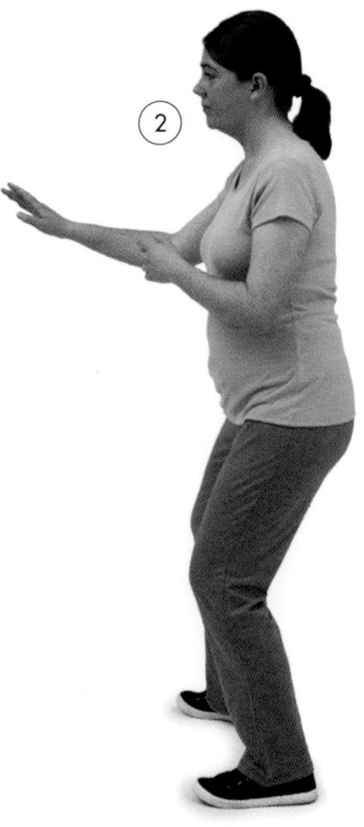

2 *Transfer your weight onto your left leg, while you turn your right palm to face forward and down and your left palm to face your body. As you transfer your weight, turn your hips to the left (east), keeping your shoulders and elbows relaxed, with your arms being carried by your body's movement. This is Rollback.*

PRESS & PUSH

As before, Rollback gives way to Press and Push. The foot stance remains the same as you shift your weight and turn your waist. This helps to loosen the hips and improve flexibility in the lower spine. It also gives the internal organs a massage.

Press

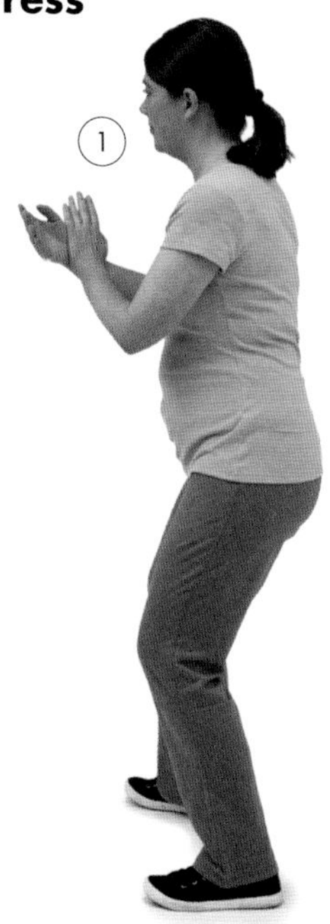

1 *Bring your right arm slightly toward you, turning your right palm to face your chest, while you raise your left arm slightly with your left palm facing outward and bring it across so that the bases of your hands touch.*

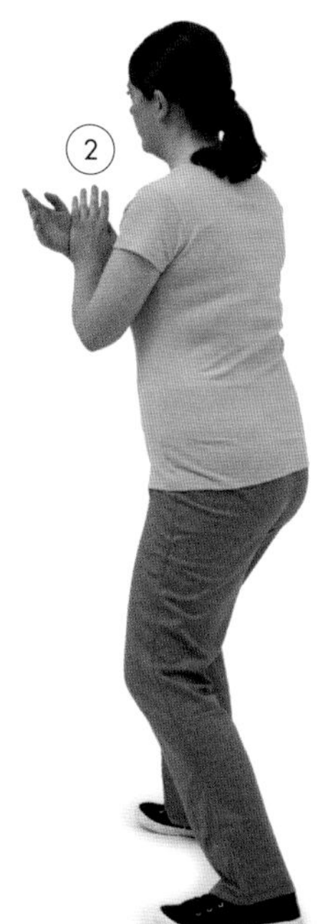

2 *As you do this, return your weight mostly to your front (right) leg so that you are facing the same direction as your right foot. This is Press.*

Push

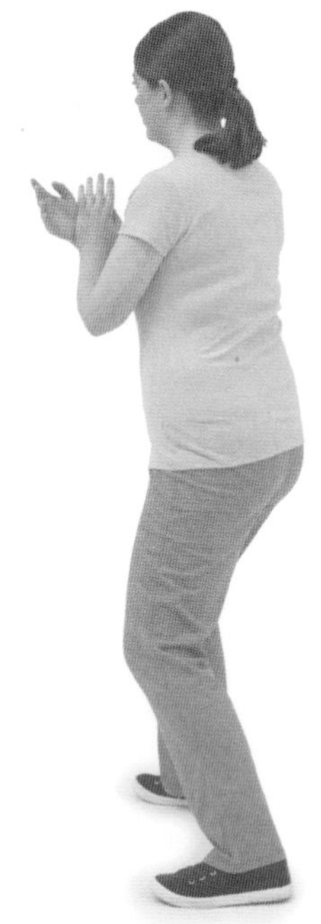

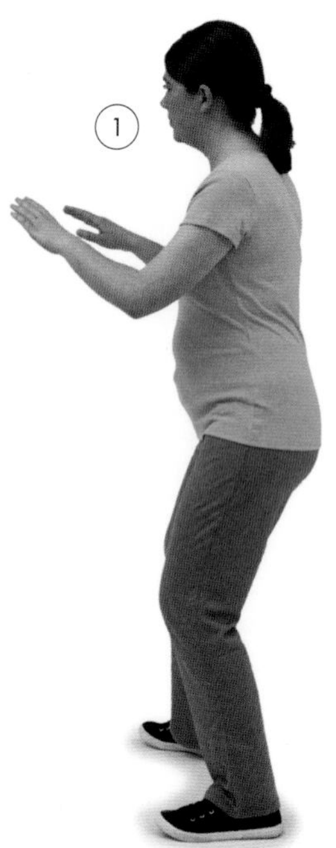

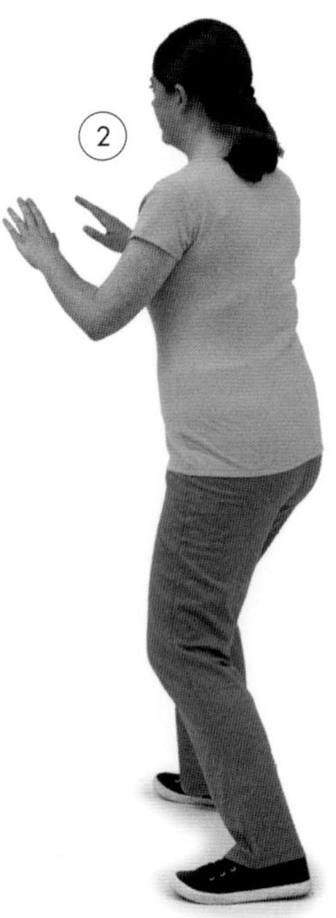

Arm Movements

As you move your arms, remember to maintain a slight space in the armpits, and to keep the wrists soft (Beautiful Hands—see page 27).

1 *Continue seamlessly into Push: Sink most of your weight into your back (left) leg as you part the wrists, bringing your elbows closer to your body with your palms facing downward but slightly frontward.*

2 *Then shift your weight back onto your front (right) leg as you push forward, raising your hands so that they are at chest height and chest-width apart in the Beautiful Hands position (see page 27). At the end of the movement, 70 percent of your weight should be on your front (right) leg and 30 percent on your back (left) leg. This is Push.*

SINGLE WHIP

Now you move into Single Whip, which this time ends with you facing the northwest corner. Keep a feeling of openness in the chest and through the arms, and remember that the fingers and thumb of your right hand should be lightly touching to create the beak, but not exerting any pressure.

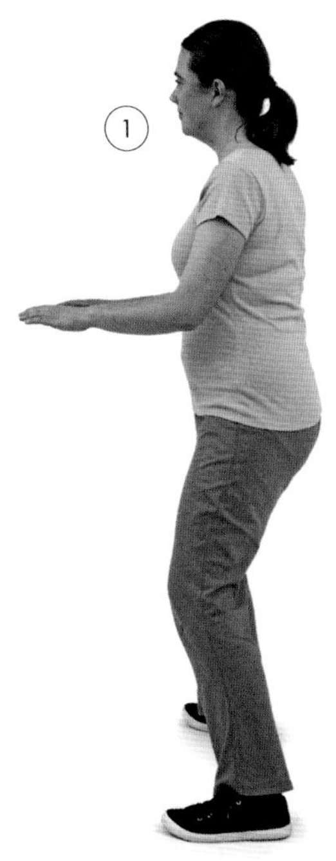

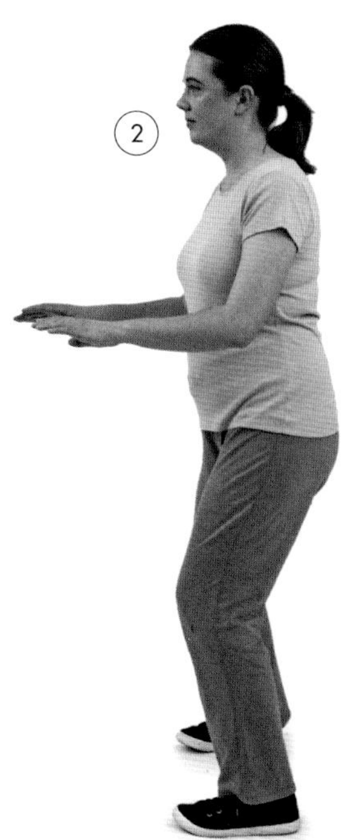

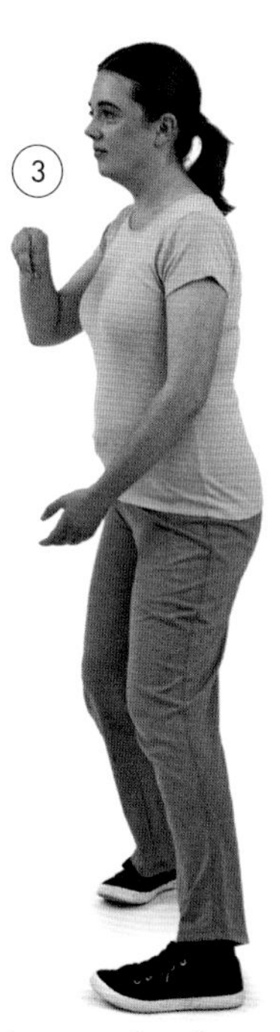

1 *Start transferring your weight back onto your left leg, lowering the forearms with a slight downward pressure so that they are parallel to the ground with the palms facing downward.*

2 *Continue shifting almost all your weight onto your left leg as you turn to the left as far as you can comfortably go by pivoting your right foot on the heel to face between east and northeast, leaving your left foot in the same position. Follow the movement of the body with your arms.*

3 *Now transfer all your weight onto your right leg and turn back to the right a little. As you do so, drop your left hand, turning the palm upward as in the Hold the Ball position (see page 87). Move your right arm in front of your chest, bending the elbow and forming a beak with your fingers (see page 96).*

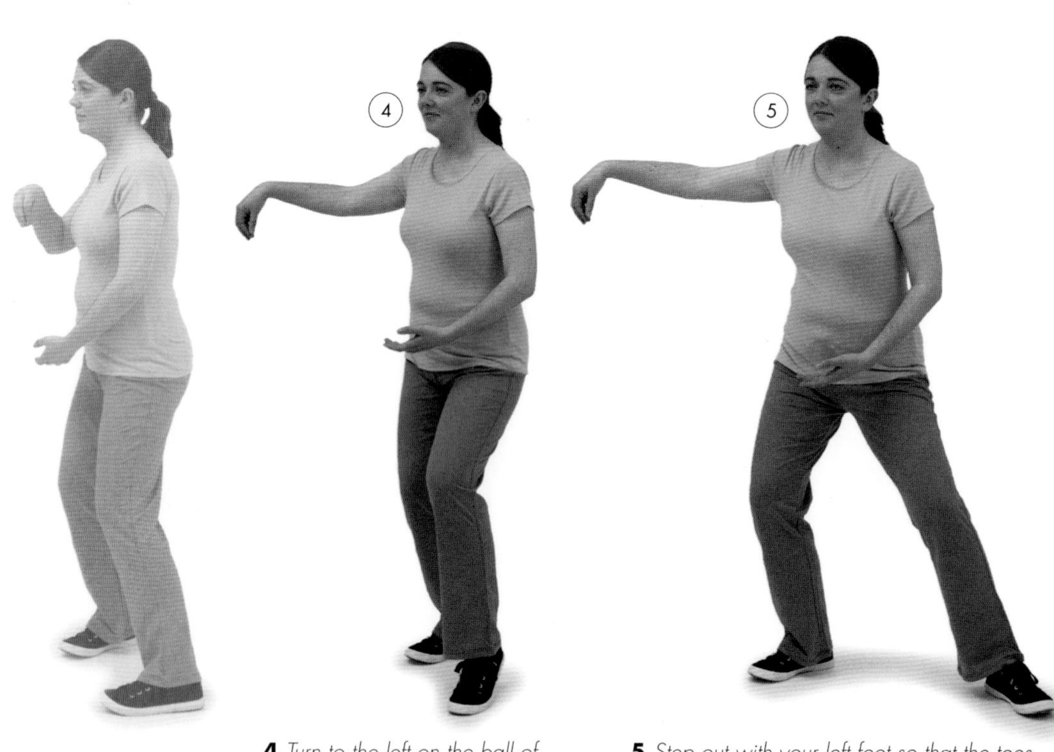

4 *Turn to the left on the ball of your left foot so that the toes are facing north while your body faces northeast. Extend your right arm out to your right, keeping your hand in the beak position and your elbow relaxed.*

5 *Step out with your left foot so that the toes are facing northwest, turning to the north as you do so, placing the heel down first and keeping the weight on your right foot (you may wish to step back briefly first to help you balance). The heels should form an L shape with a shoulder-width distance between them.*

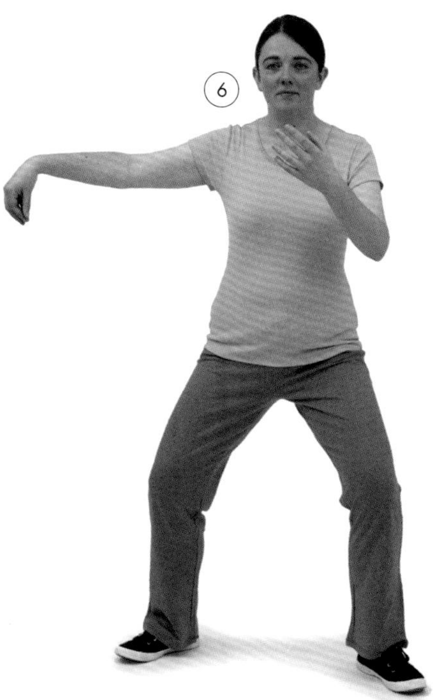

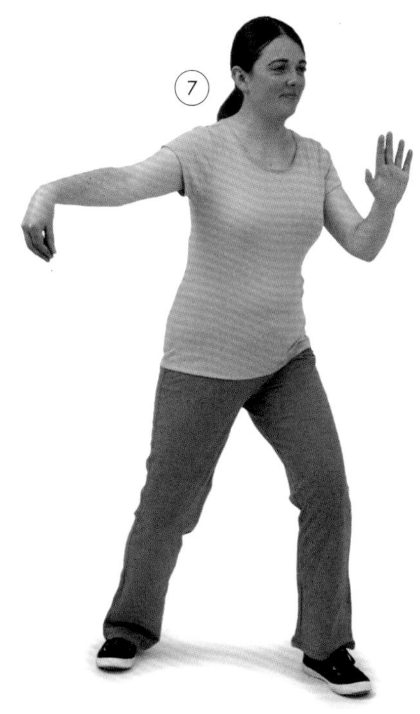

6 *Now shift about 70 percent of your weight onto your left leg and bring your left hand up so that the palm is facing your chest.*

7 *Pivot on your right heel so that the toes are pointing north and turn your body to the left to face northwest in Bow Stance again (see page 74). As you end the movement, turn your left palm to face outward in the Beautiful Hands position (see page 27). This is Single Whip.*

FIST UNDER ELBOW

This is a good movement for promoting coordination and balance. When you step back, ensure that you keep your weight on your front leg

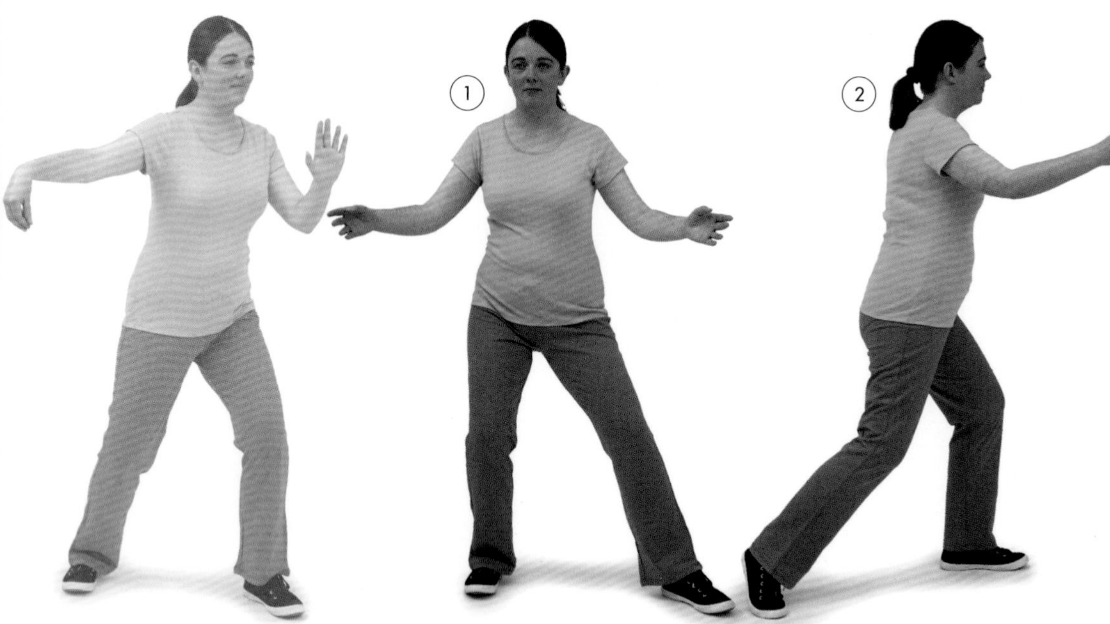

1 *Pour all your weight into your right leg, relaxing your arms and softly opening them wide with your palms facing inward.*

2 *Step your left foot out to the left (facing west), placing the heel down first, with your left hand following the movement to the left. Transfer all your weight to your left leg as you turn to the left (west), your right arm being carried by the movement of your body, while you drop and relax your left arm outside your left thigh.*

as you place your back foot down. Only when your back foot has made good connection with the ground can you start to shift your weight back.

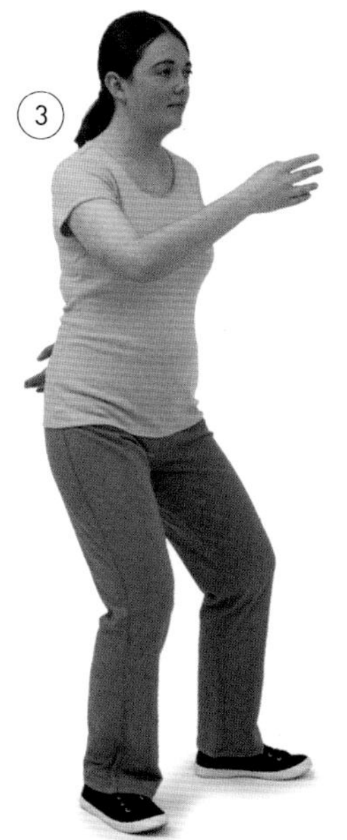

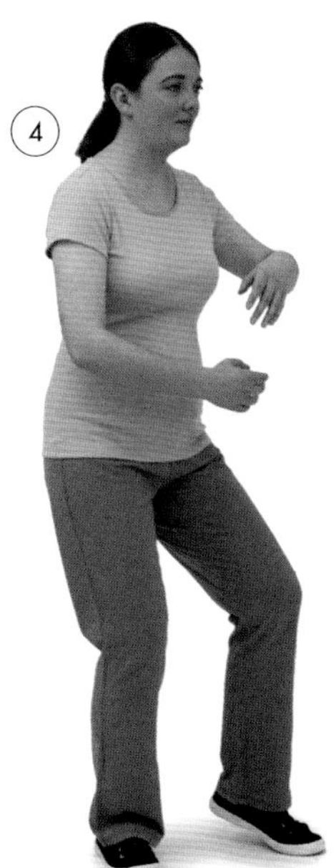

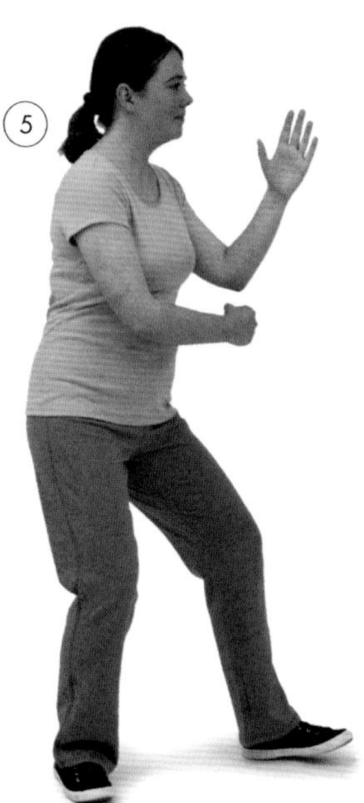

3 *Step up with your right foot, the toes pointing to the northwest, and drop the back of your left hand near the tailbone.*

4 *Sink your weight into your right foot, while the back of your left hand brushes lightly up the sacrum to the back of your waist and then around to the front of your body and the right arm drops down to the front of the stomach. Raise your left heel slightly so that you are resting on the ball of the foot.*

5 *Adjust your left foot to Heel Stance (see page 77). Drop your left elbow and point the fingers of your left hand to the ceiling in a straight line with the forearm. Form a Tai Chi Fist (see page 115) with your right hand and bring it under (or comfortably near) your left elbow. Look to the west.*

STEP BACK TO REPULSE MONKEY (RIGHT)

This is a long sequence in which you step back three times—to the right, to the left, and then to the right again. It is a useful movement to practice by itself because it both requires and

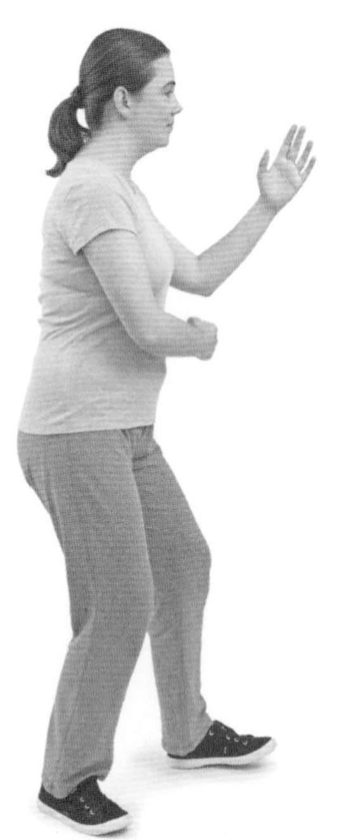

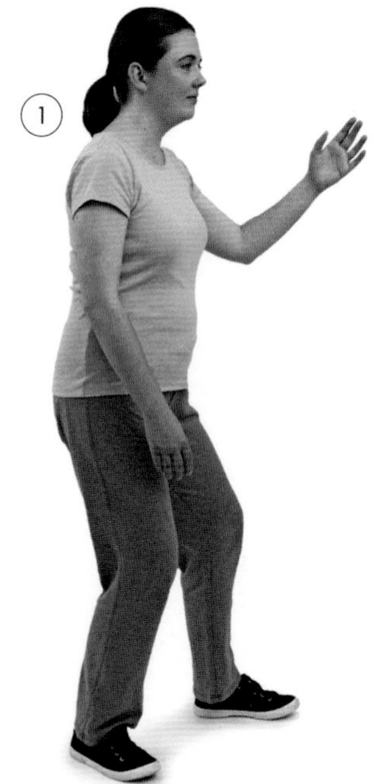

1 *Roll your left foot down from Heel Stance and then turn to the right, keeping your weight on your right leg. Let your left arm relax at shoulder height with your palm facing upward as you turn. At the same time, open up your right-hand fist and relax your right shoulder so that your right arm hangs by your right hip*

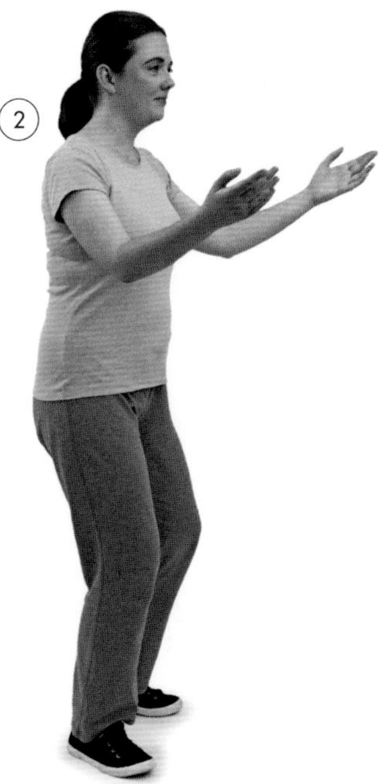

2 *Draw your left foot back so that it is level with your right foot and simultaneously raise your right hand to shoulder height, palm facing upward.*

promotes good balance and coordination. It also improves flexibility in the lower spine, and the extended arm movements help to open up the chest. Maintain a straight spine, keeping your tailbone tucked in, as you step back.

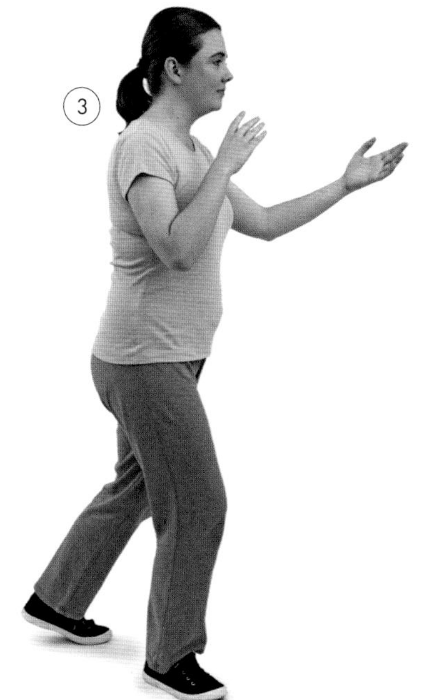

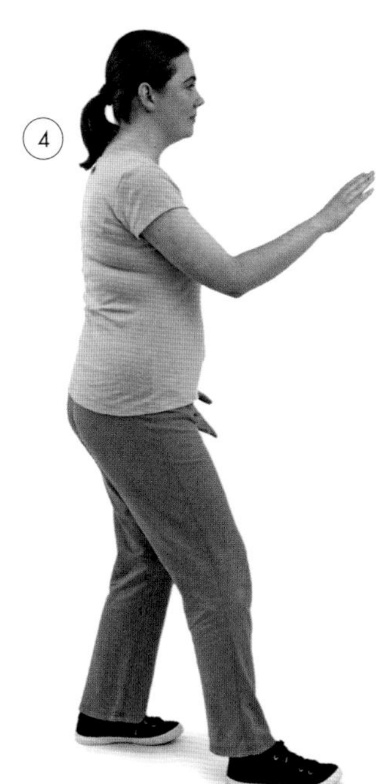

3 *Fold your right arm inward toward your right shoulder with your palm facing slightly downward and to the left, ready to push, then take a backward step with your left foot.*

4 *Shift most of your weight—about 80 percent—onto your left foot and turn to the center to face west. Pivot on your right heel so that the toes are facing west. Bring your right arm forward, palm facing outward in the Beautiful Hands position (see page 27), and let your left hand drop down outside your left thigh, palm forward. Relax your shoulders.*

STEP BACK TO REPULSE MONKEY (LEFT)

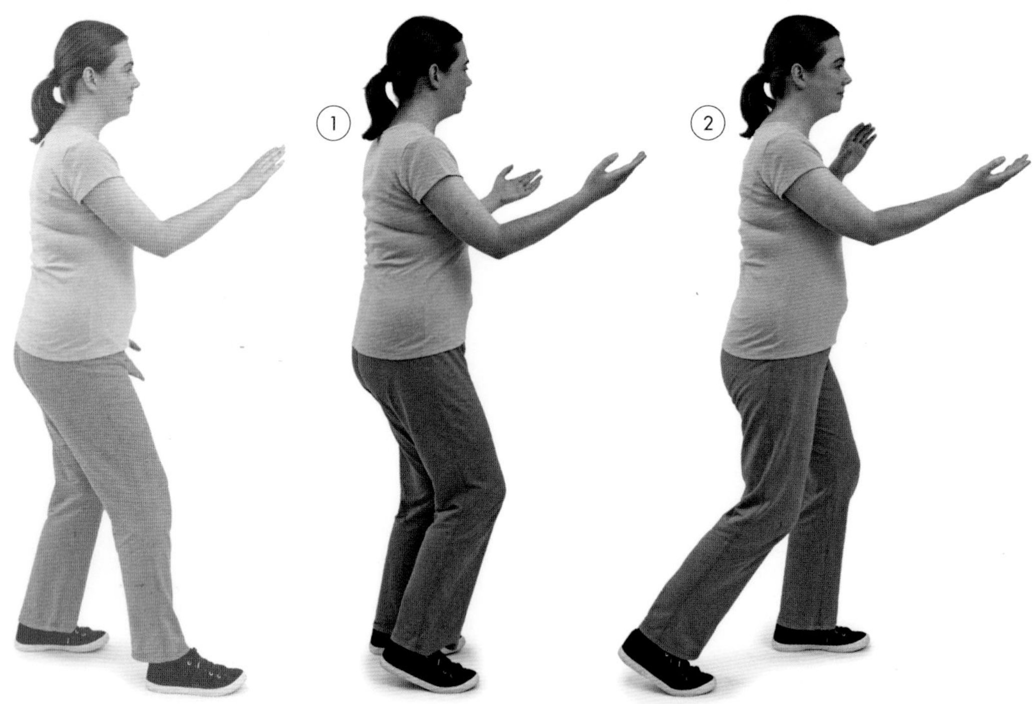

1 *Raise your left hand to shoulder height, palm facing upward, and rotate your right hand until the palm is also facing upward, drawing your right foot back so that it is level with your left foot.*

2 *Fold the left arm inward toward your left shoulder with your palm facing slightly downward and to the right, then take a backward step with your right foot.*

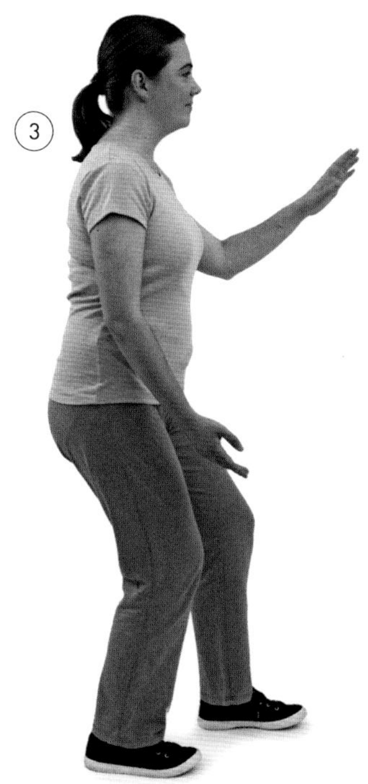

3 *Let your right hand drop down outside your right thigh, palm forward. Shift most of your weight—about 80 percent—onto your right foot. Bring your left arm forward, palm facing outward in the Beautiful Hands position (see page 27). Relax your shoulders.*

Backward Stepping

Whenever you step back in tai chi, always put the toes and ball of the foot down first. Make sure you step back far enough to maintain a shoulder-width distance between your feet—it is easy to make this step too narrow. In this movement, aim to keep your feet facing forward and parallel to each other.

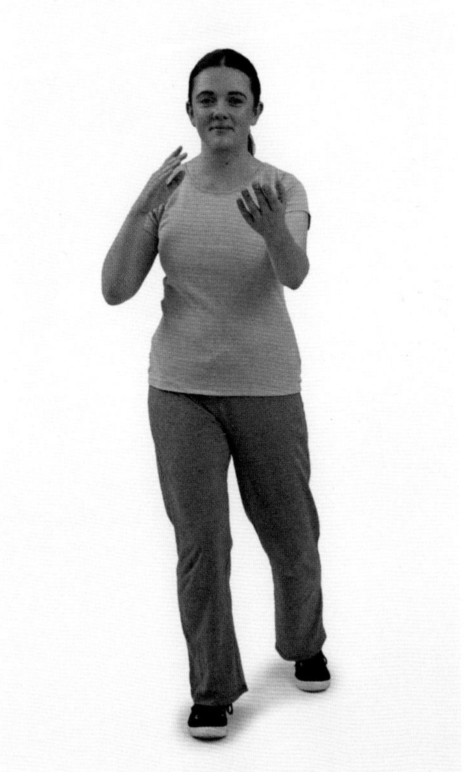

STEP BACK TO REPULSE MONKEY (RIGHT)

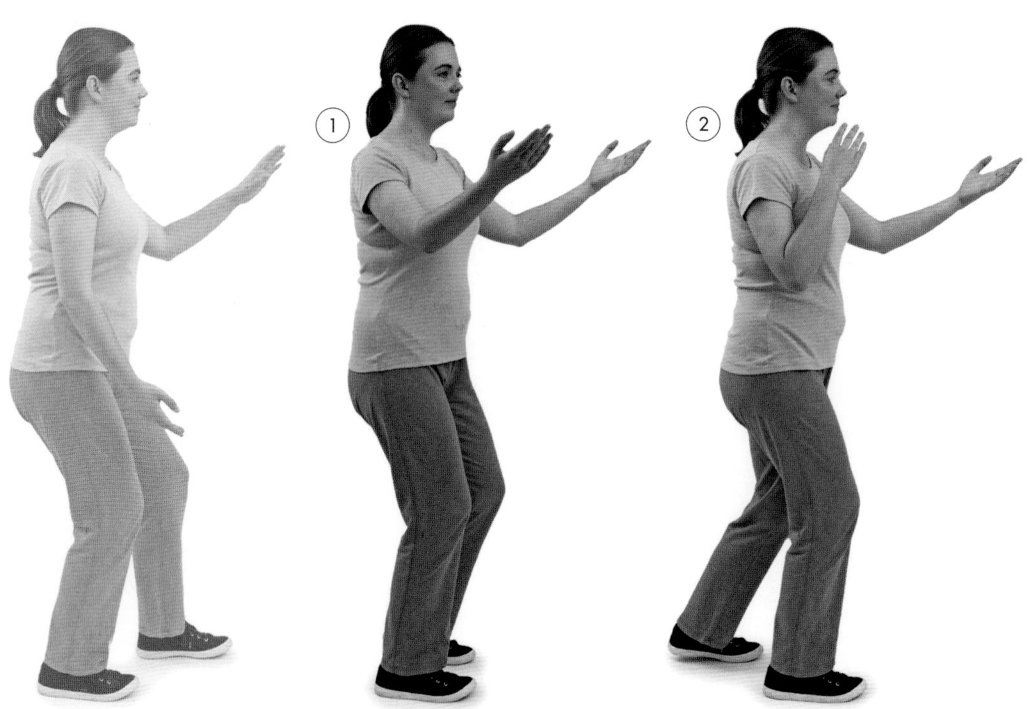

1 *Raise your right hand to shoulder height, palm facing upward, and rotate your left hand until the palm is also facing upward, drawing your left foot back so that it is level with your right foot.*

2 *Fold the right arm inward toward your right shoulder with your palm facing slightly downward and to the left, then take a backward step with your left foot.*

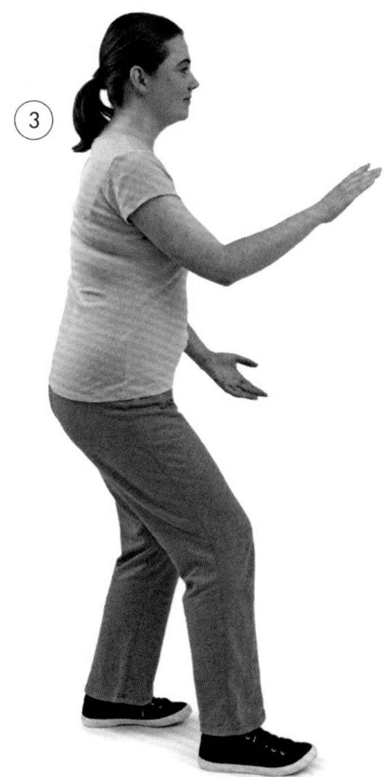

3 *Let your left hand drop down outside your left thigh, palm forward. Shift most of your weight—about 80 percent—onto your left foot. Bring your right arm forward, palm facing outward in the Beautiful Hands position (see page 27). Relax your shoulders.*

Whole-Body Movement

As this sequence becomes more familiar, you can focus on creating smooth and integrated movements, especially in step 2 when you have both to step the foot back and move the arms. Watch that you keep your elbow dropped here because it is tempting to let it rise when you fold in your arm. Keep breathing naturally throughout.

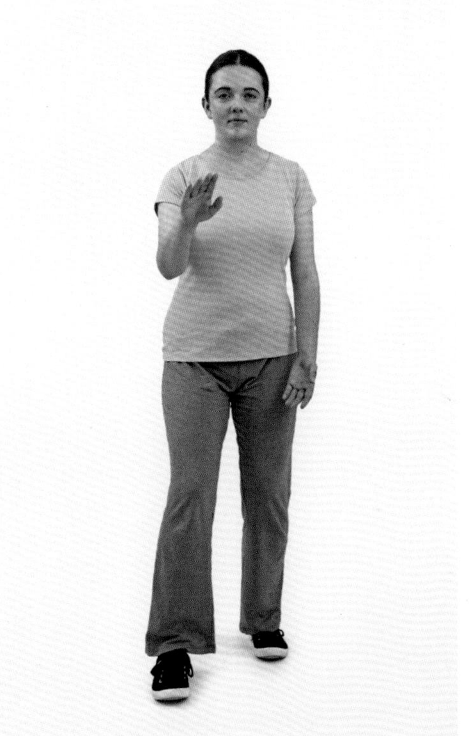

DIAGONAL FLYING

This movement involves taking a wide step around. It is relatively tricky to do, and you need to ensure that your spine stays straight. The right

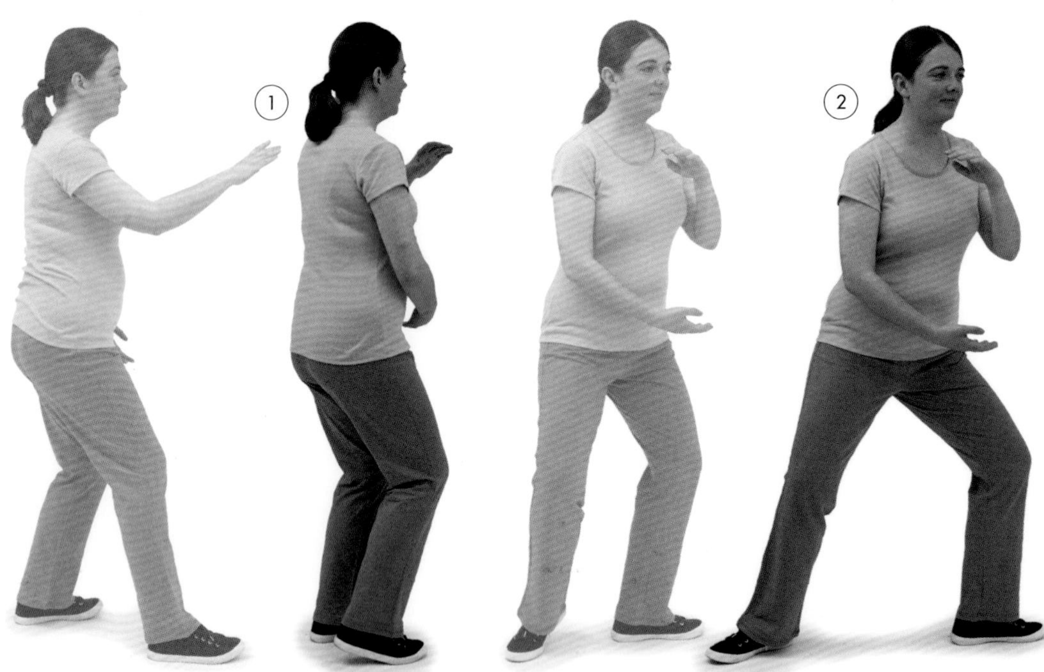

1 *Bring a little more weight onto your left leg—about 90 percent—and turn to the left. At the same time, bring your arms into the Hold the Ball position (see page 87): Let your right arm circle down, turning the palm of your right hand up, and bring your left arm up, turning the palm of your left hand down. Step back with the toes of your right foot.*

2 *Pivoting on the ball of the foot, turn your hips to the right. Step out with your right heel to the northeast and put your foot down. As you step with the right leg, make sure that the left knee does not move inward. Keep it facing in the same direction as the left foot.*

arm extends up and out, while the left one extends downward, creating a feeling of expansion and openness in the front of the body.

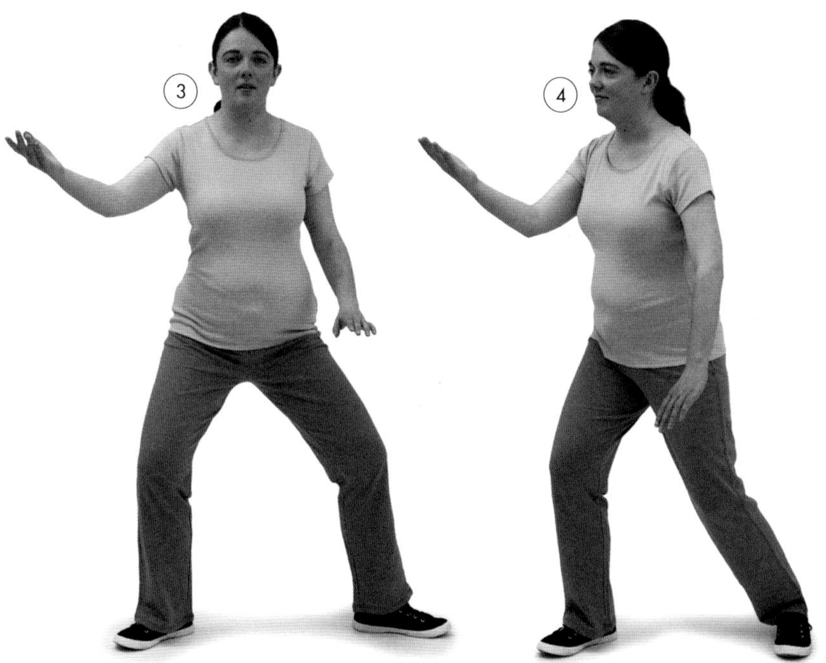

3 *Shift most of your weight onto your front (right) leg, parting your arms, keeping the palm of your right hand up and the palm of your left hand down.*

4 *Lift the toes of your back (left) foot and pivot on the heel to bring your feet into the correct position for Bow Stance (see page 74). At the same time, relax your left arm so that it drops down with the palm facing downward and behind you. Make sure that your left hand is in the Beautiful Hands position (see page 27) and your body, right foot, and right hand are all in alignment with the northeast. Your weight should be distributed so that 70 percent is on the right leg and 30 percent is on the left leg. This is Diagonal Flying.*

Focus on Wave Hands Like Clouds

Wave Hands Like Clouds, also known as Cloud Hands, is one of the best-known tai chi movements. It combines sidestepping and turning with beautiful circular movements of the arms. The hands are the clouds of the movement's name, and the turns and steps can be seen as the breeze that sends them scudding across the sky.

It is important that your arms are rounded in this movement, with a space between the arms and the body, and that the hands and wrists are relaxed (Beautiful Hands—see page 27).

Remember that in tai chi, arm movements are directed from the body, so your arms should only be moving when being carried along by the momentum of the body. You will need to turn the waist as fully as you are able (without pulling the spine out of alignment) in order to facilitate this. The arm movements should be flowing and seamless; try to have a sense of your hands floating through the air, like clouds floating across the sky. Watch that your shoulders do not rise when your arms come up—keep them relaxed.

Going with the breath

More advanced practitioners like to integrate the breath with the movement, inhaling as the hands change position and exhaling as the body turns. But the key thing for beginners is simply to breathe naturally and deeply into the abdomen—being aware of the breath will ensure that you do not inadvertently hold it by concentrating too hard on the movements.

Solo exercise

Cloud Hands is said to be one of the best movements for promoting the flow of chi through the body, and is often practiced as a solo exercise. As you gain mastery of the physical movements, you can begin to concentrate on the feeling of energy flow, and may notice feelings of warmth and relaxation through the body. Try to maintain a sense of connection with the ground through the feet, and then up the legs, into the waist, down the arms, and through the fingertips as you move. You can play with the pace of the sequence, going faster and then slower again.

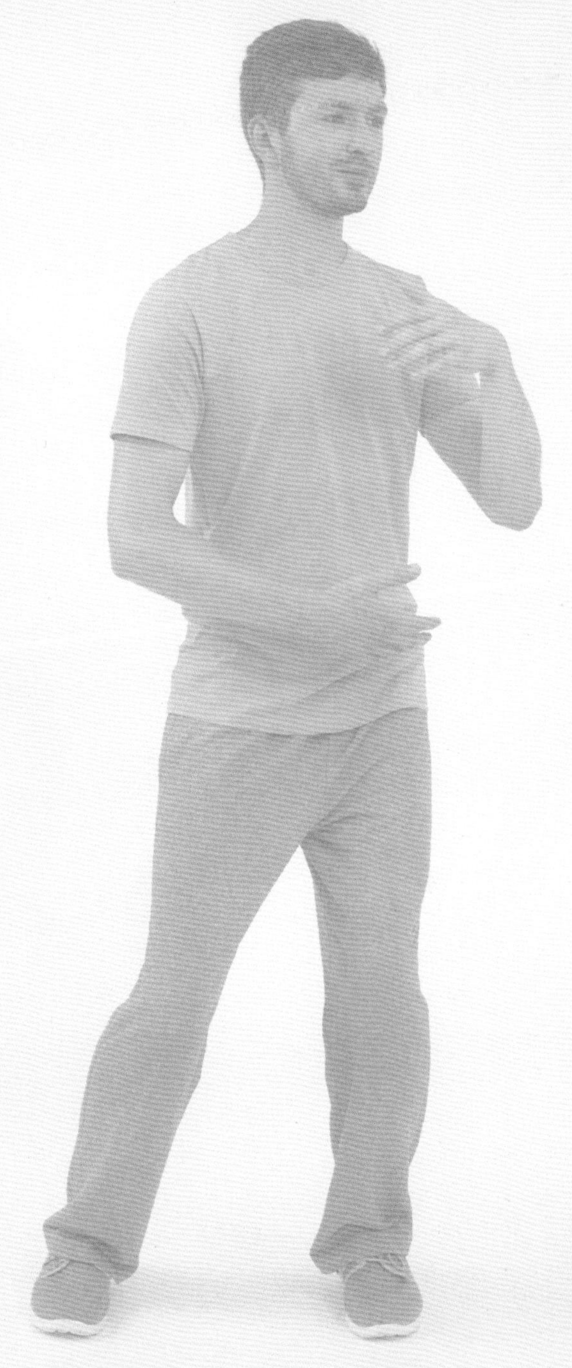

WAVES HANDS LIKE CLOUDS

This elegant movement introduces sidestepping to the form, and incorporates repeated waist turns that encourage spinal flexibility, relax tight back muscles, and provide a massage for the kidneys. Here you

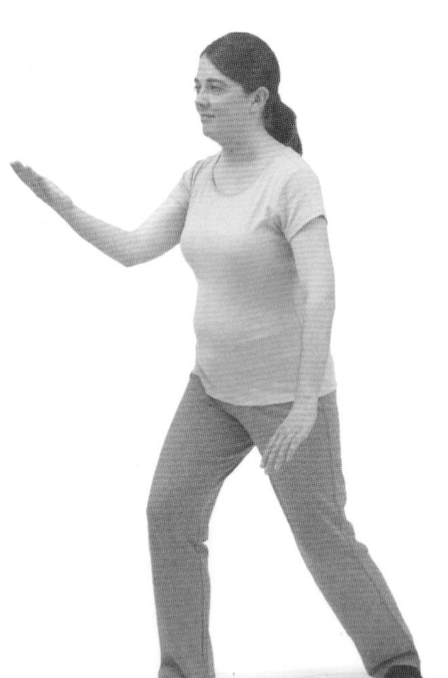

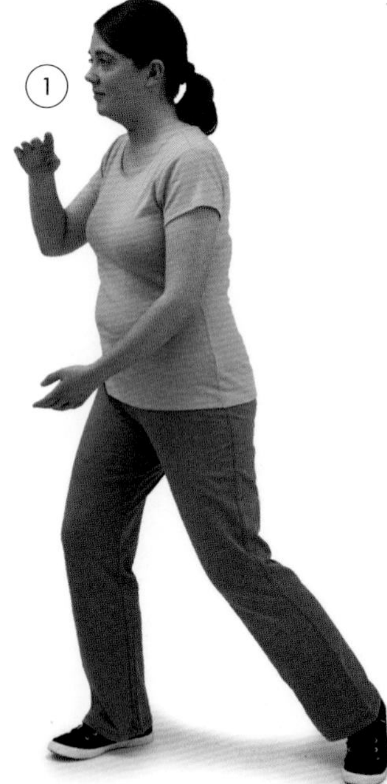

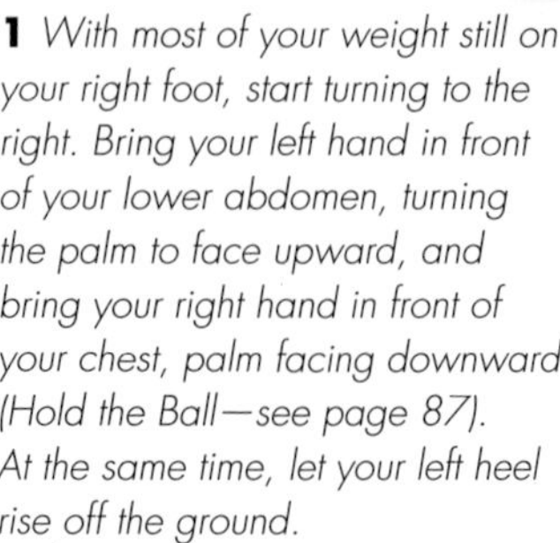

1 *With most of your weight still on your right foot, start turning to the right. Bring your left hand in front of your lower abdomen, turning the palm to face upward, and bring your right hand in front of your chest, palm facing downward (Hold the Ball—see page 87). At the same time, let your left heel rise off the ground.*

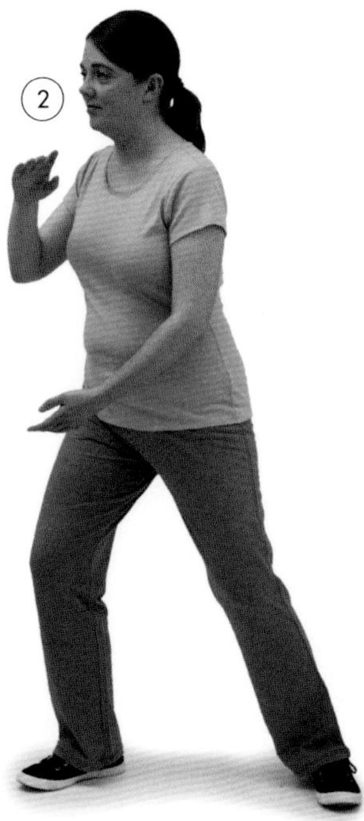

2 *Then take a slight step forward with your left foot so that the heel is in line with the heel of your right foot along the east–west axis (the toes of your left foot should still face to the north).*

turn first to the right and then to the left, before performing three more turns (left, right, left—see pages 146–147)

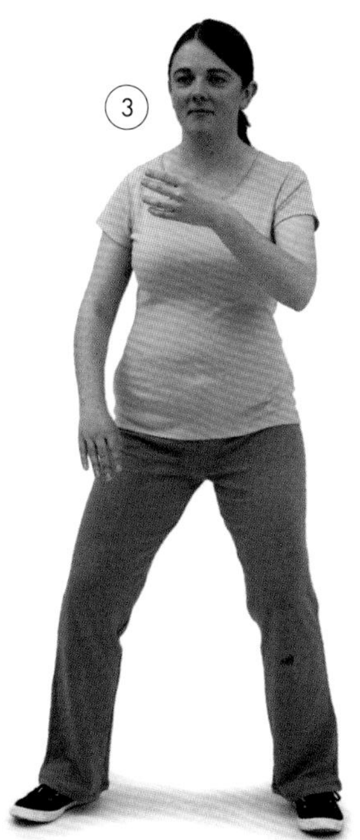

3 *Shift your weight so that it is evenly distributed between your legs. As you do so, lower your right arm and raise your left one, keeping your left hand close to your body and letting your right hand pass over it.*

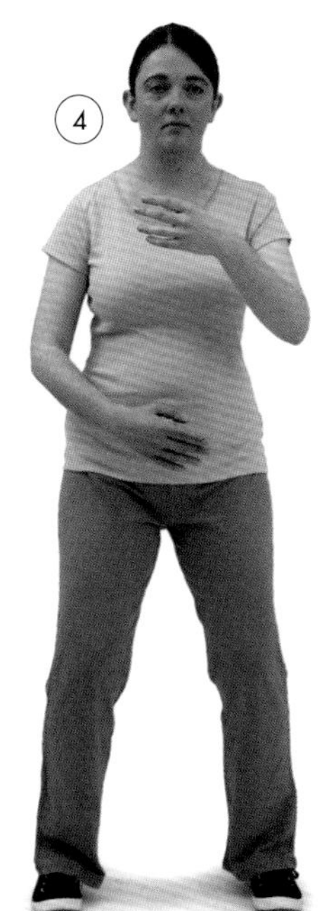

4 *Raise the toes of your right foot and turn your right foot and your body to face north, the same direction as your left foot. Turn your palms to face your body.*

Step to the Left

In Cloud Hands, the sidestepping is always to the left, whether the right or left foot is performing the movement.

Continued overleaf

Turning to the left

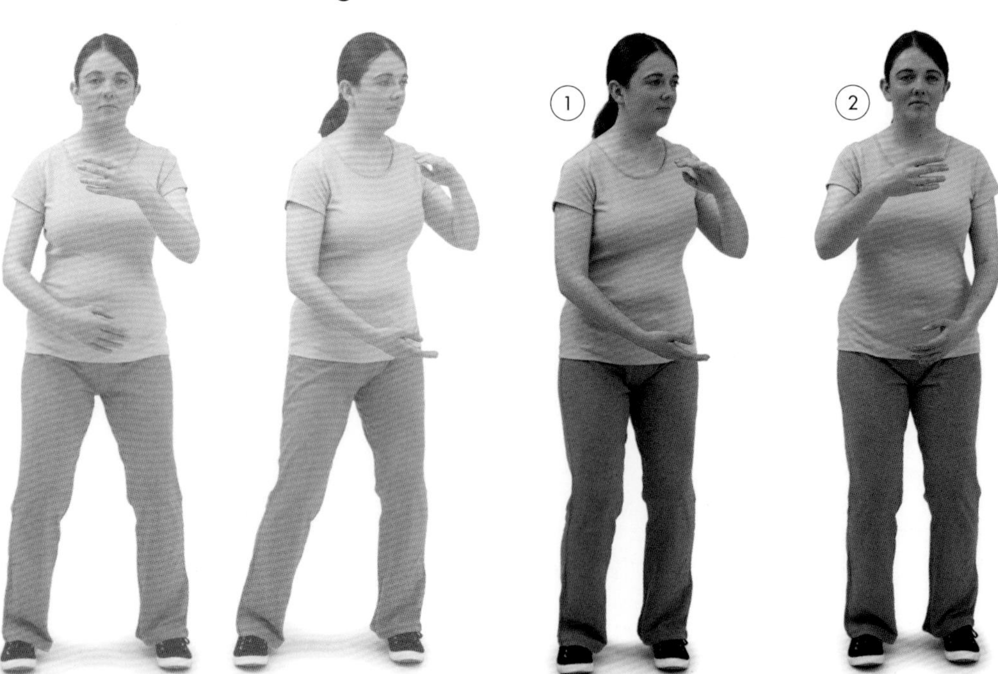

1 *Shift all your weight onto your left leg, turning your hips to the left as you do so, and turn your palms so that they are facing each other as in Hold the Ball (see page 87). Step your right foot in toward your left so that your feet are parallel and about half a shoulder width apart.*

2 *Shift your weight so that it is evenly distributed between your legs. At the same time, change the position of your arms, lowering your left arm and raising your right arm, keeping your right hand close to your body this time and letting your left hand pass over it. Turn your palms to face your body.*

Turning to the right

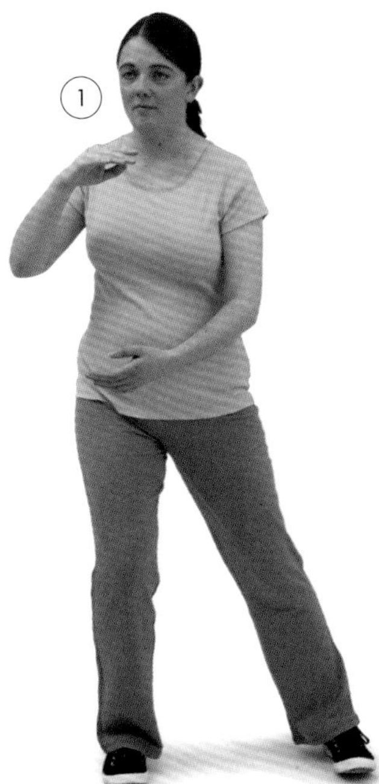

1 *Transfer all your weight onto your right leg, turning your hips to the right as you do so, and turn your palms so that they are facing each other as in Hold the Ball (see page 87). Step your left foot to the left so that your feet are shoulder-width apart again.*

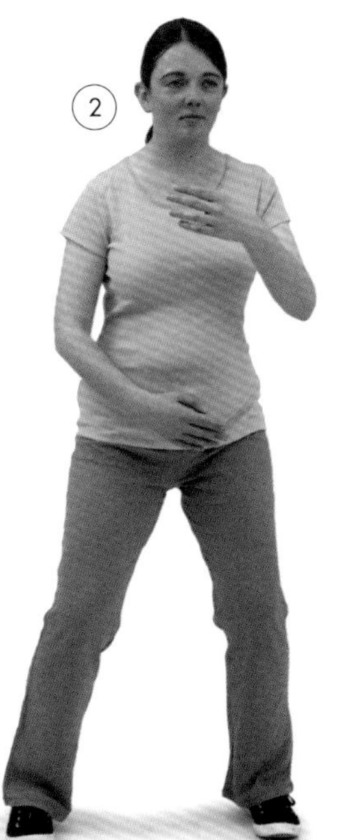

2 *Shift your weight so that it is evenly distributed between your legs. At the same time, change the position of your arms again so that your left arm floats up and your right arm floats down, keeping your left hand close to your body and letting your right hand pass over it. Turn your palms to face your body.*

Turning to the left

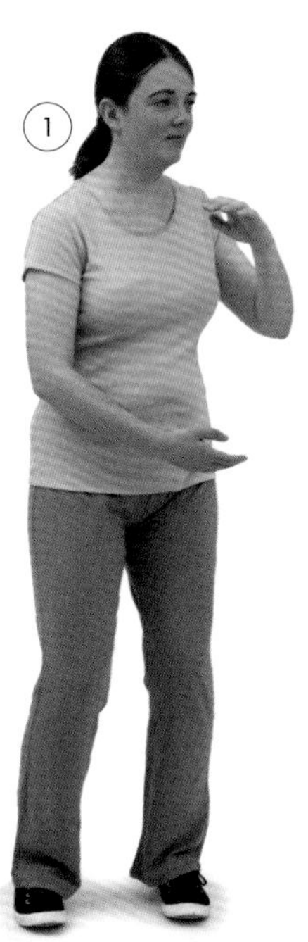

1 *Transfer all your weight onto your left leg, turning your hips to the left as you do so, and turn your palms so that they are facing each other as in Hold the Ball (see page 87). Step your right foot in toward your left so that your feet are parallel and about half a shoulder width apart.*

SINGLE WHIP

The form now repeats Single Whip for the third time. As in the first rendition of this movement, you face west.

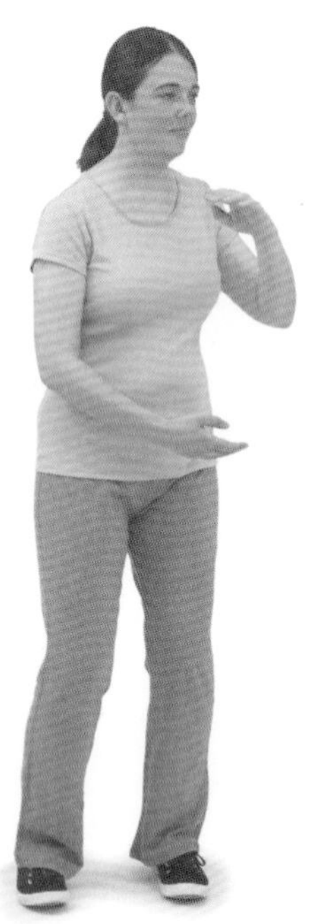

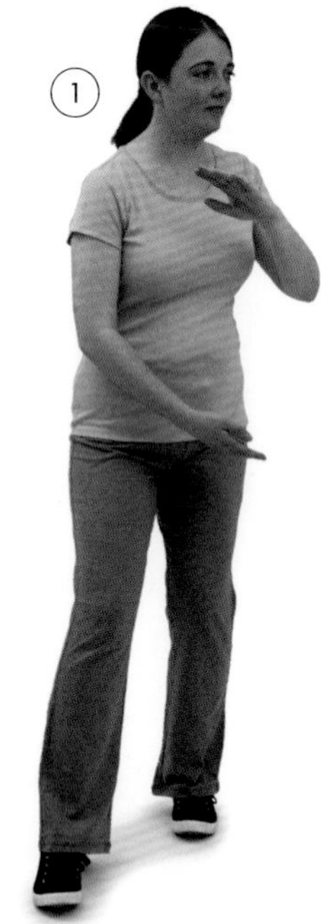

1 *Step forward, toward the north, with your right foot, placing the heel down first and then rolling down the rest of the foot.*

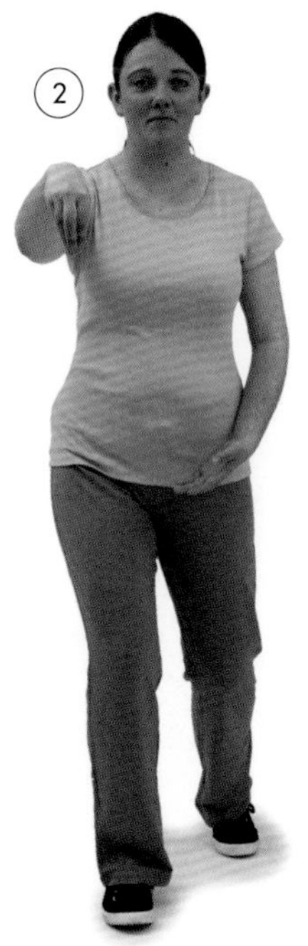

2 *Transfer your weight onto your right leg, turning your body to face the north. As you do so, extend your right arm upward and outward, with the wrist at shoulder height and the hand forming the beak (see page 96), while you lower the left arm to rest in front of you, palm facing upward.*

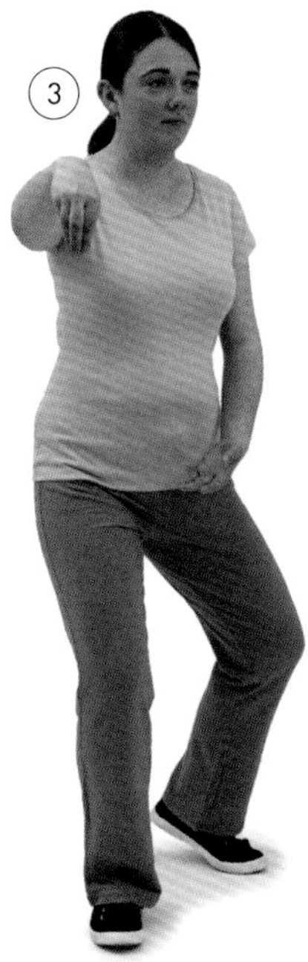

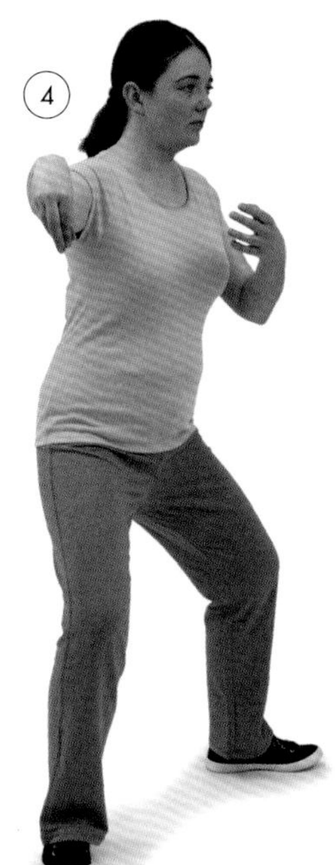

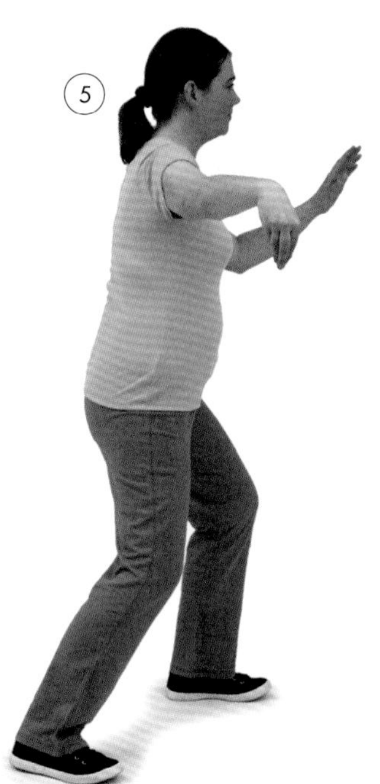

3 *Lift the heel of your left foot and pivot on the ball to bring the toes to face west.*

4 *Take a step to the left, placing the heel down first and then rolling down the rest of the foot. Shift about 70 percent of your weight onto your left leg and bring your left hand up so that the palm is facing your chest, keeping the elbow dropped.*

5 *Raise the toes of your right foot and pivot on the heel to bring them in by 45 degrees as you turn to the left so that you are facing west. Turn the palm of your left hand to face outward. This is Single Whip.*

THE YANG SHORT FORM PART 3

This section deals with the most challenging movements of the form. It begins with a variation of Single Whip known as Descending Single Whip where you sink down toward the ground. It also includes the posture Golden Rooster Stands on One Leg, which is good preparation for the toe and heel kicks that follow. These postures help build your understanding and execution of single-weightedness—something that can inform the rest of your practice.

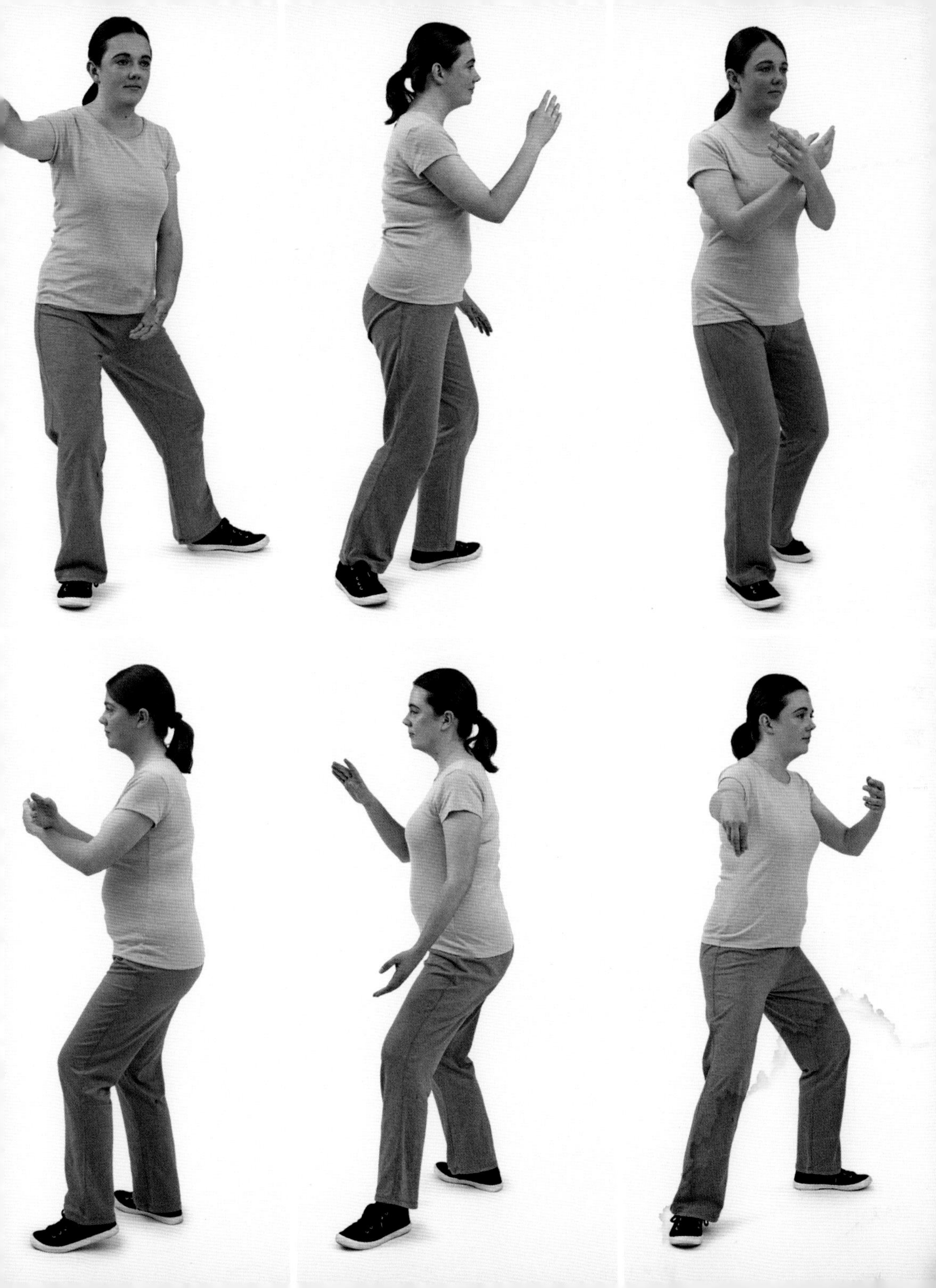

Squatting & One-Legged Postures

Descending Single Whip appears twice in the form, each time following seamlessly on from Single Whip. For most people this squatting posture is one of the hardest to execute because of its physical demands.

The posture is also known as Snake Creeps Down. In tai chi, "snake" is a term for the spine, and the name conveys the slow downward squat of the movement. Make sure that your stance is wide enough to manage this comfortably—if your feet are too close together it will be harder to maintain good posture. Take care not to sink down lower than you can manage because you want to maintain continuous graceful movement both in the descent and then in the ascent that leads into the following posture, Golden Rooster.

One-legged rooster

After Descending Single Whip comes a corresponding upward movement, Golden Rooster Stands on One Leg, or, to give it its full name, Golden Rooster Stands on One Leg to Greet the Dawn. It is also known as Golden Pheasant.

Balancing on one leg is difficult for some people. The natural response to such difficulty is to tense up, but the consequence is to lose your balance. To do Golden Rooster well, you need to root strongly into the foot, relax the body downward ("sinking"), and maintain your good alignment. Golden Rooster is a foundational posture for the toe-and-heel kicks that follow it.

Practitioners sometimes find this posture frustrating, but frustration has a value in tai chi. It helps us bring a quality of patience to our practice, respecting our limitations and struggles as part of the process. You may need to make some practical adaptations to this pose. In particular, do not try to raise your knee too high and keep it low if you need to, or with your toes touching the ground. In time, your balance will improve.

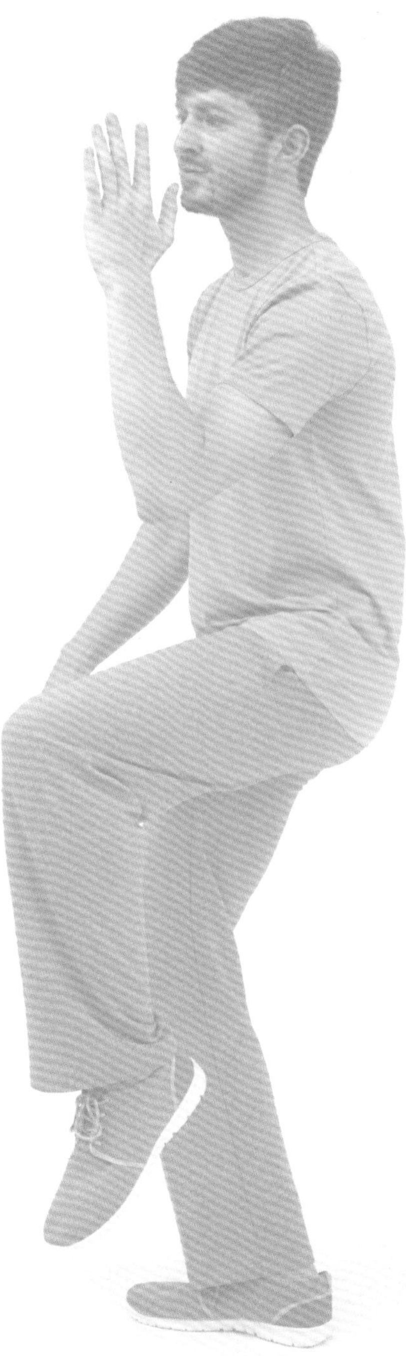

Benefits of Balance

Being able to stand on one leg is a useful indicator of general fitness and brain health, so try practicing this one-legged stance daily—you can do it in spare moments, such as waiting for coffee to brew. As well as building strength in the ankles and lower legs, it has an additional benefit—it is very hard to maintain balance while standing on one leg without focusing on what you are doing, and if your mind wanders, you start to wobble. So it also has a built-in mindfulness detector.

DESCENDING SINGLE WHIP

The first move of this section of the form follows straight on from Single Whip (see page 148) and is a variation of this posture. It is also known more poetically as Snake Creeps Down. The full posture

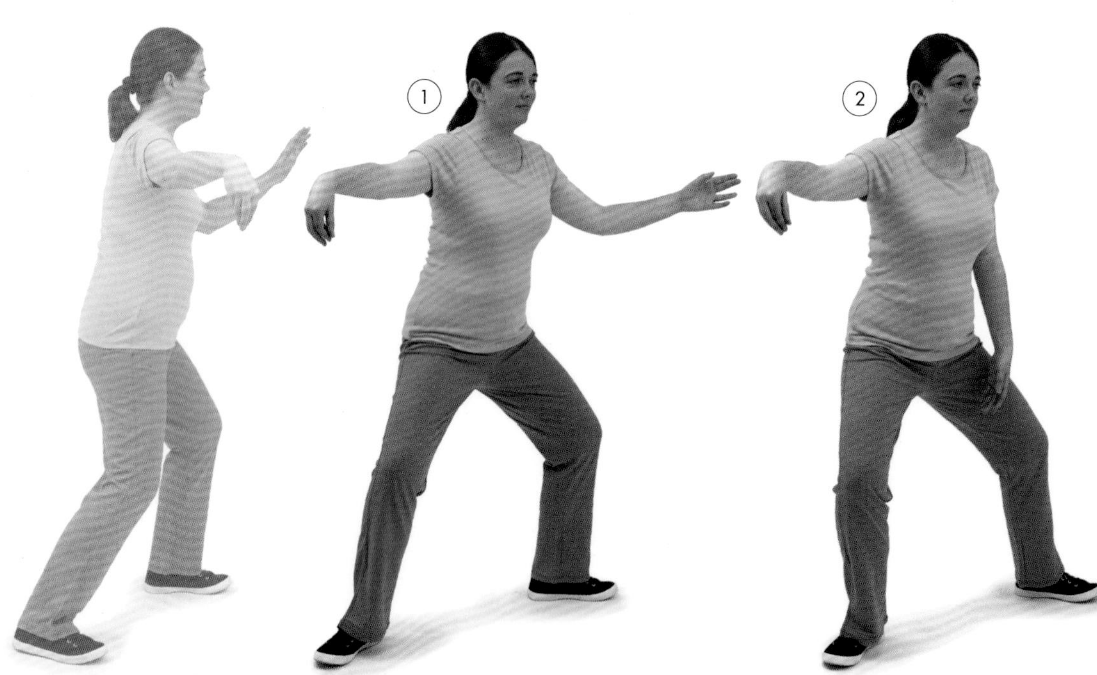

1 *Turn to the right. Raise the toes of your right foot off the ground and turn your foot through a 135-degree angle so that the toes are pointing northeast. At the same time, turn the palm of your left hand to the right, while the right hand remains in its beak position with the right arm out to the side.*

2 *Transfer most of your weight onto your right leg, sinking toward the ground as you draw your left arm back and then downward, fingers pointing toward the ground. As you do so, turn in the toes of your left foot a little.*

develops excellent balance and flexibility. You do not need to go as far down as shown here—maintain awareness of your spine and ensure that you feel relaxed throughout the movement. Your gaze follows the arc of your left arm.

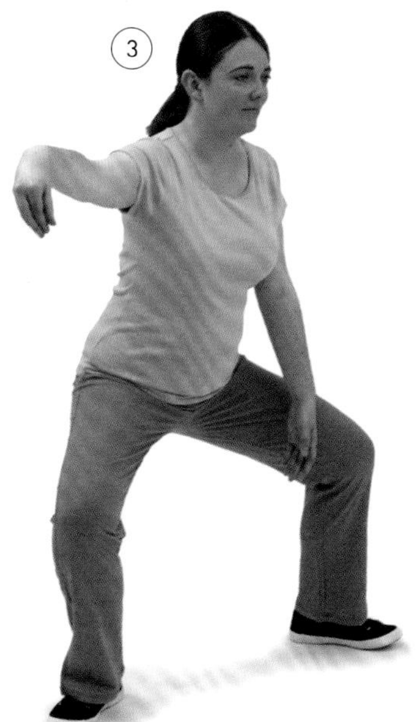

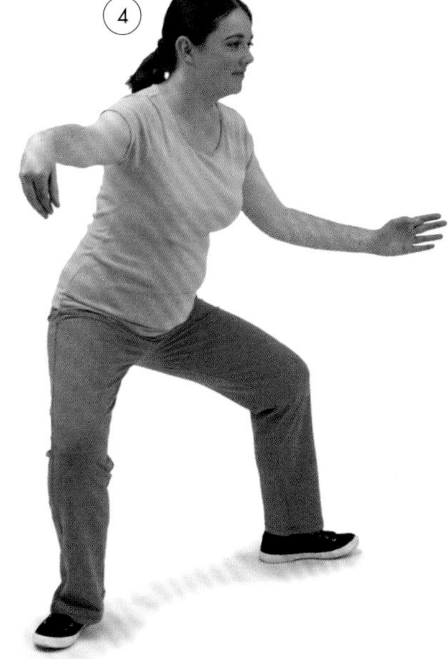

Slide the Foot

If you need to spread your feet wider to squat comfortably, slide your right foot along the ground or take a step when you turn your toes in step 1. Both feet should maintain good contact with the ground throughout this move.

3 *Continue sinking downward with the weight mostly on your right leg without overreaching with the knee or tensing the back or shoulders.*

4 *Lower your left elbow to point the fingers forward, relaxing your shoulders as you do so to avoid leaning, then turn the toes of your left foot back to the west and shift forward so that 60 percent of your weight is on your left leg. This is Descending Single Whip.*

GOLDEN ROOSTER STANDS ON ONE LEG (LEFT)

After the descending movement of the previous posture, there is a corresponding upward movement in which you come up from the squat and then continue the momentum into a knee lift. The right hand rises in harmony with the right knee, ready to deliver a chop to an imaginary opponent's chin as the knee strikes. Focus on synchronizing the movements of the arms and the leg.

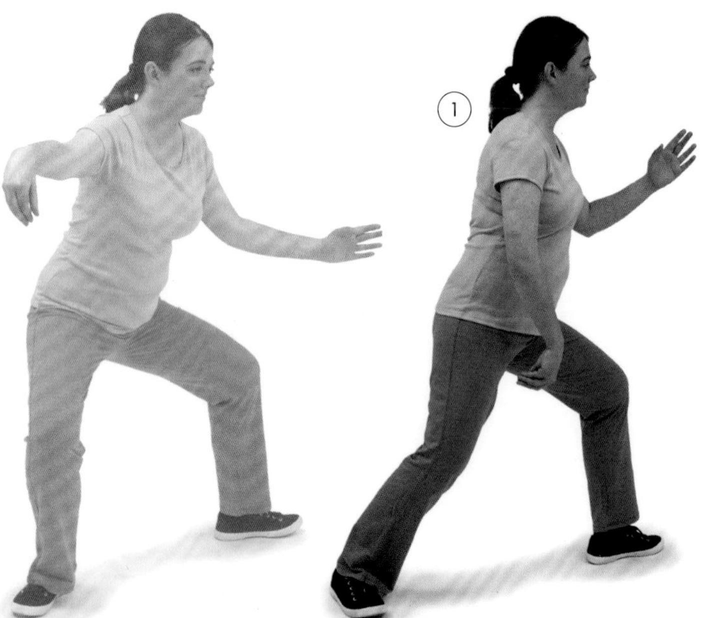

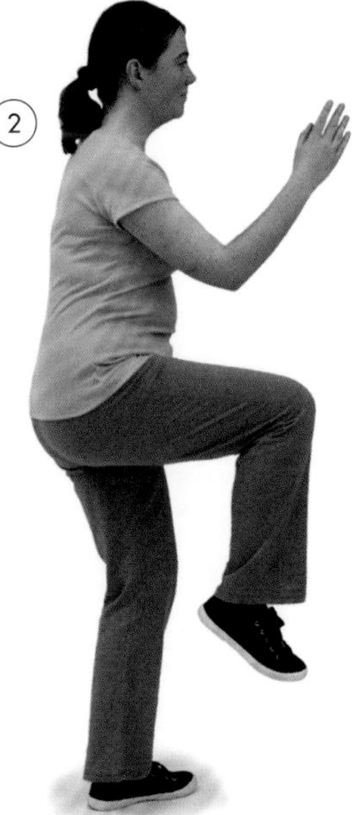

Raise the Knee

In the final posture, the thigh is parallel with the ground with the toes pointing downward. Only go as high as feels comfortable. Remember that in tai chi there is no straining or forcing, and you do not work to the limit of your ability but stay well within it.

1 *Pivot on the heel of your right foot to turn the toes to face northwest. Pivot on the ball of your left foot so that the toes face southwest. Start to transfer the rest of your weight to your left leg. The right hand floats down with the back of it facing west, remaining in its beak, while the left hand rises slightly, palm stll facing to your right.*

2 *Step forward with your right foot. Bring the toes briefly to rest by your left heel before bending your knee and lifting the foot from the ground. As you raise your foot, bend your right elbow to bring your right hand in front of your face, releasing the beak so that the fingers point upward. Lower your left hand, palm facing backward.*

GOLDEN ROOSTER STANDS ON ONE LEG (RIGHT)

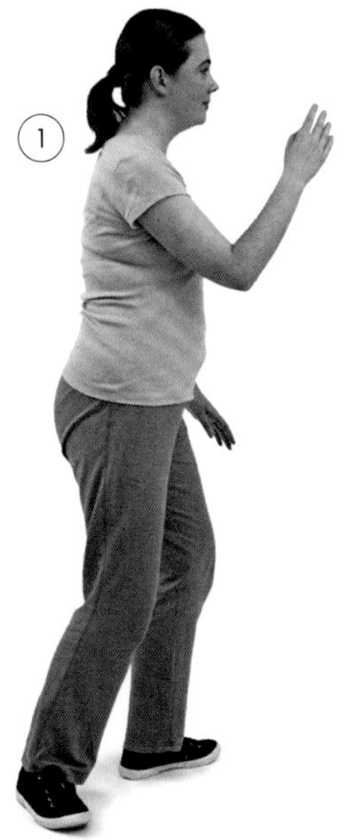

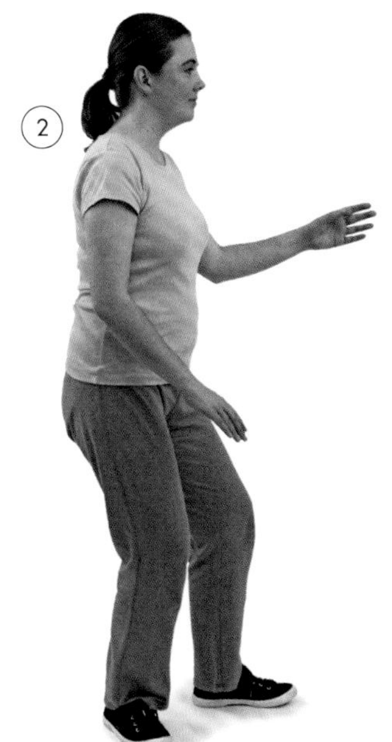

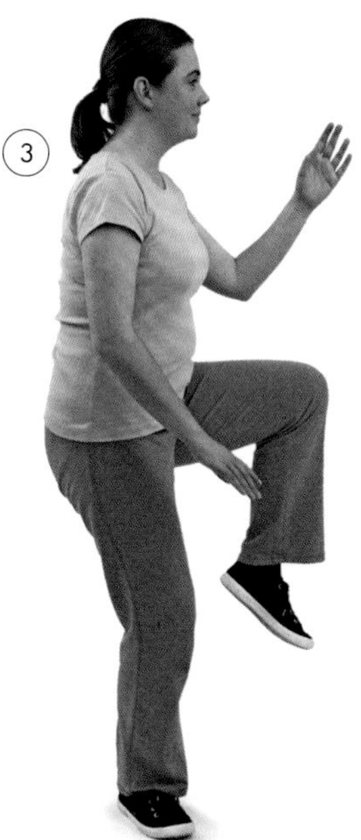

1 *Bring your right leg down, stepping it behind and to the right. Place the toes down first, pointing away from the body to face northwest, and then roll down the rest of the foot.*

2 *Transfer all your weight onto your right leg. Let your right hand press downward and turn the left palm to face the right. Turn the toes of your left foot and pivot on the heel to turn them in by 45 degrees so that they face west.*

3 *Raise your left knee, bringing your left thigh parallel to the ground or as high as you can comfortably manage. At the same time, bend your left elbow to bring your left hand in front of your face, fingers pointing upward. As before, point the toes of your raised foot downward.*

RIGHT TOE KICK

This posture is also known as Separate Right Foot, which is the literal translation of its Chinese name. Make sure that the kicking leg remains relaxed and that you control the movement through its entirety—the "kick" is very

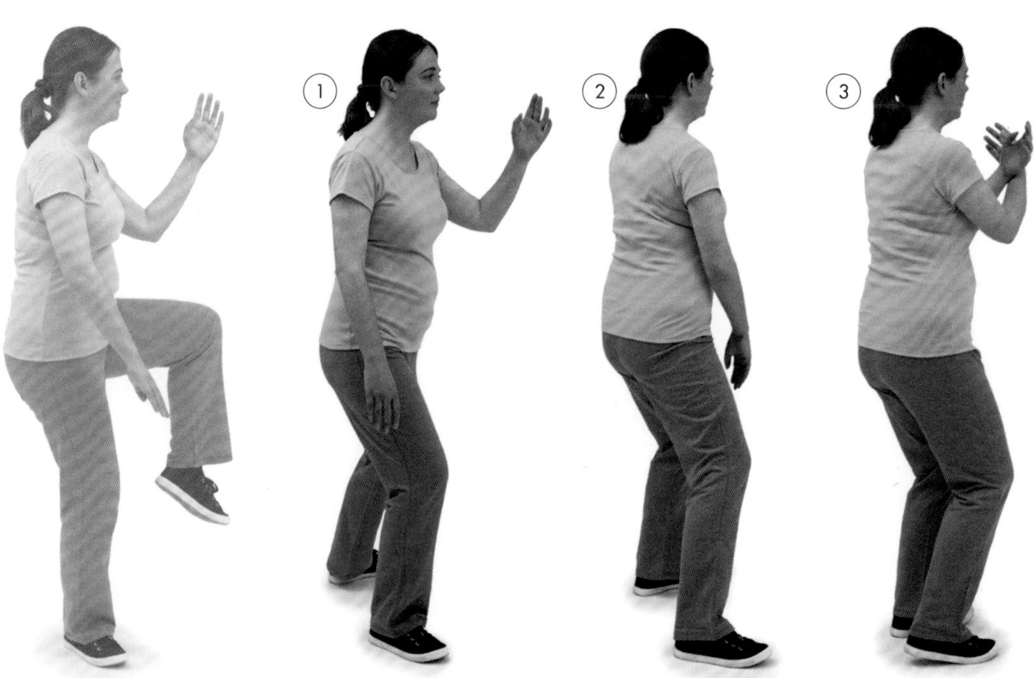

1 *From the raised knee lift of Golden Rooster (see page 156), bring your left leg down and to the back and left, placing the ball of the foot down first, with the toes pointing outward to face southwest. Relax the shoulders.*

2 *Start transferring your weight onto your left leg and relax your arms so that they hang down either side of your left thigh with the palms facing toward it.*

3 *As you continue the turn to the left, bring all your weight onto your left leg, and draw in the toes of your right foot to rest by the heel of your left foot. Bring your arms up and cross your wrists in front of you with your left hand outside your right hand.*

slow and controlled. This is the first kick in the short form; there are two more. You kick first with the right foot and then repeat the move on the other side with a Left Toe Kick (see page 160).

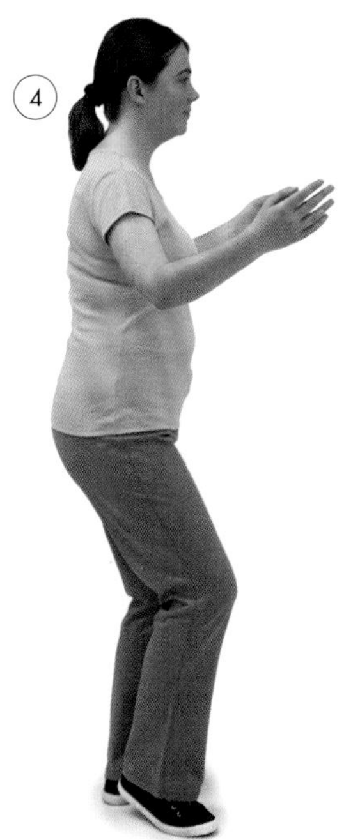

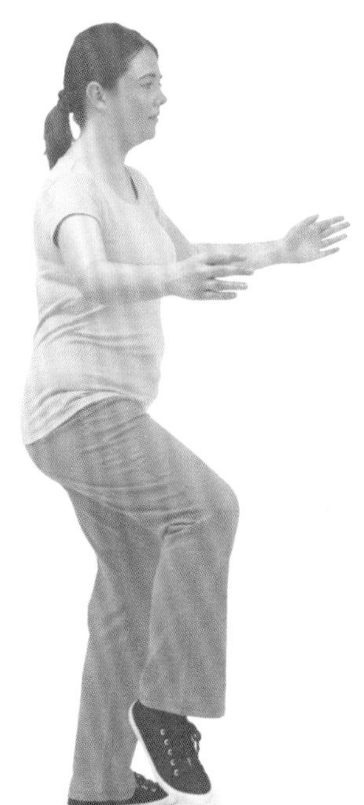

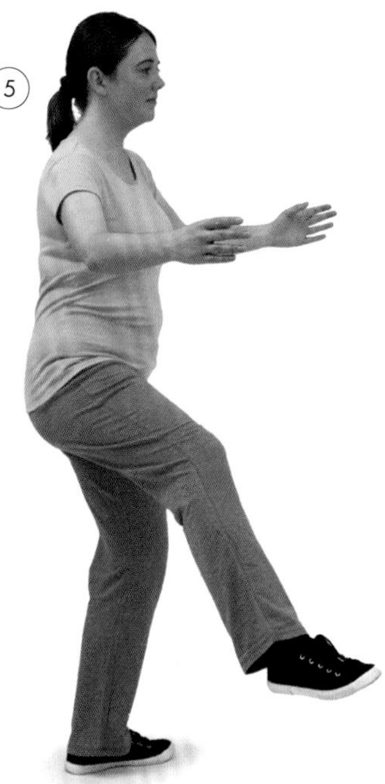

4 *Softly relax and open your shoulders and hips so that your arms open with the palms facing inward. Raise your right heel to prepare to kick.*

5 *Kick softly outward to a comfortable height to the northwest with your right foot. To help you keep your balance, make sure that you relax into your left foot, and be aware of your arms through to your fingertips, keeping your hands alive but not stiff.*

LEFT TOE KICK

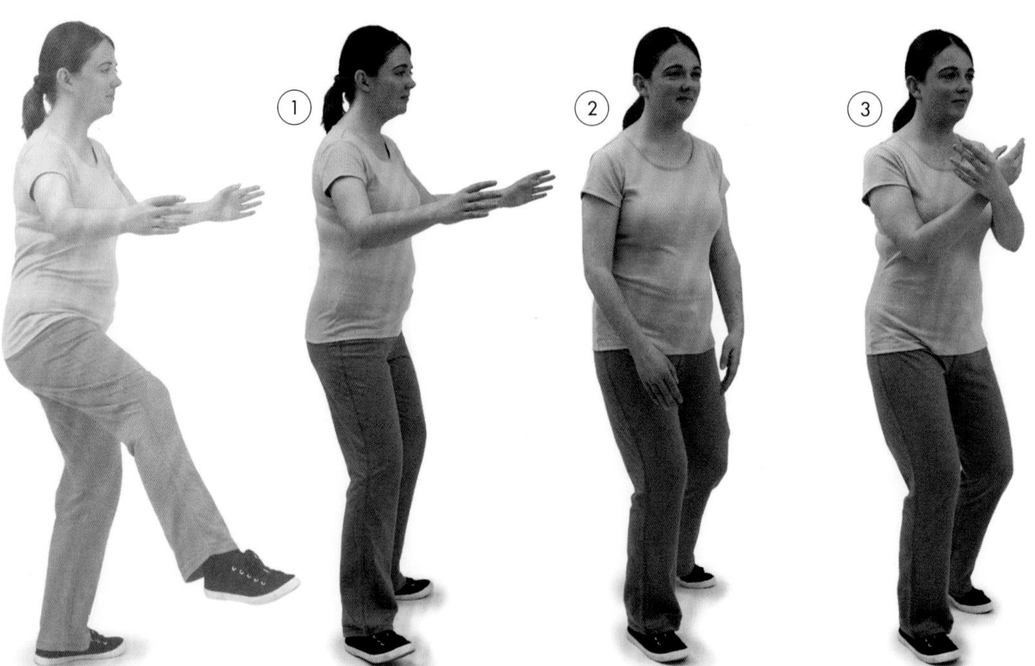

1 *Relax the right foot and step back and to the right, toes pointing outward to face northwest. Start transferring your weight to your right leg.*

2 *Continue bringing your weight onto your right leg and relax the arms so that they hang down either side of your right thigh with the palms facing toward it.*

3 *As you continue the turn to the right, bring all your weight onto your right leg, and draw in the toes of your left foot to rest by the heel of your right foot. Bring your arms up and cross your wrists in front of you with your left hand outside your right.*

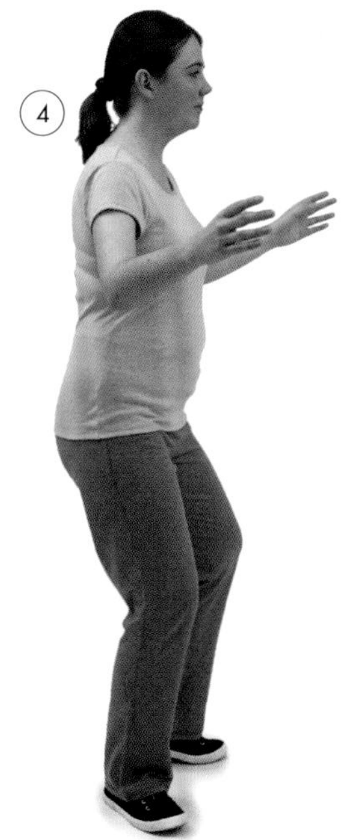

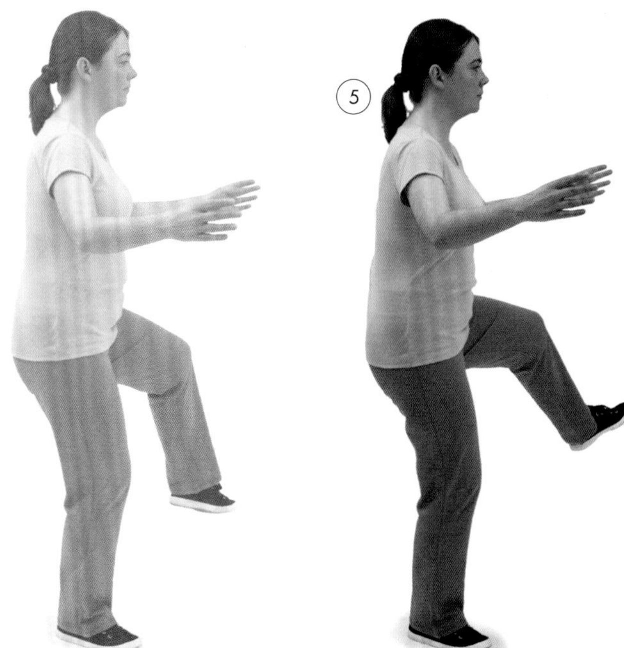

4 *Softly relax and open your shoulders and hips so that your arms open with the palms facing inward. Raise your left heel to prepare to kick.*

5 *Kick softly outward to a comfortable height to the southwest with your left foot. To help you keep your balance, make sure that you relax into your right foot, and be aware of your arms through to your fingertips, keeping your hands alive but not stiff.*

TURN & KICK WITH LEFT HEEL

This is the most challenging maneuver of the form because you have to pivot on your right heel right through a 180-degree turn while your left foot rests on the toes by your right heel, or remains

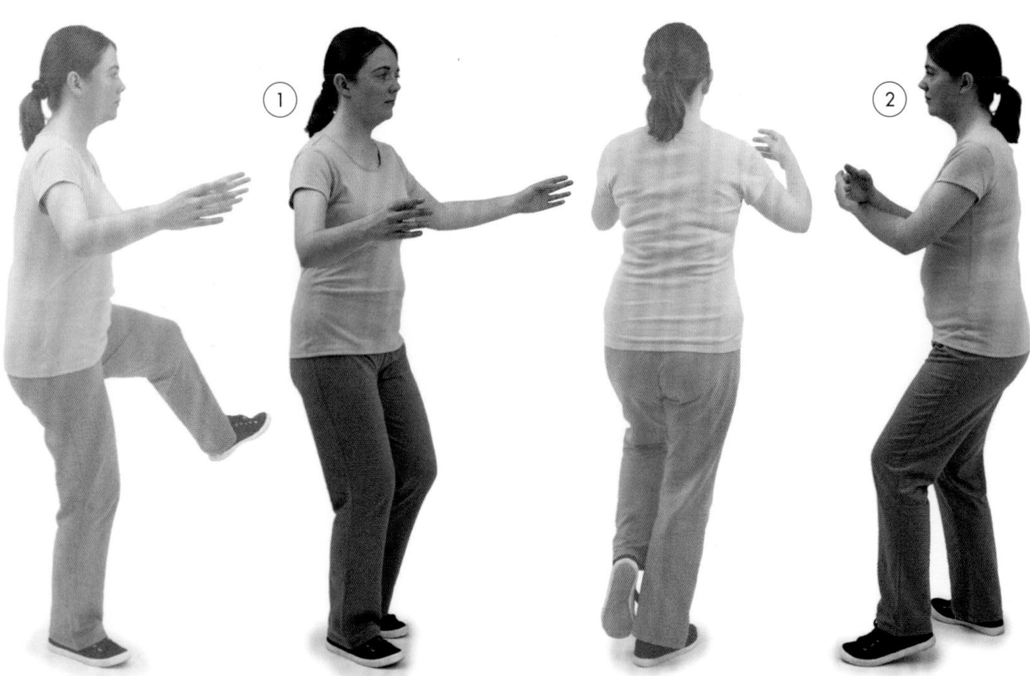

1 *Lower your left leg ready to spin.*

2 *Bring your left hand to face your chest and drop your right hand down by your thigh as you start to turn to the left and quickly swing your right arm to cross inside your left wrist as you pivot on your right heel. The toes of your right foot now face southeast. Keeping relaxed throughout this movement is the secret to managing the turn.*

suspended in the air if your balance is good enough. Expect to invest in some sustained practice to master this posture.

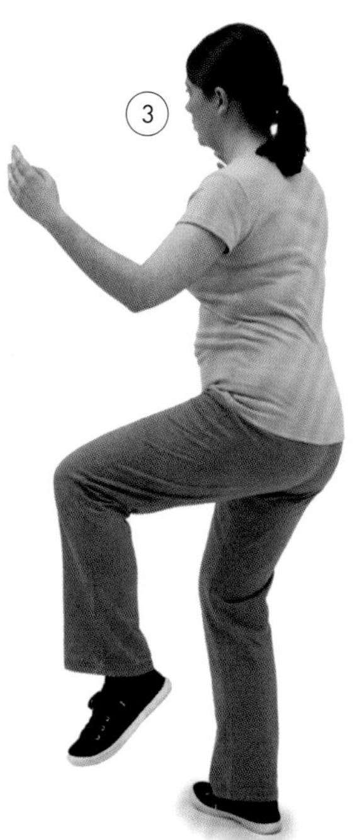

3 *Bringing all your weight onto your right leg, raise your left knee into a heel kick. At the same time, start to fan your arms outward, extending your left arm out in tandem with your left leg at about shoulder height, and extending your right arm up and out.*

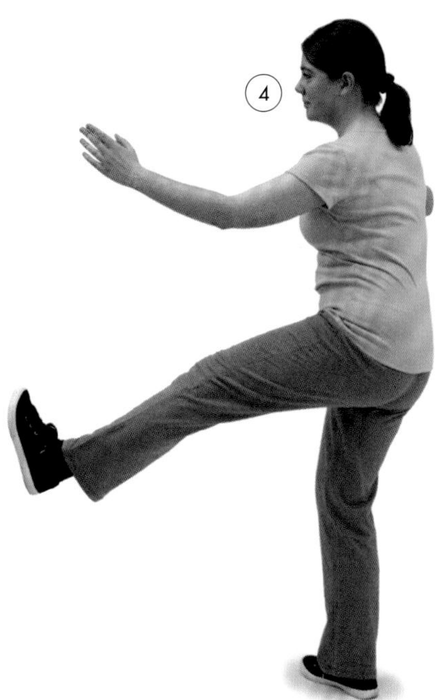

4 *Kick your left heel away, straightening the leg completely.*

BRUSH LEFT KNEE & PUSH

After the demanding balance postures that precede it, this movement can feel like an old friend, since this is the third time it appears in the form. It is tricker than before because the left foot is in the kick position.

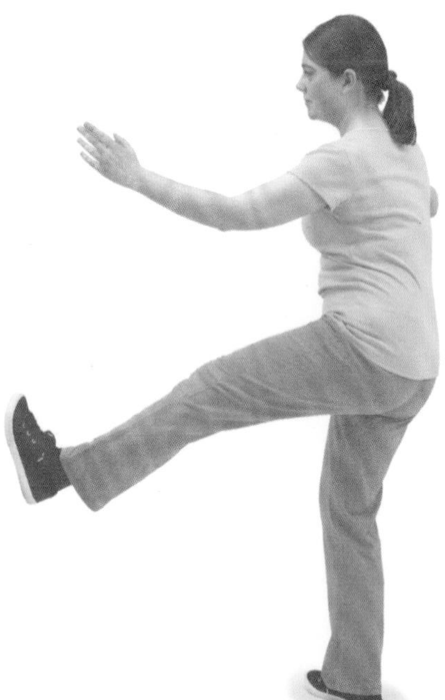

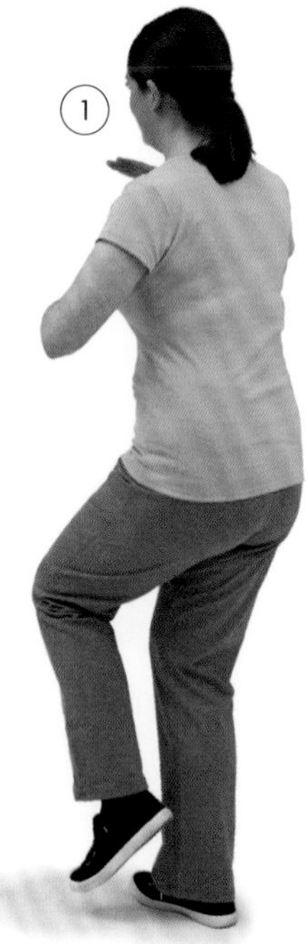

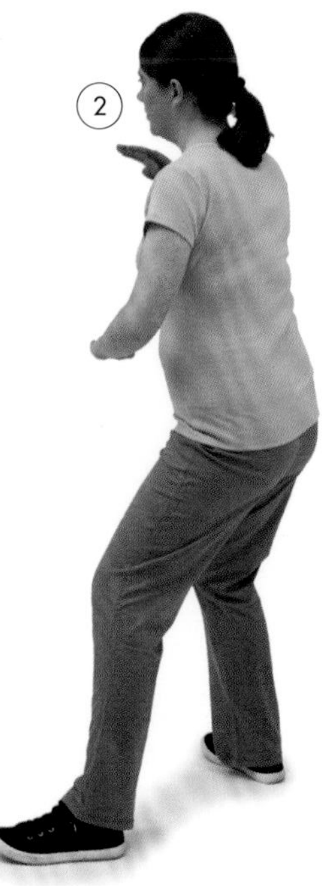

1 *Relax your left leg and turn to the right. Bring your left arm toward you, bending it at the elbow, and start to fold in your right arm, bending this elbow, too, and turning the palm to face downward.*

2 *Now step your left foot to the left, placing the heel down first and ensuring that there is a shoulder-width distance between the heels, with the toes pointing east.*

Lower the foot slowly and with control; it is momentarily suspended in the air before you step outward. To help you balance, touch the toes of your left foot on the ground before stepping out.

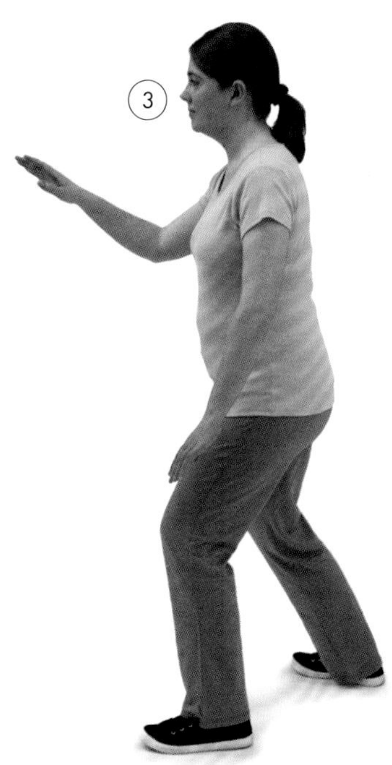

3 *Bring 70 percent of your weight onto your front (left) foot. Turn to the left, then raise the toes of your right foot and pivot on the heel to bring them in for Bow Stance (see page 74). Extend your right arm forward, dropping the elbow, and bring your left hand over your left thigh, finishing just outside it. This is Brush Left Knee and Push.*

Lifting the Toes

When you raise the toes off the ground, avoid lifting them very high, otherwise it will cause tension in the shin and ankle. Just lift them to the point where you can pivot smoothly on the heel.

BRUSH RIGHT KNEE & PUSH

This is the same posture as the preceding one, but performed on the other side. When making the pushing movement with the left hand, watch that you do not lean the body too far forward or lose the

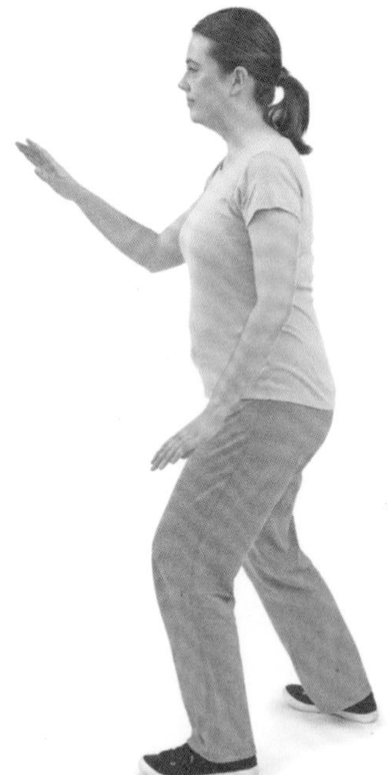

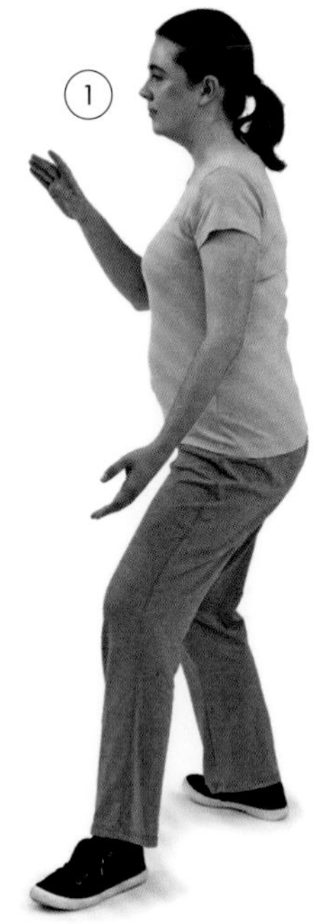

1 *Transfer your weight to your back (right) leg. Lift the toes of your left foot and pivot on the heel to turn the toes out by 45 degrees. Draw the right hand toward you, bending the elbow, as you rotate the left arm so that the palm faces upward.*

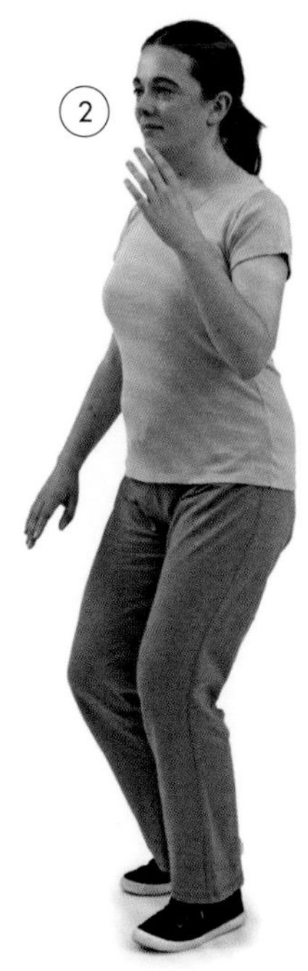

2 *Transfer your weight to your left foot as you step in with your left foot. Turn your right palm down in front of your body while you bend your left arm at the elbow until the palm is facing forward near the shoulder.*

relaxation in the shoulders—the power comes from the legs. Maintain the feet's connection with the ground.

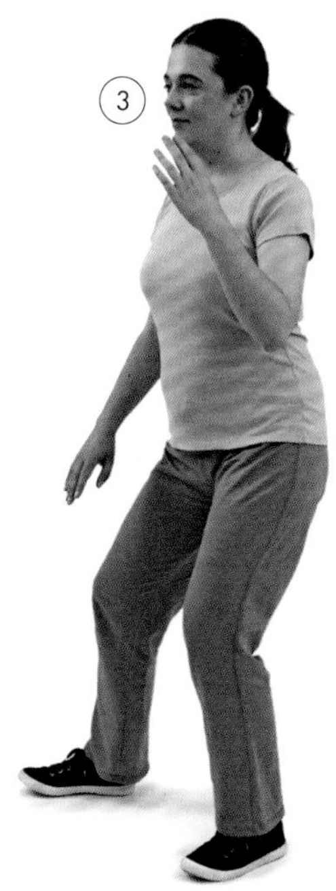

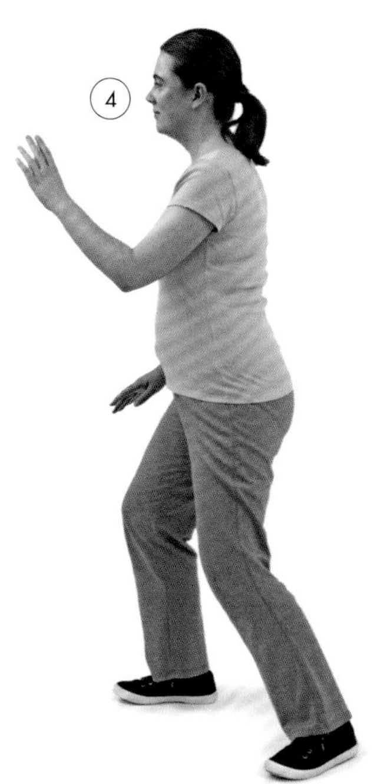

3 *Step forward with the right foot, placing the heel down first with the toes pointing forward and ensuring that there is a shoulder-width distance between your feet.*

4 *Transfer 70 percent of your weight onto your front (right) leg and turn to face in the same direction (east). Raise the toes of your left foot and pivot on the heel to turn them inward (Bow Stance—see page 74). Extend the left arm forward, dropping the elbow, and bring your right hand over your right thigh, finishing just outside it. This is Brush Right Knee and Push.*

BRUSH LEFT KNEE & PUNCH DOWNWARD

In this posture, you repeat the Brush Left Knee movement, but instead of the Push, you Punch Downward with your right hand. Remember that the Tai Chi Fist is firm but relaxed, and the thumb always rests on the outside of the fingers.

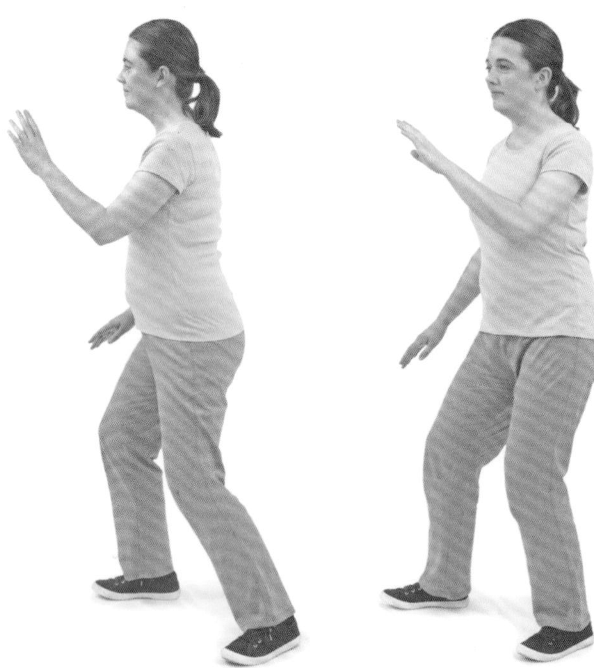

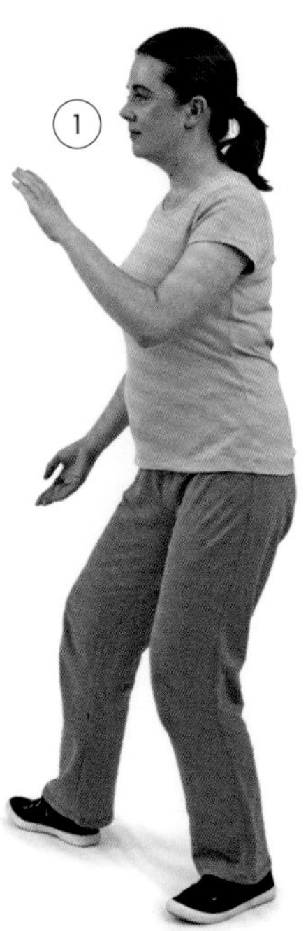

1 *Transfer most of your weight onto your back (left) leg. Pivot on the toes of your right foot to turn them out by 45 degrees, while rotating your right arm so that the palm faces upward.*

Hold the Line

Keep your back straight as you perform the Punch. Note the straight line created by the back leg, spine, and neck.

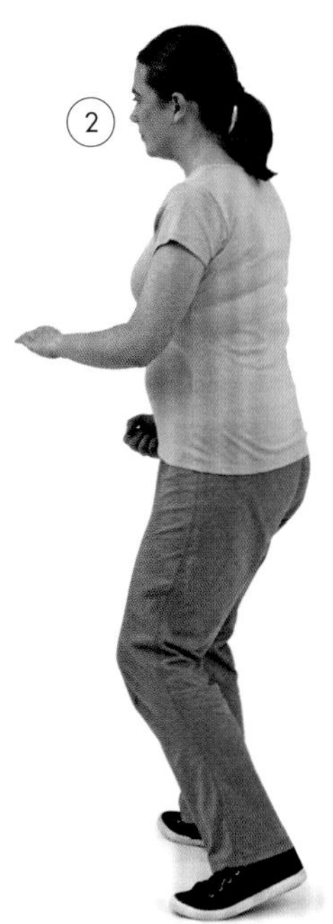

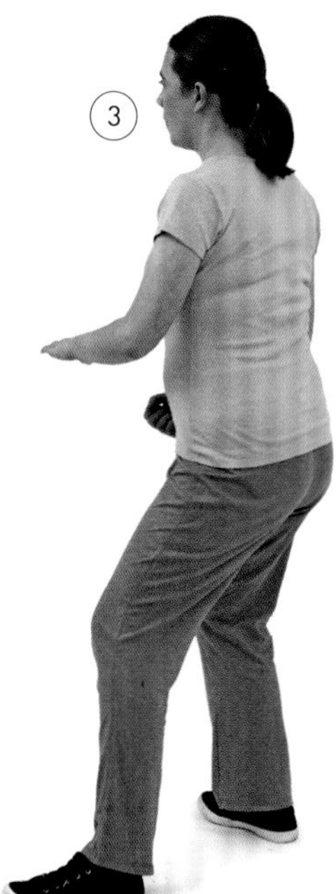

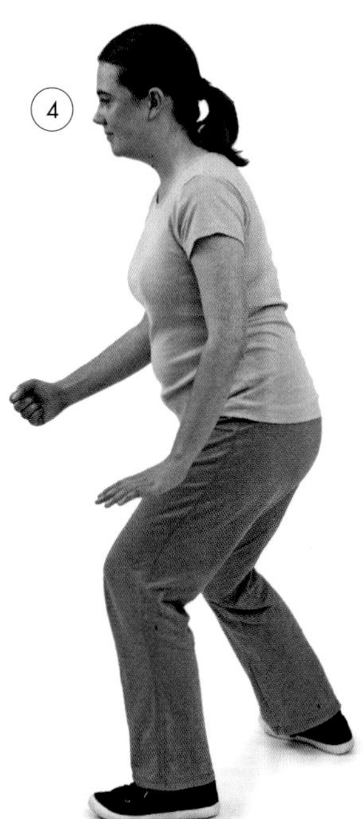

2 *Roll your right foot down and shift most of your weight onto your front (right) leg and step in with your left foot. Bring your right hand into a soft Tai Chi Fist (see page 115) in front of your stomach and lower your left arm, palm facing downward.*

3 *Step your left foot forward, placing the heel down first, so that it faces east, with a shoulder-width distance between your heels.*

4 *Transfer about 70 percent of your weight onto your front (left) foot. Brush your left hand over your left knee (without touching) and move your right hand forward and down in a low punch, as you squat gently into your left leg.*

WARD OFF RIGHT

The form now returns to the familiar postures of Grasp the Sparrow's Tail, beginning here with Ward Off Right, which appears for the second

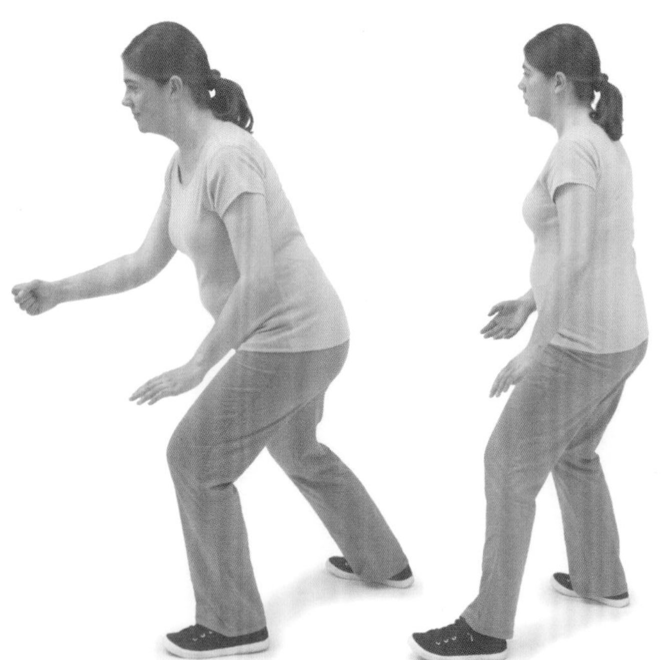

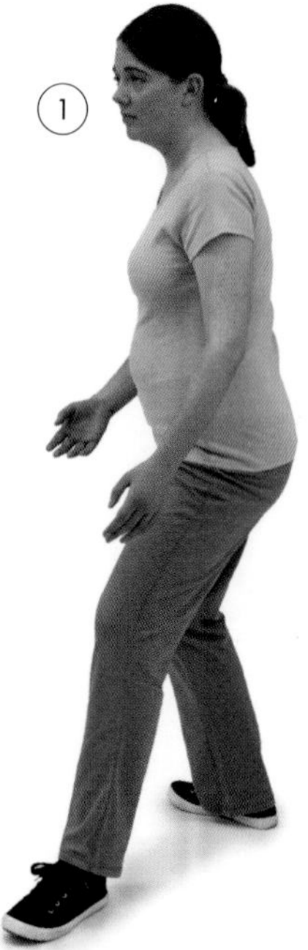

1 *Transfer your weight to your back (right) foot as you come up from the low punch of the previous posture. Raise the toes of your left foot and pivot on the heel to turn them out by 45 degrees. Open your right-hand fist.*

Rising Straight

As you rise up, watch that your back maintains its straightness and that your shoulders remain relaxed with the elbows dropped.

time. The start of the movement differs from the previous rendition because you need first to rise up from the Punch Downward position and then take a step forward.

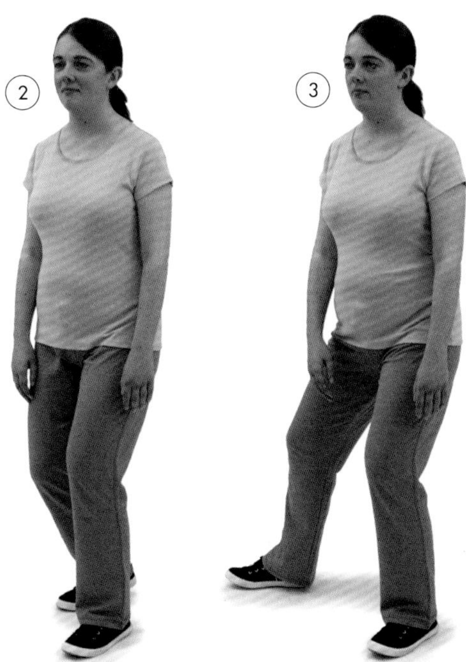

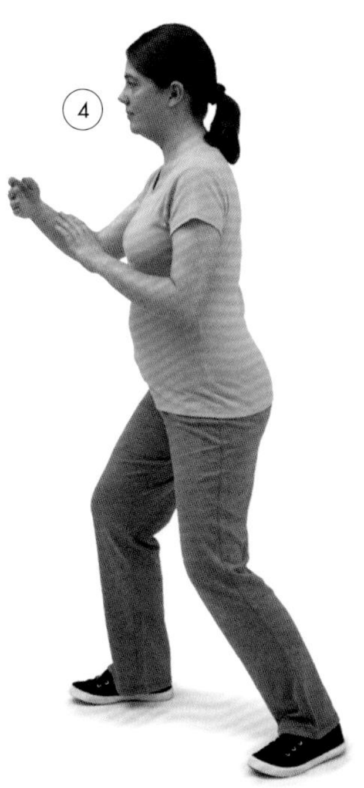

2 *Bring your weight onto your left leg. Draw the right foot forward toward the left foot ready to step out, with your hands hanging either side of your left thigh.*

3 *Step your right foot forward to face east, placing the heel down first before rolling down the rest of the foot.*

4 *Shift 70 percent of your weight onto your right leg (Bow Stance—see page 74) as you complete the right turn to face east. At the same time, raise both hands so that the fingers of your right hand are facing left and the fingers of your left hand are pointing to your right wrist. This is Ward Off Right.*

ROLLBACK You probably feel comfortable with this beautiful, defensive posture now. Make a point of sinking into the final position and take this opportunity to mentally check through the key points of tai chi posture (see page 28). Your feet do not move as the weight shifts first to the right leg and then to the left leg.

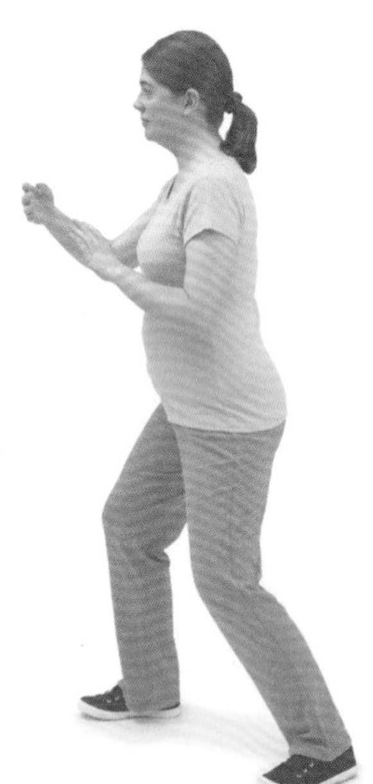

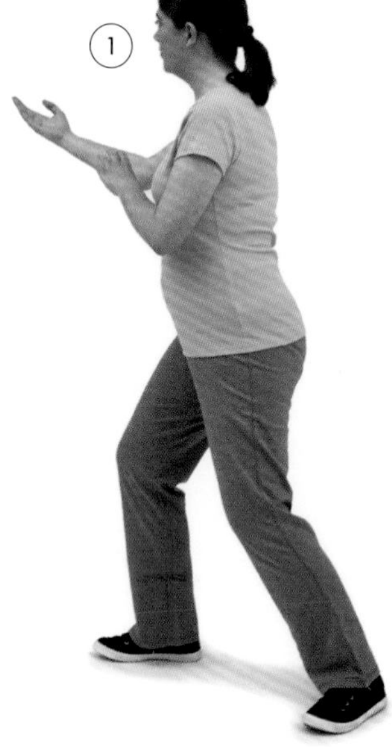

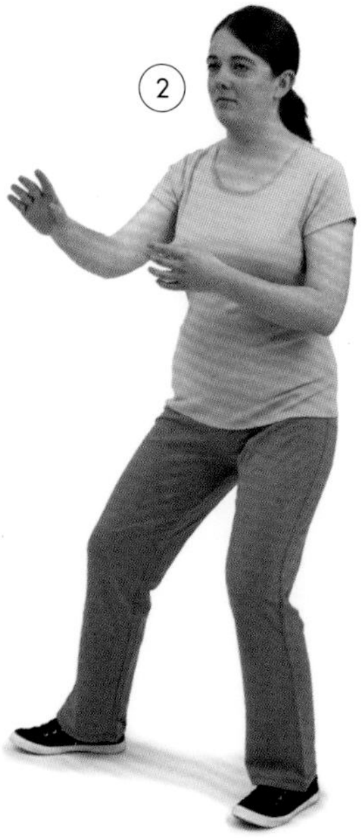

1 *Turn a little to the right, shifting more of your weight onto your right leg. As you do so, turn your right palm upward, keeping the fingers of your left hand pointing to your right wrist.*

2 *Transfer your weight onto your left leg, while you turn your right palm to face forward and down and your left palm to face your body. As you transfer your weight, turn your hips to the left (northeast), keeping your shoulders and elbows relaxed, letting your arms be carried by your body's movement. This is Rollback.*

PRESS & PUSH

From Rollback, you move back into Press and Push, transmitting power from the legs up through thc body and into the hands. Remember that the spine stays straight even when pushing forward. Keep the pace of your movcments slow enough for you to execute them accurately and mindfully.

Press

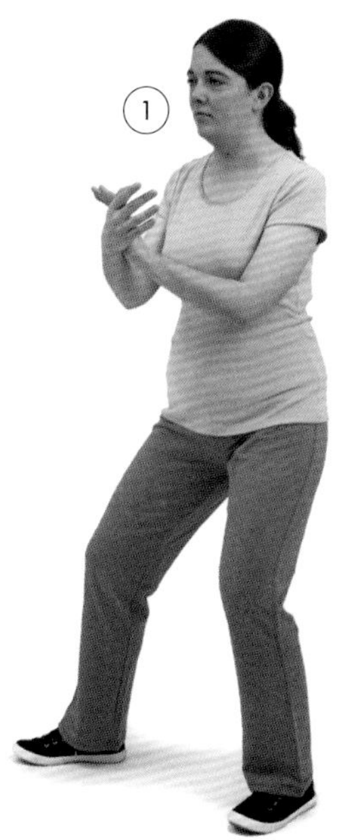

1 *Bring your right arm slightly toward you, turning your right palm to face your chest, while you raise your left arm slightly with your left palm facing outward and bring it across so that the bases of your hands touch.*

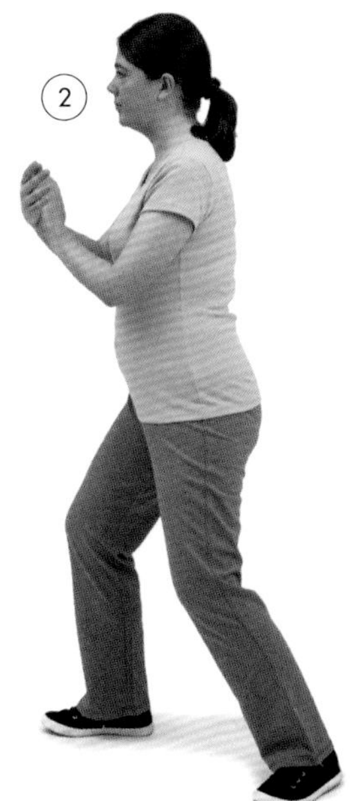

2 *As you do this, return your weight mostly to your front (right) leg so that you are facing the same direction as your right foot. This is Press.*

Push

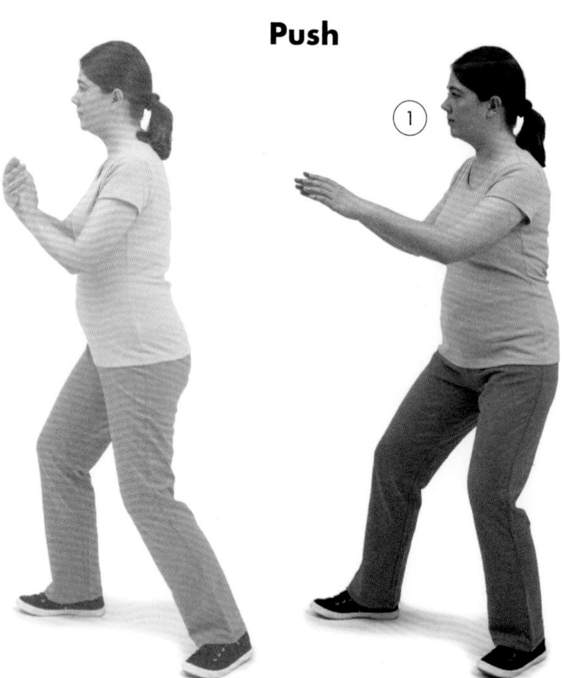

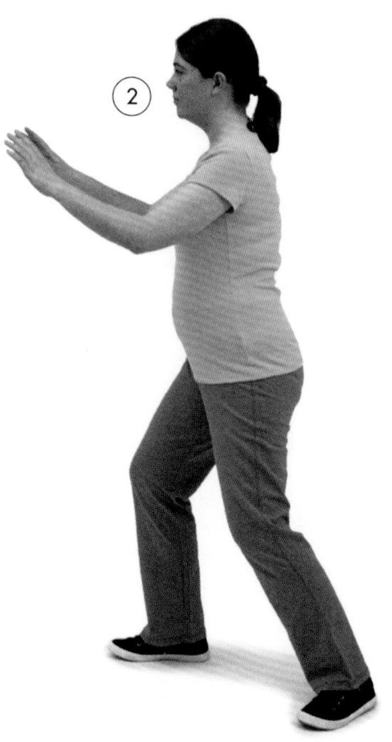

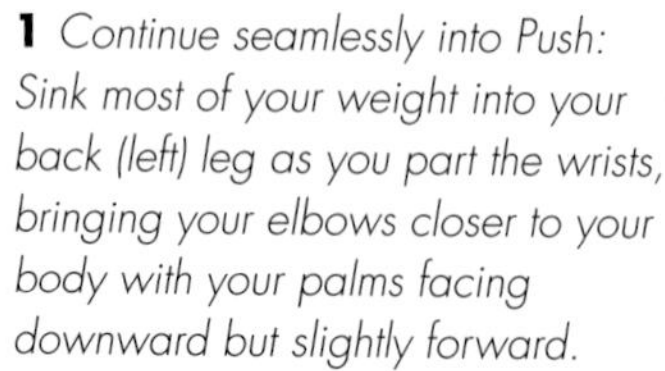

1 *Continue seamlessly into Push: Sink most of your weight into your back (left) leg as you part the wrists, bringing your elbows closer to your body with your palms facing downward but slightly forward.*

2 *Then shift your weight back onto your front (right) leg as you push forward, raising your hands so that they are at chest height and chest-width apart in the Beautiful Hands position (see page 27). At the end of the movement, 70 percent of your weight should be on your front (right) leg and 30 percent on your back (left) leg. This is Push.*

SINGLE WHIP

Here is Single Whip again, the final posture in this section of the form and one that brings you back to face west again. Remember that the fingers in the beak should be just touching but not exerting any pressure.

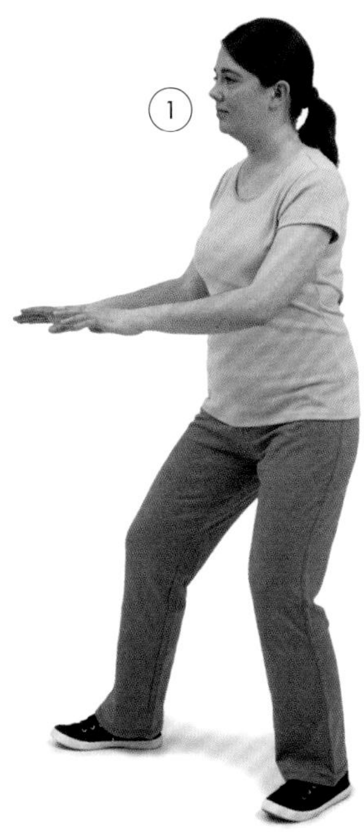

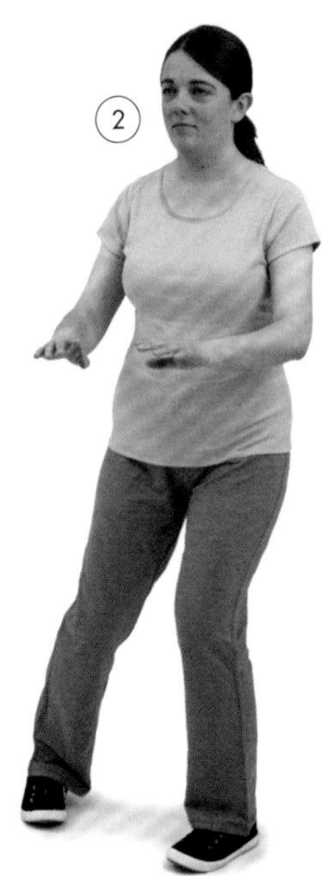

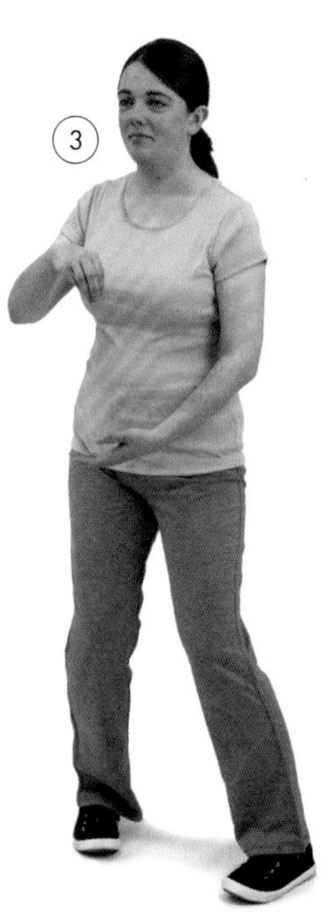

1 *Start transferring your weight back onto your left leg, lowering your forearms with a slight downward pressure so that they are parallel to the ground with the palms facing downward.*

2 *Continue shifting almost all your weight onto your left leg as you turn to the left as far as you can comfortably go by pivoting the right foot on the heel to face forward (north), leaving your left foot in the same position. Follow the movement of your body with your arms.*

3 *Now transfer all your weight onto your right leg and turn back to the right. As you do so, drop your left hand, turning the palm upward as in Hold the Ball position (see page 87). Move your right arm in front of your chest, bending the elbow and forming a beak with your fingers (see page 96).*

Continued overleaf

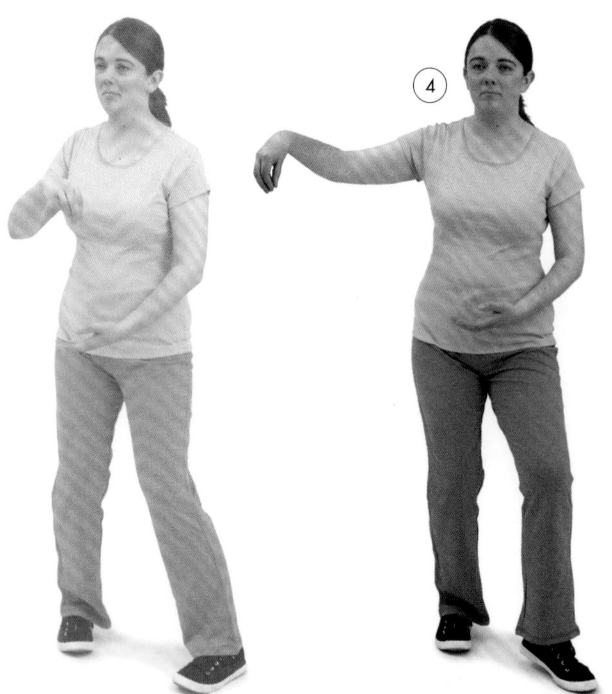

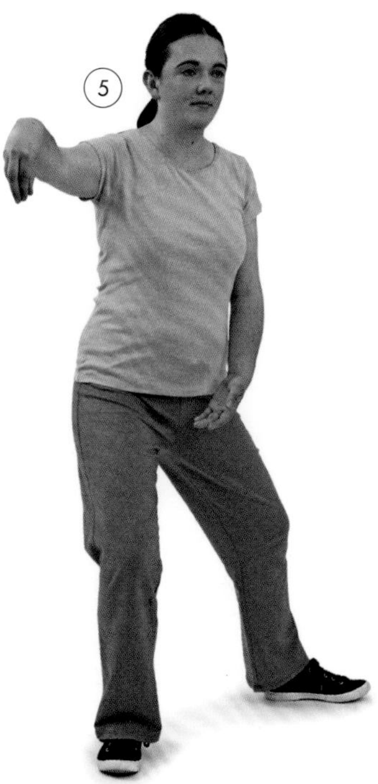

4 *Turn to the left on the ball of your left foot so that the toes are facing northwest while your body faces north. Extend your right arm out to the right, keeping your hand in the beak position and your elbow relaxed.*

5 *Step out with your left foot so that the toes are facing west, turning to the northwest as you do so, placing the heel down first and keeping the weight on your right foot (you may wish to step back briefly first to help you balance). Your heels should form an L shape with a shoulder-width distance between them.*

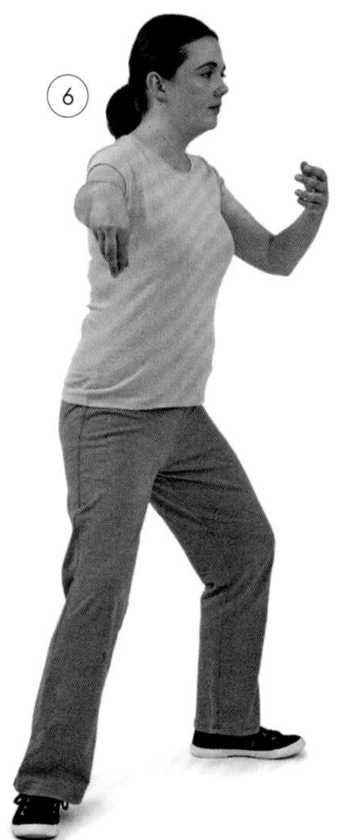

6 *Now pour about 70 percent of your weight into your left leg and bring your left hand up so that the palm is facing your chest.*

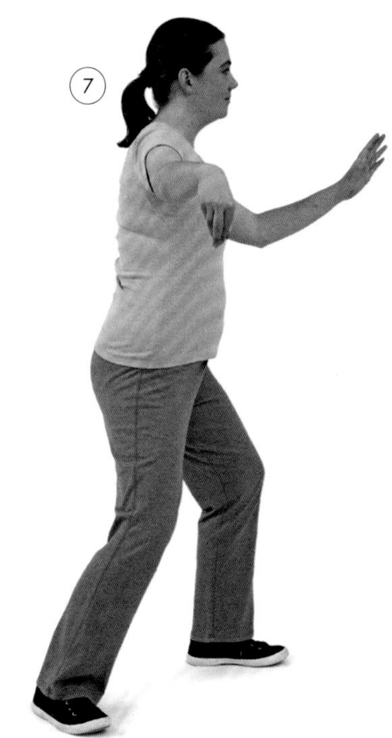

7 *Pivot on your right heel so that the toes are pointing northwest and turn your body to the left to face west in Bow Stance again (see page 74). As you end the movement, turn your left palm to face outward in the Beautiful Hands position (see page 27). This is Single Whip.*

THE YANG SHORT FORM PART 4

Some of the most difficult sequences of the form are contained within this final section, but it also features some familiar exercises. Cheng Man Ching used to recommend that his students practiced the form as if they were swimming through air. Keeping this image in mind will encourage you to move as if encountering slight resistance, which both slows your movements and also helps you to bring the desired quality of relaxed power to them.

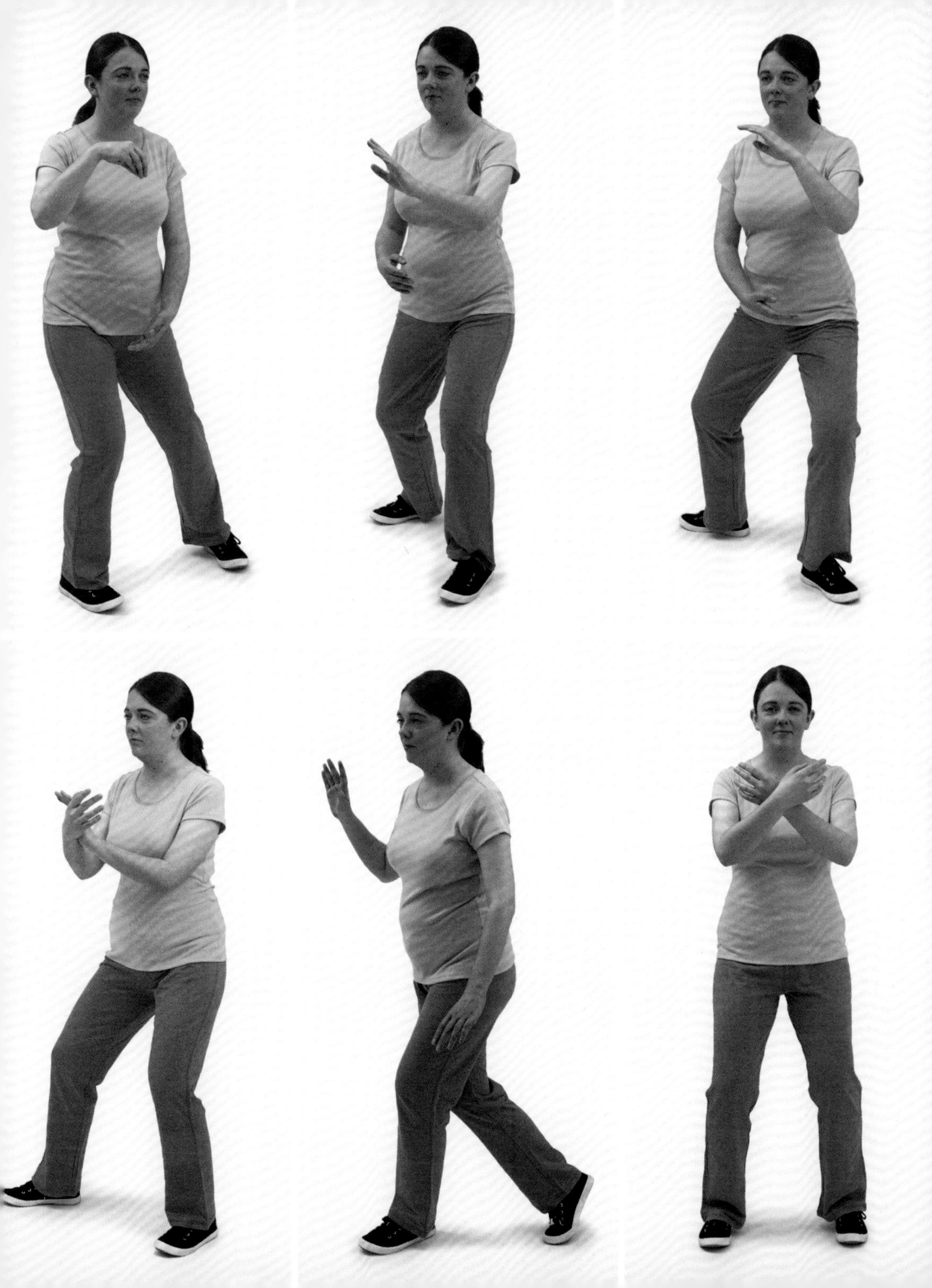

Fair Lady & Onward

This section of the form begins with a long sequence called Fair Lady Weaves the Shuttle, which involves a back-and-forward movement that is reminiscent of the action of working the shuttle on a loom.

The posture is performed four times, in four directions, and is sometimes named simply Four Corners because each movement is performed to the corner (or diagonal) in the following order: northeast, northwest, southwest, southeast.

Understanding the move

In this move, one hand is raised near to the head, and the other is pushing forward at chest height. From the martial art point of view, this is intended as a movement to deal with attackers from various directions. The upper hand absorbs the force of a blow and deflects it, while the lower arm moves forward to deliver a palm strike to the opponent's now-unprotected chest.

Many people find this a confusing sequence to learn, so expect to take your time with it. It is helpful to remember that the hand that is raised is on the same side as the front leg. Make sure that the shoulders are relaxed, especially the shoulder of your raised arm, and that your elbows do not stick out.

Embracing the familiar

The form continues with the final repetition of Grasp the Sparrow's Tail followed by Descending Single Whip, which occurs here for the second time. Enjoy the smoothness of action that comes when a posture is well known and well practiced, and try to maintain the same sense of conscious awareness of your movements as with a new and more complicated sequence. You come up from Descending Single Whip into a new posture, Step Forward to the Seven Stars. This is named for the Big Dipper or Plough constellation, which the body is said, somewhat fancifully, to resemble in this posture—your elbows and fists form the upper part of the constellation, with the hip, knee, and foot of the right leg forming the tail.

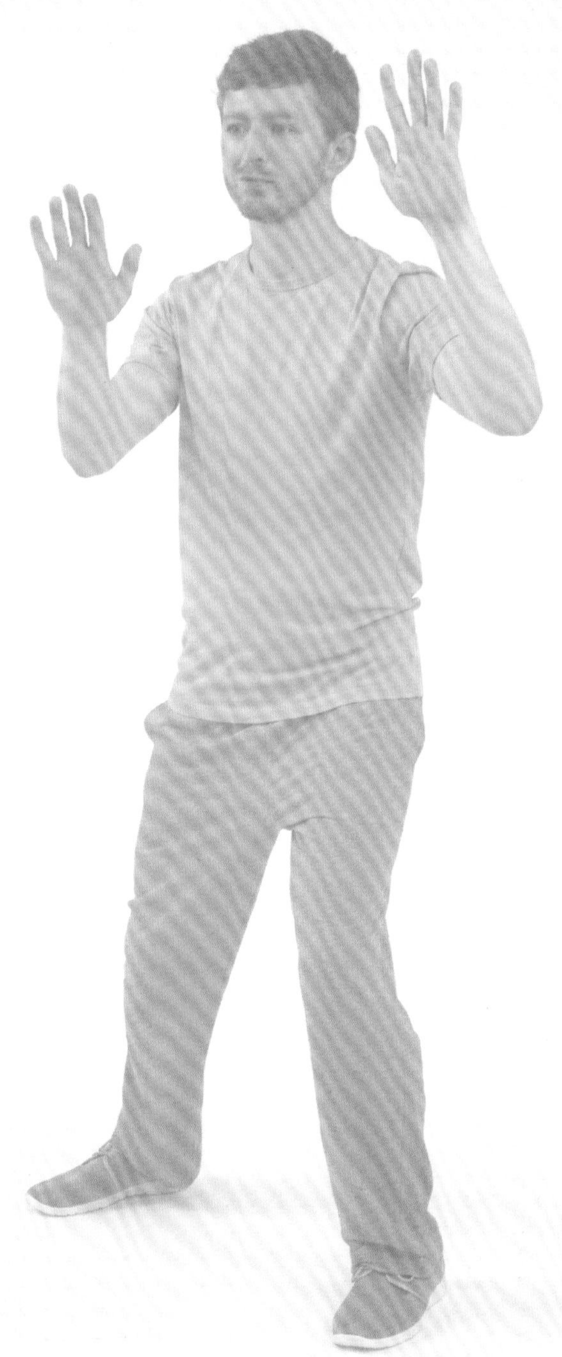

FAIR LADY WEAVES THE SHUTTLE (1, NORTHEAST)

This first rendition of the posture ends with you facing northeast. It is repeated three more times—always to the corner. Many practitioners find this the trickiest sequence

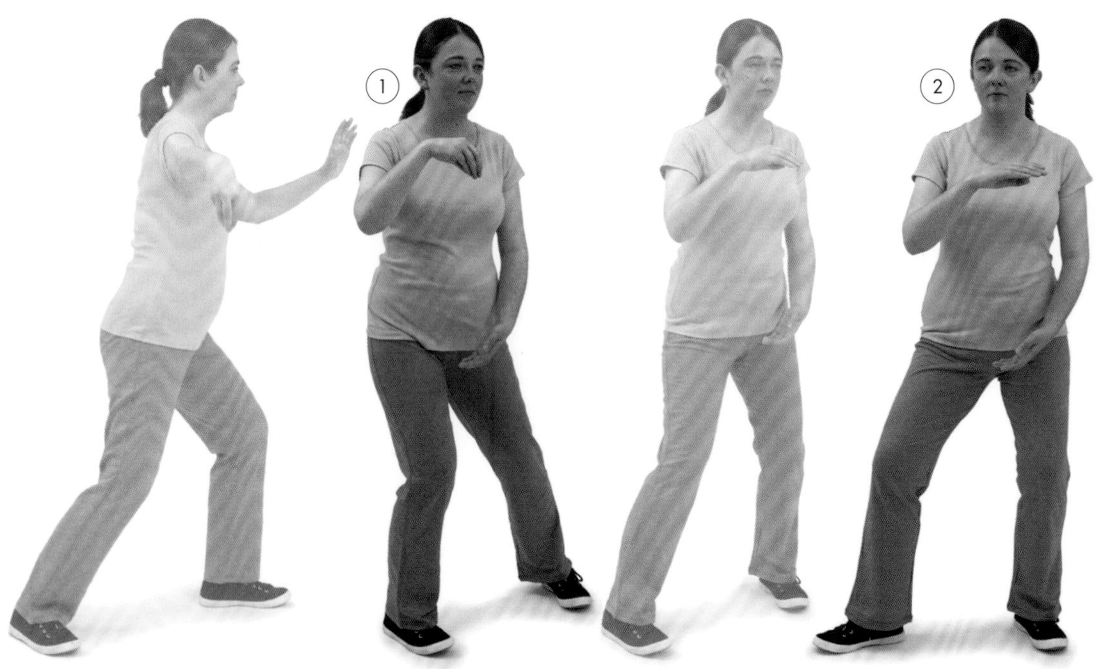

1 *Bring your weight onto your right leg as you turn to the right. At the same time, drop your right elbow, keeping your right hand in its beak, and lower your left arm, turning the palm upward under your navel.*

2 *Transfer your weight back onto your left leg, then open the beak of your right hand. Pivot on the ball of your right foot, toes facing east. Take a small step with your right foot, placing the right heel in line with the left heel on the east-west axis and with the toes of the right foot facing to the east.*

of the form because it involves many shifts of weight and some large turns, so be patient with yourself while you are learning it.

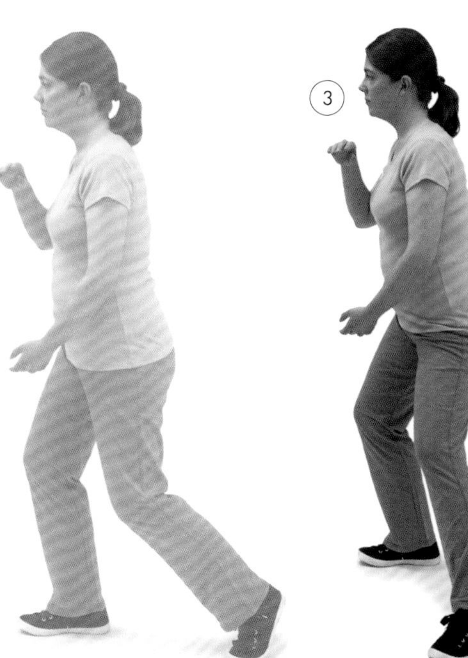

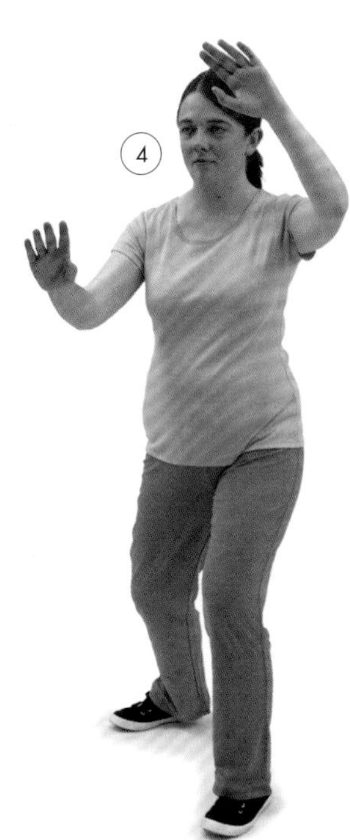

3 *Shift your weight to your right foot, turning to the right as you do so. Step with your left foot to the north, toes pointing northeast.*

4 *Transfer 70 percent of your weight onto your left leg, raising your left arm as you do so, then turn the palm outward. Push the palm of your right hand forward as you turn on your left leg to face northeast. You can pivot the back foot a little to make the stance more comfortable. This is Fair Lady Weaves the Shuttle 1.*

FAIR LADY WEAVES THE SHUTTLE (2, NORTHWEST)

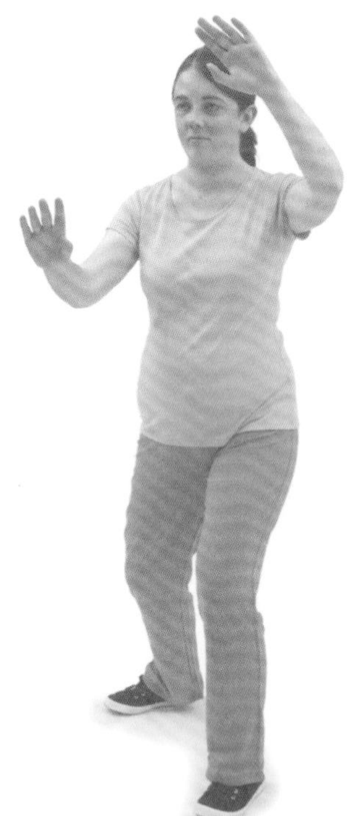

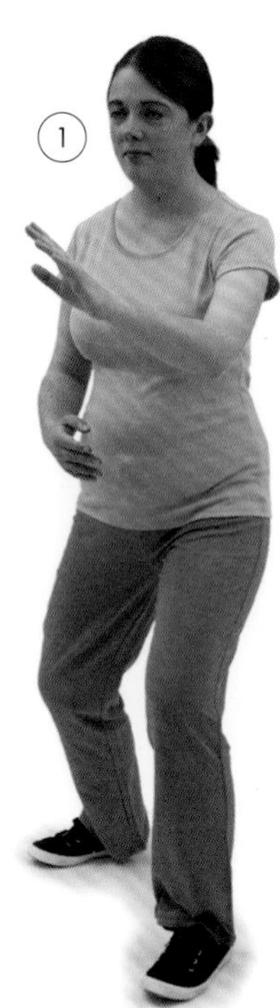

1 *Relax your arms as you begin to transfer your weight onto your right leg, with the palm of your right hand facing your body and the palm of your left hand facing outward.*

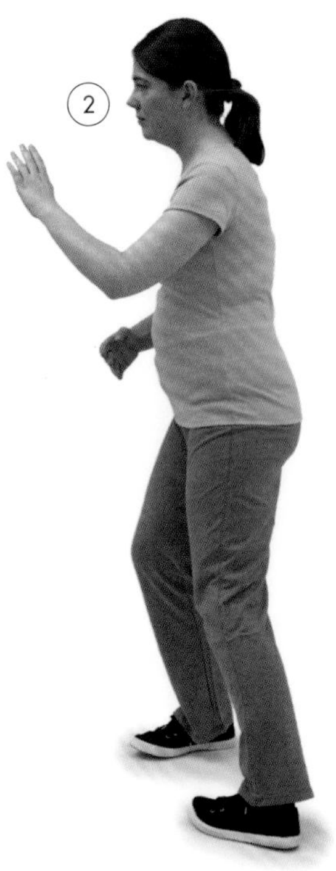

2 *Carry your arms with you, turning your body, as you continue to shift your weight onto your right leg, then pivot on the ball of your left foot to turn the heel out and the toes in as far as is comfortable.*

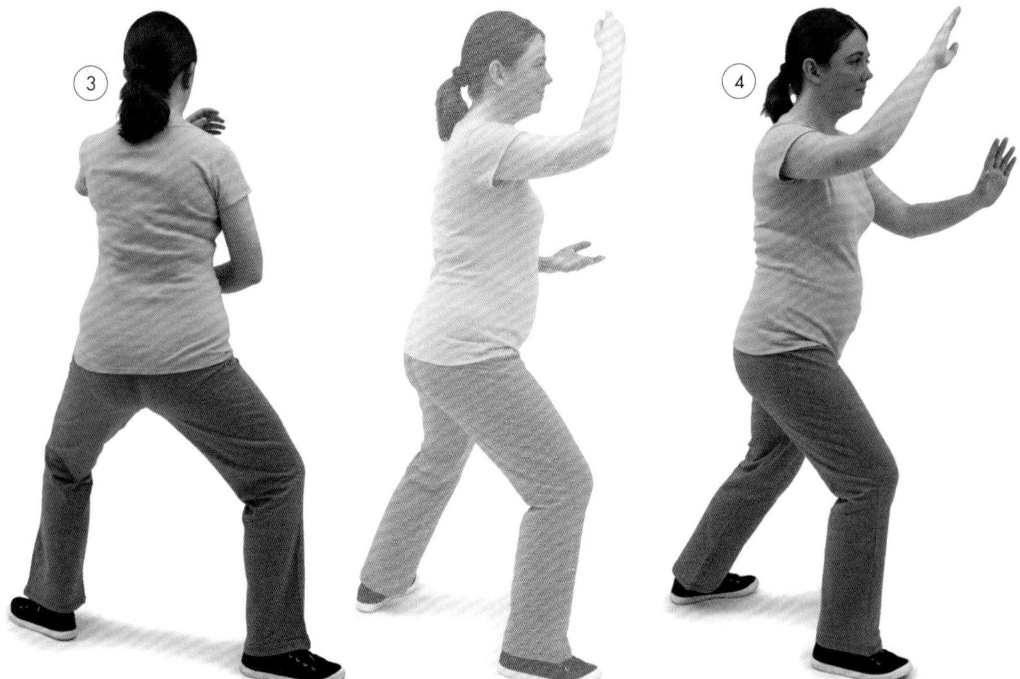

3 *Shift your weight onto your left leg and turn your palms to face each other as in Hold the Ball (see page 87). To step behind, first draw back your right foot so that the toes are level with your left heel. Pivot on the ball of your right foot before stepping, heel first, to the northwest with the toes pointing in the same direction.*

4 *Transfer 70 per cent of your weight onto your right leg while raising your right hand to head height, passing to the outside of your left arm, turning the palm of your left hand outward to prepare for the push. As you transfer your weight, turn from the hips to face northwest and turn the palm of your right hand outward while you push forward with your left. This is Fair Lady Weaves the Shuttle 2.*

FAIR LADY WEAVES THE SHUTTLE (3, SOUTHWEST)

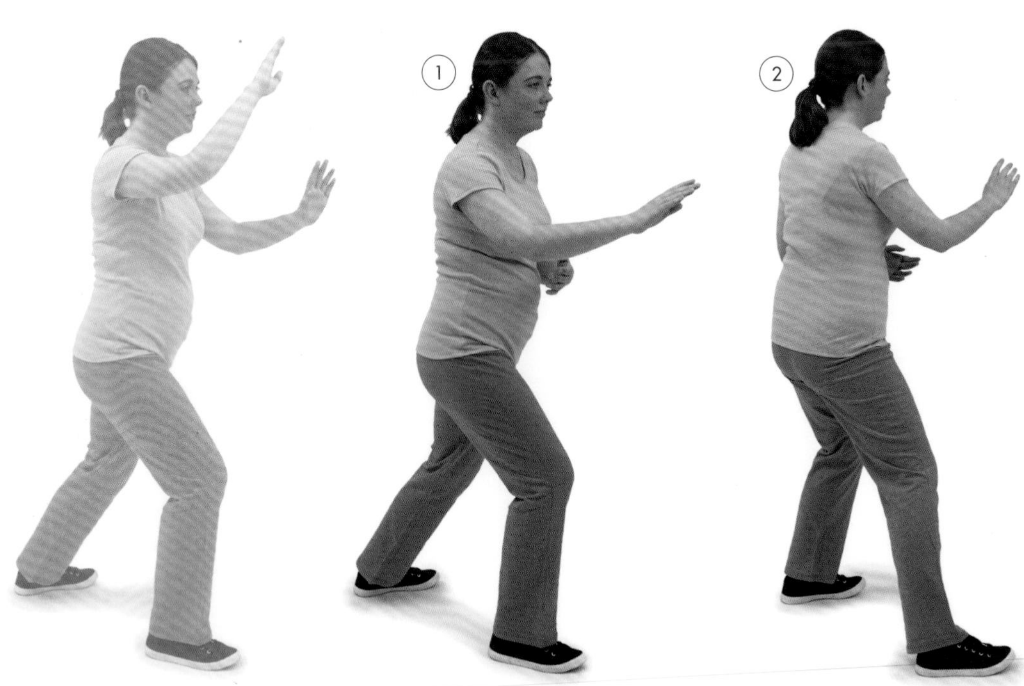

1 *Relax your arms as you begin to transfer your weight onto your left leg, with the palm of your left hand facing your body and the palm of your right hand facing outward.*

2 *Carry your arms with you, turning your body, as you continue to shift your weight onto your left leg, then turn the toes of your right foot in to face west.*

Relax the Body

This corner is easier to accomplish than the previous or next one because the step is shorter. Watch that your elbows remain dropped and your shoulders relaxed throughout in order to keep the arm movements continuous and flowing. Remember to coordinate the arms with the movements of the feet and the turns of the waist.

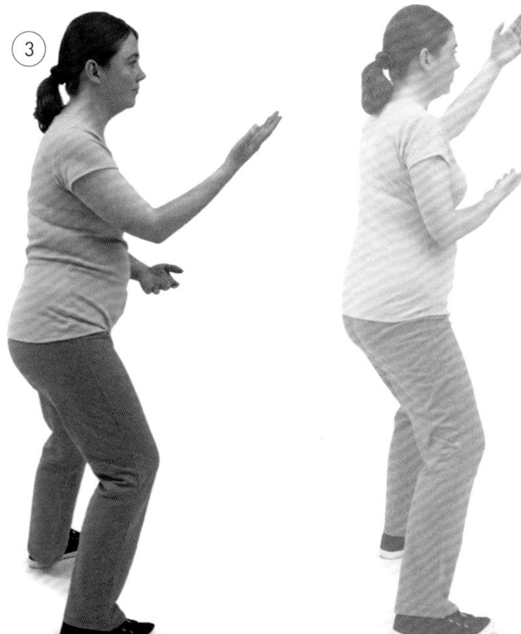

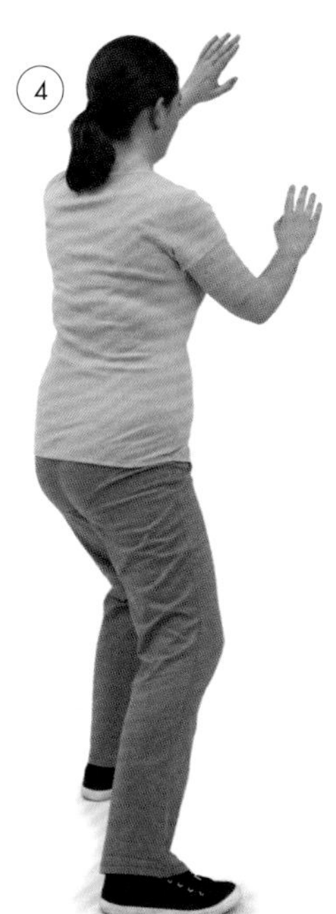

3 *Shift your weight onto your right leg, then step with your left heel to the south of the right heel, toes facing southwest. As you do so, turn your right palm to face toward you.*

4 *Transfer 70% of your weight onto your left leg while raising your left hand to head height, passing to the outside of your right arm, turning the palm of your right hand outward to prepare for the push. As you transfer your weight, turn from the hips to face southwest and turn your left palm outward while you push forward with your right. This is Fair Lady Weaves the Shuttle 3.*

FAIR LADY WEAVES THE SHUTTLE (4, SOUTHEAST)

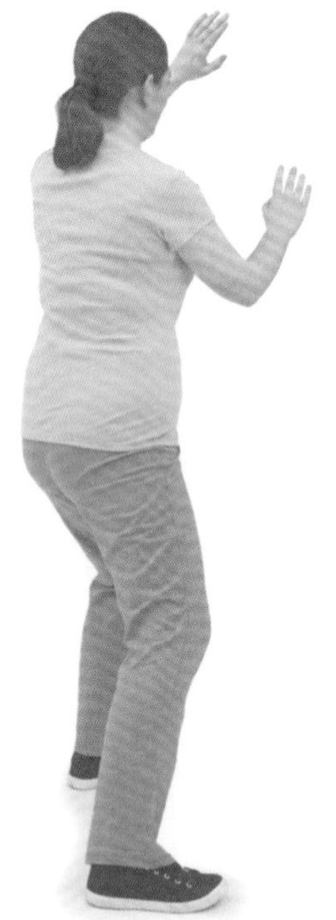

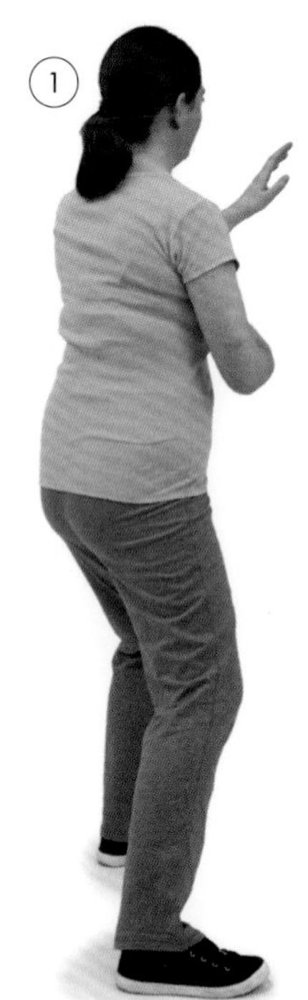

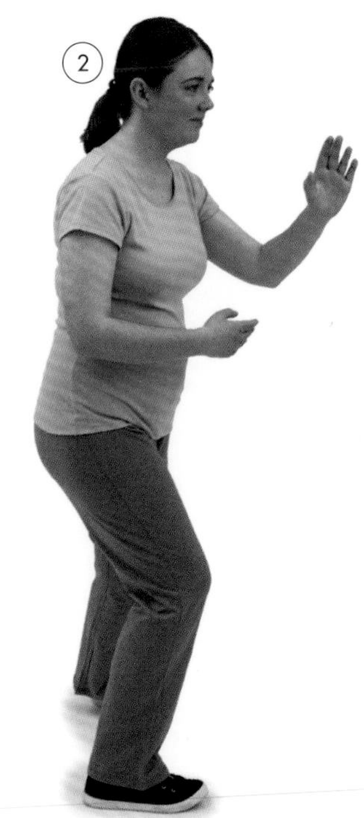

1 *Relax your arms as you begin to transfer your weight onto your right leg, with the palm of your right hand facing your body and the palm of your left hand facing outward.*

2 *Carry your arms with you, turning your body, as you continue to shift your weight onto your right leg, then pivot on the ball of your left foot to turn the heel out and the toes in as far as is comfortable.*

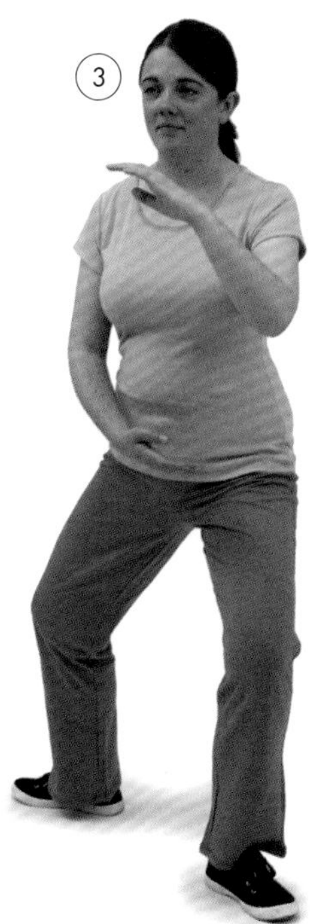

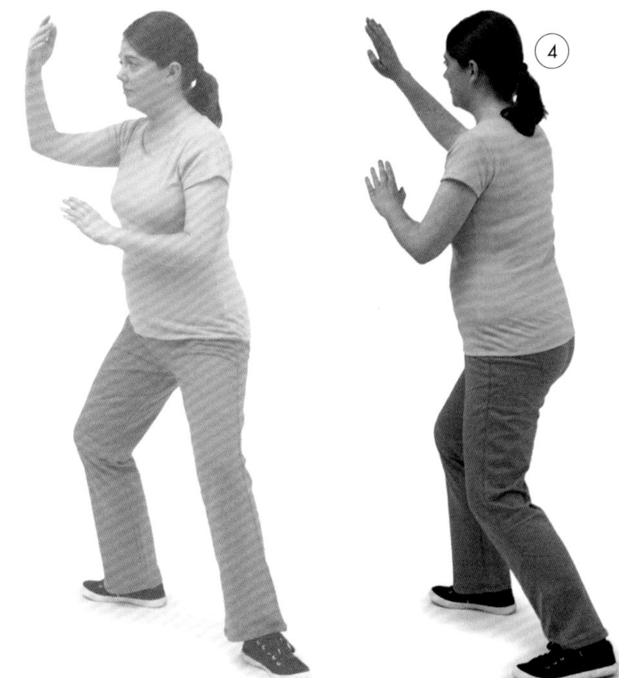

3 *Shift your weight onto your left leg and turn your palms to face each other as in Hold the Ball (see page 87). To step behind, first draw back your right foot so that the toes are level with your left heel, then pivot on the ball of your right foot before stepping, heel first, to the southeast with the toes pointing in the same direction.*

4 *Transfer 70 per cent of your weight onto your right leg while raising your right hand to head height, passing to the outside of your left arm, turning the palm of your left hand outward to prepare for the push. As you transfer your weight, turn from the hips to face southeast and turn your right palm outward while you push forward with your left. This is Fair Lady Weaves the Shuttle 4.*

WARD OFF LEFT

After the complex movements of Fair Lady Weaves the Shuttle, the form returns to the familiar territory of Grasp the Sparrow's Tail, beginning

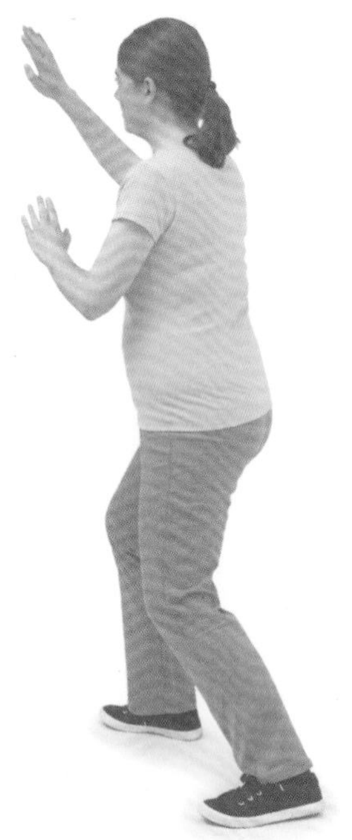

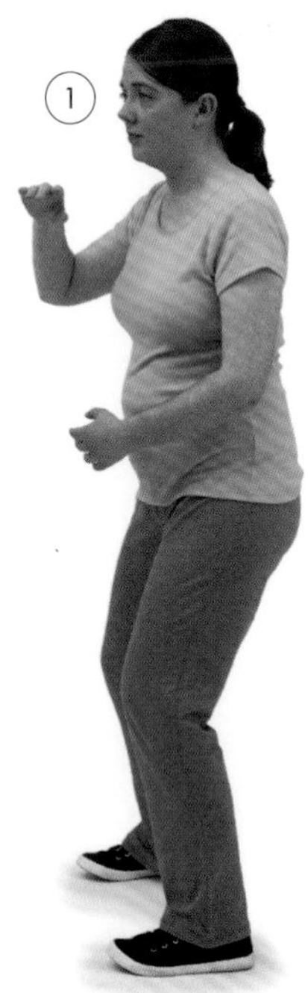

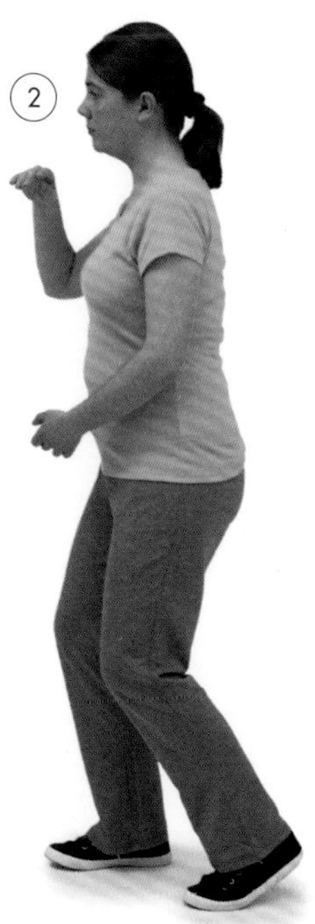

1 *From Fair Lady 4, transfer your weight to your back (left) leg and turn to the left. Raise the toes of your right foot and pivot on the heel through 45 degrees to bring the foot to face directly east. At the same time, bring your hands into the Hold the Ball position (see page 87), right hand above with the palm facing downward, and the left hand below with the palm facing upward.*

2 *Bring your weight onto your right leg, turning to face east. Draw back your left foot to bring the toes to rest on the ground near the heel of your right foot, then pivot on the ball of your right foot, opening the hips and stepping out with your left foot, heel first, to the northwest.*

with Ward Off Left and Ward Off Right (see page 192), and followed by Rollback, Press, and Push (see pages 194–196).

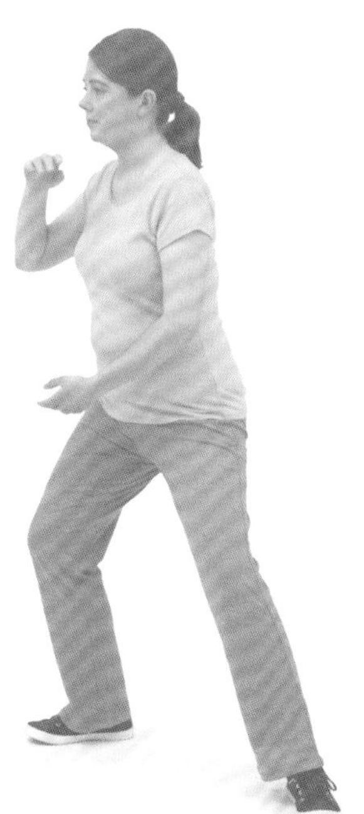

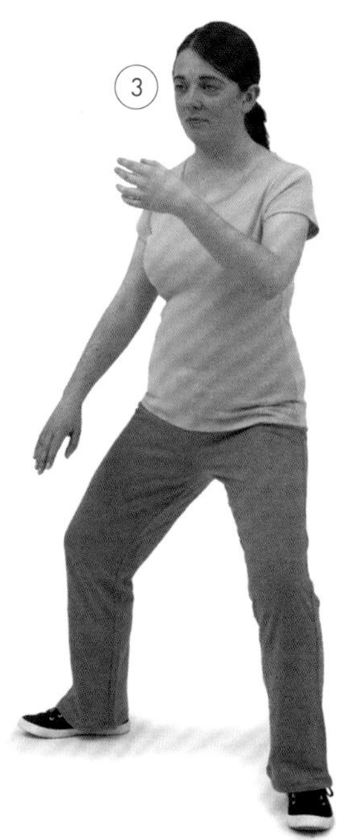

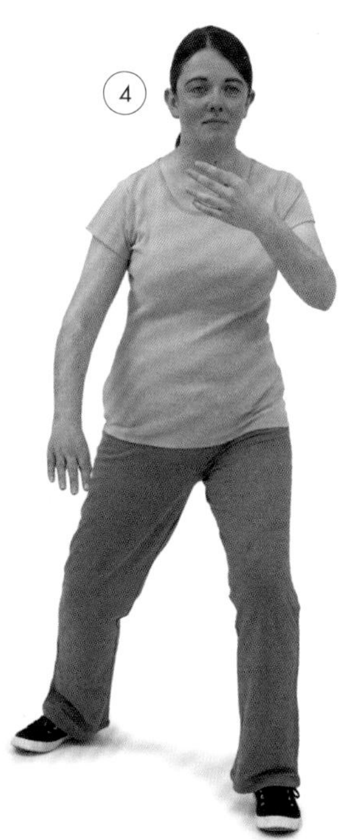

3 *Start shifting your weight onto your left foot, floating your left hand up to chest height with the palm facing in, and letting your right hand float down, palm facing behind you.*

4 *When the weight is roughly equal between your feet, turn your body to face forward and bring the toes of your right foot in by 45 degrees. Continue shifting your weight as you do so, ending with it about 70 percent on your left leg (Bow Stance—see page 74). This is Ward Off Left.*

WARD OFF RIGHT

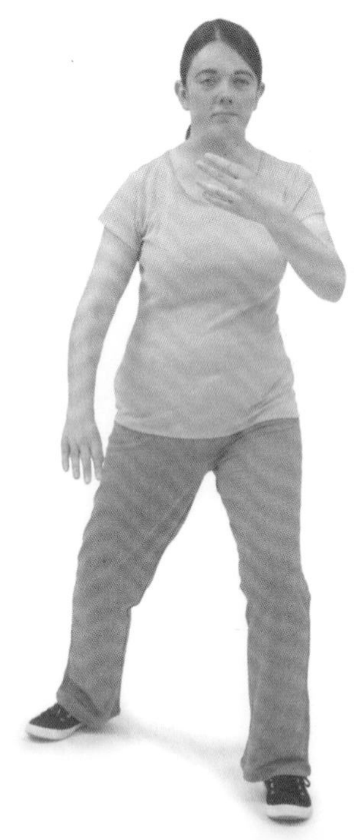

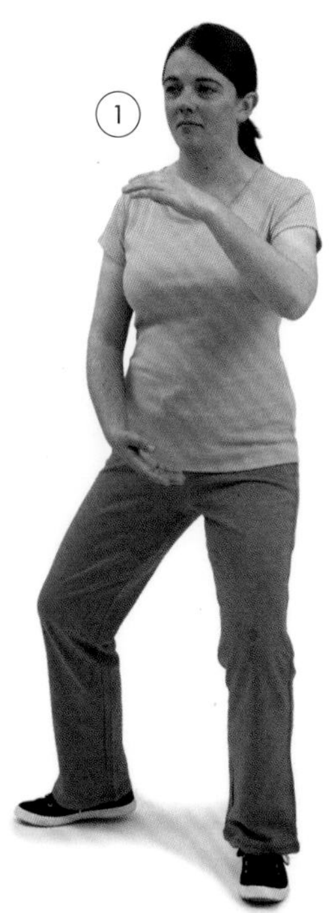

Moving the Ball

When the hands are in the Hold the Ball position, try to move as if there is a sphere of energy between them. Note that the position of the hands in the final posture is different from that of Ward Off Left (see page 191).

1 *Transfer all your weight onto your left leg, letting your right heel rise up from the ground. Turn your body to the right, as you pivot on the ball of your right foot through 45 degrees, to face northeast. At the same time, bring your hands into the Hold the Ball position (see page 87), this time with your left hand at chest height, palm facing downward, and your right hand underneath, palm facing upward.*

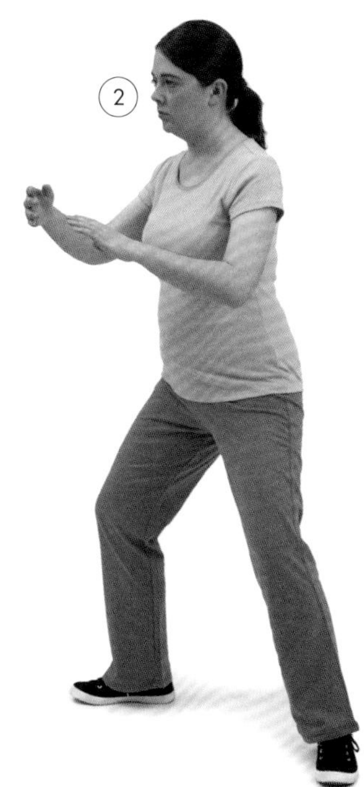

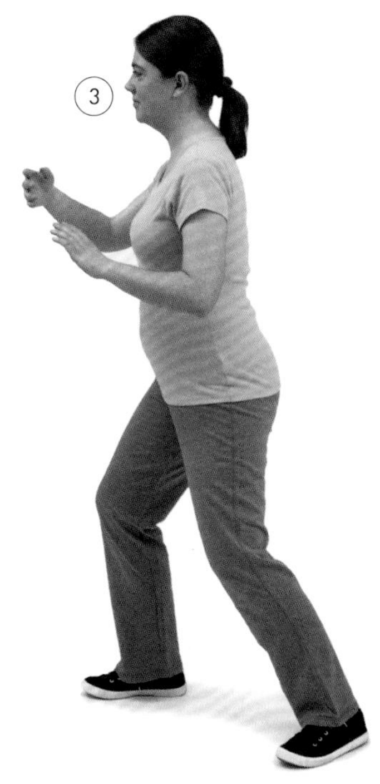

2 *Step your right foot out to the right, placing the heel down first, so that your foot points to the right (east). Your feet should be at right angles to each other, with a shoulder-width distance between your heels. Continue turning to the right, with your arms following your body and your right hand beginning to rise with the fingers facing left, while the fingers of your left hand point toward the palm of your right hand.*

3 *Transfer about 70 percent of your weight onto your right leg. Turn your body to the right so that it is facing the same direction as your right foot, and bring the toes of your left foot in by 45 degrees (Bow Stance—see page 74). This is Ward Off Right.*

ROLLBACK

The same Bow Stance is maintained from Ward Off Right, through Rollback and the following moves of Press and Push (see opposite). Take care not to turn too far in Rollback—a common error—and keep the toe, knee, and hip in alignment. As always, make sure that the knees do not extend farther than the toes at any point.

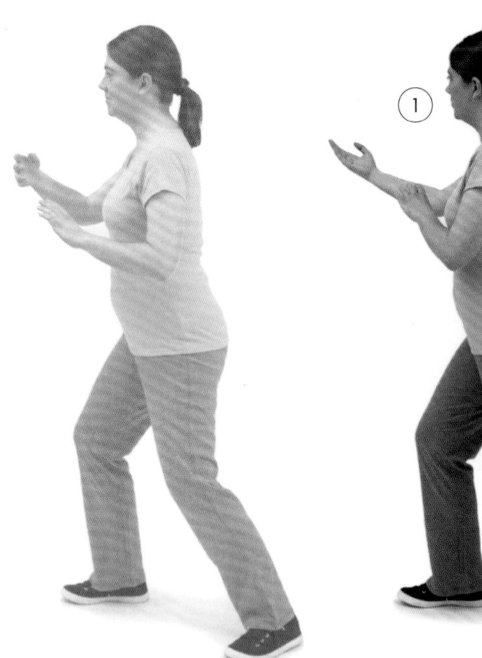

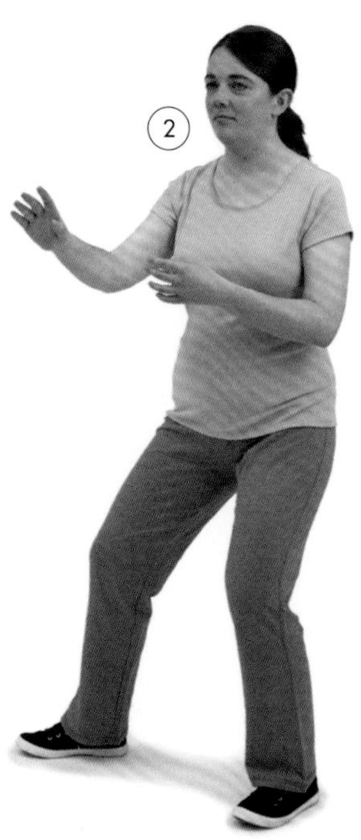

1 *Turn a little to the right, bringing more of your weight onto your right leg. As you do so, turn your right palm upward, with the fingers of your left hand pointing toward your right wrist.*

2 *Transfer your weight onto your left leg, turning your right palm to face forward while your left palm continues to face your body. As you transfer your weight, turn your hips to the left (northeast), keeping your shoulders and elbows relaxed, with your arms being carried by your body's movement. This is Rollback.*

PRESS & PUSH

Keep the feet well connected to the ground as you turn your waist and pour your weight from one leg to the other, the weighted leg bending as the other straightens, maintaining a soft knee. The spine does not lean into the Press or Push but remains upright.

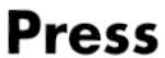

Press

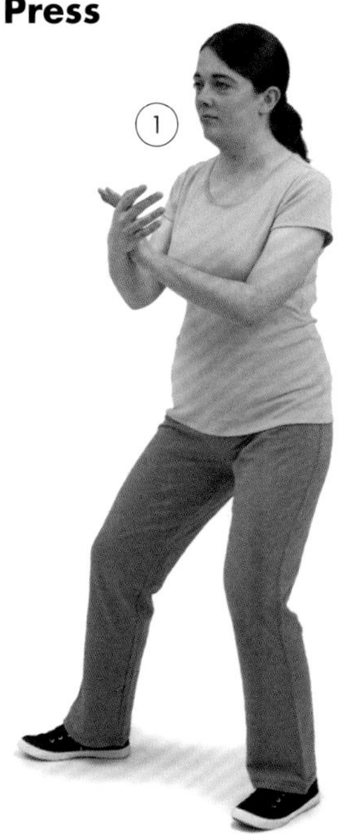

1 *Bring your right arm slightly toward you, turning the palm to face your chest, while you raise your left arm slightly with your left palm facing outward and bring it across so that the bases of your hands touch.*

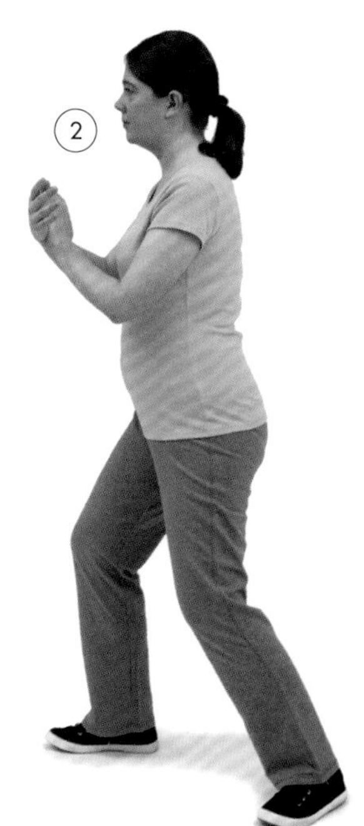

2 *As you do this, return your weight mostly to your front (right) leg so that you are facing the same direction as your right foot. This is Press.*

Push

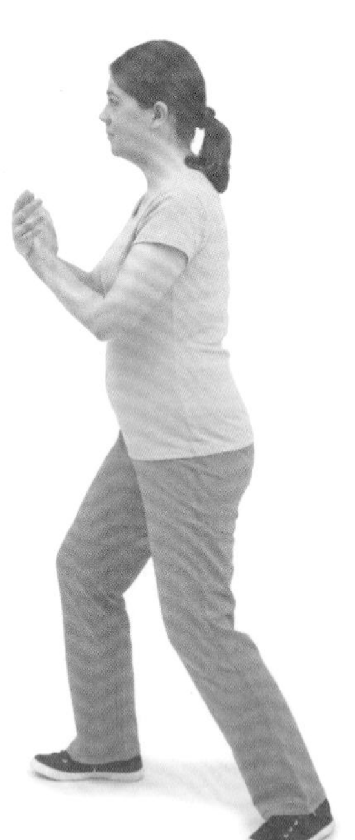

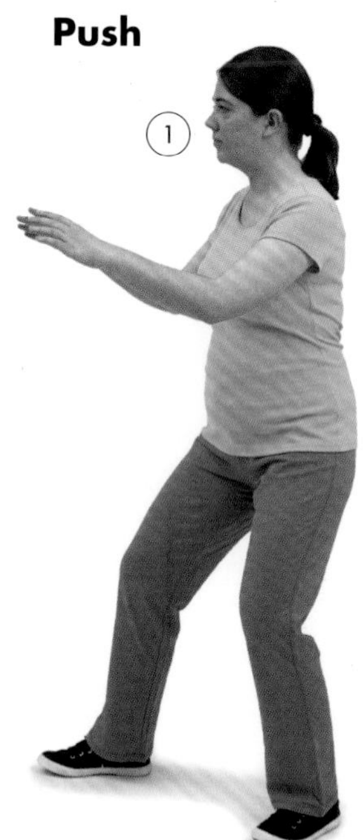

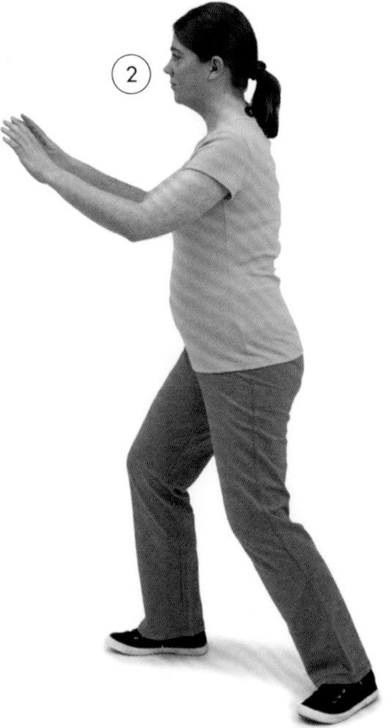

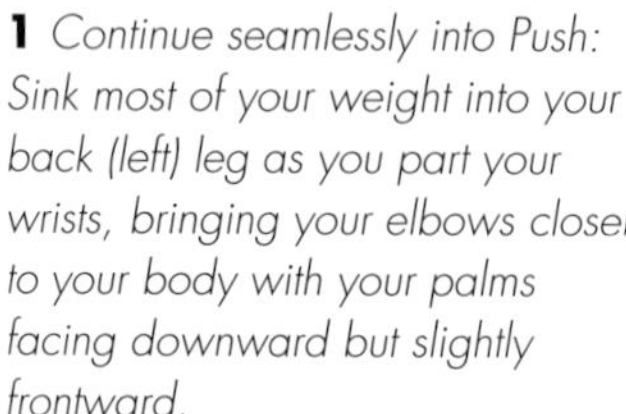

1 *Continue seamlessly into Push: Sink most of your weight into your back (left) leg as you part your wrists, bringing your elbows closer to your body with your palms facing downward but slightly frontward.*

2 *Then shift your weight back onto your front (right) leg as you push forward, raising your hands so that they are at chest height and chest-width apart in the Beautiful Hands position (see page 27). At the end of the movement, 70 percent of your weight should be on your front (right) leg and 30 percent on your back (left) leg. This is Push.*

SINGLE WHIP The Grasp the Sparrow's Tail sequence is succeeded by the elegant Single Whip. If Descending Single Whip, the following posture, is difficult for you, then you may want to make your stance in this pose wider than usual—step out your left foot to create a distance one and a half times your shoulder width in step 5.

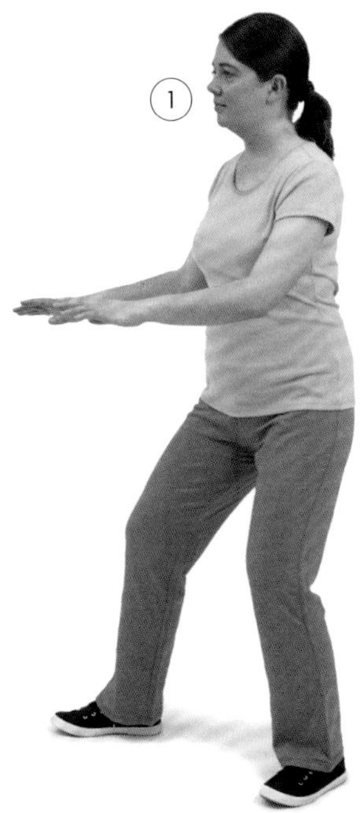

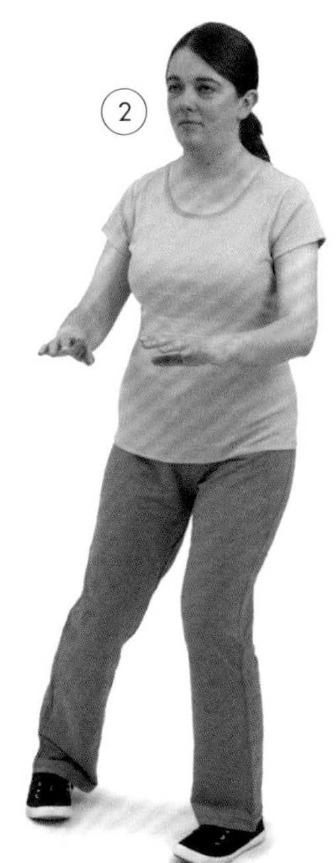

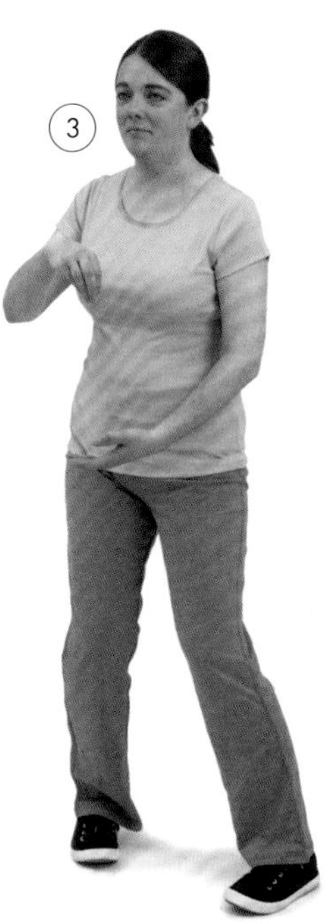

1 *Start transferring your weight back onto your left leg, lowering your forearms with a slight downward pressure so that they are parallel to the ground with the palms facing downward.*

2 *Continue shifting almost all your weight onto your left leg as you turn to the left as far as you can comfortably go by pivoting your right foot on the heel to face forward (north), leaving your left foot in the same position. Follow the movement of your body with your arms.*

3 *Tansfer your weight onto the right leg and turn to the right. As you do so, drop your left hand, turning the palm upward as in the Hold the Ball position (see page 87). Move your right arm in front of your chest, bending the elbow and forming a beak with your fingers (see page 96).*

Continued overleaf

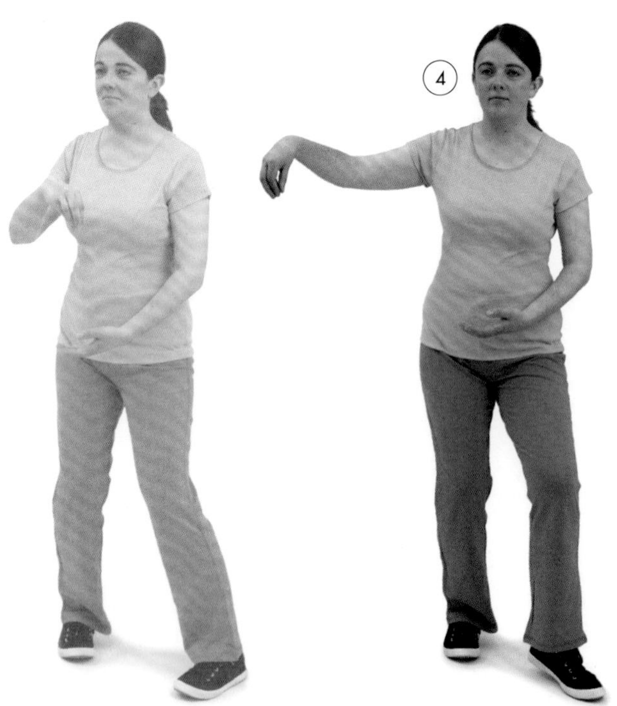

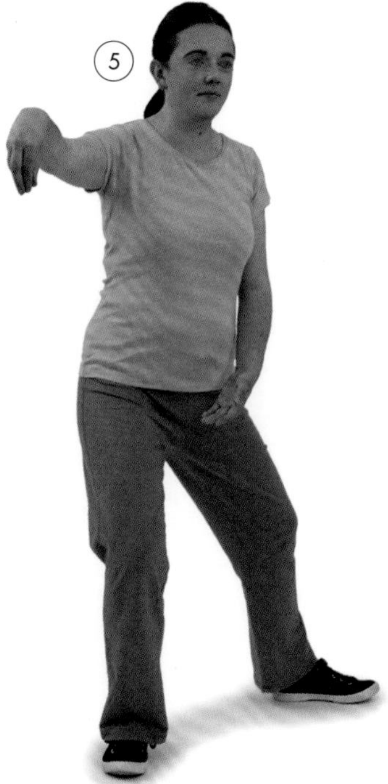

4 *Turn to the left on the ball of your left foot so that the toes are facing northwest while your body faces north. Extend your right arm out to the right, keeping your hand in the beak position and your elbow relaxed.*

5 *Step out with your left foot so that the toes are facing west, turning to the northwest as you do so, placing the heel down first and keeping the weight on your right foot (you may wish to step back briefly first to help you balance). Your heels should form an L shape with a shoulder-width distance between them.*

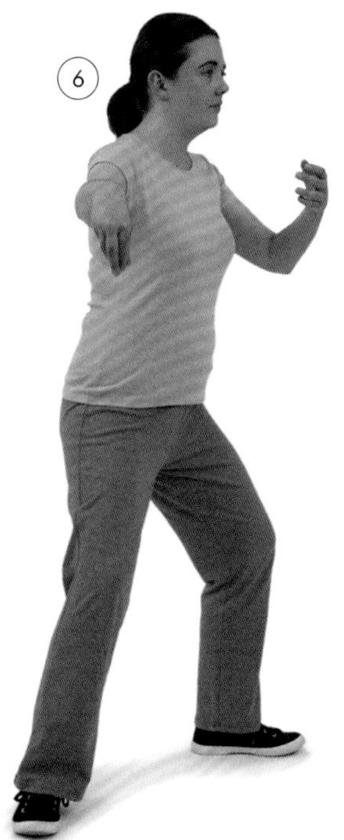

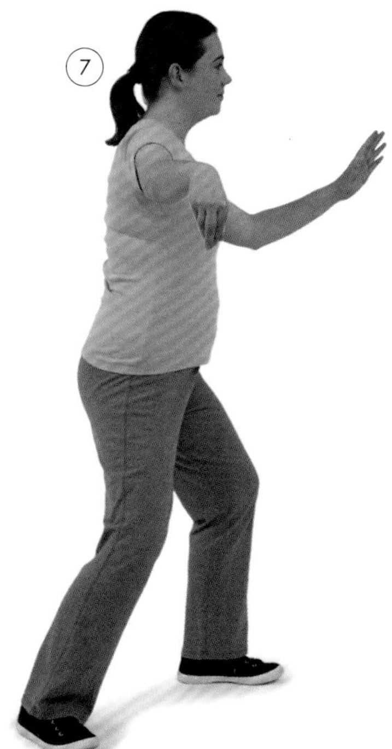

6 *Now pour about 70 percent of your weight into your left leg and bring your left hand up so that the palm is facing your chest.*

7 *Pivot on your right heel so that the toes are pointing northwest and turn your body to the left to face west in Bow Stance again (see page 74). As you end the movement, turn your left palm to face outward in the Beautiful Hands position (see page 27). This is Single Whip.*

DESCENDING SINGLE WHIP

After Single Whip, you sink down into the squatting variation of this move for the second time in the form. The key thing here, and in tai chi generally, is to respect your limitations. If you do not have the

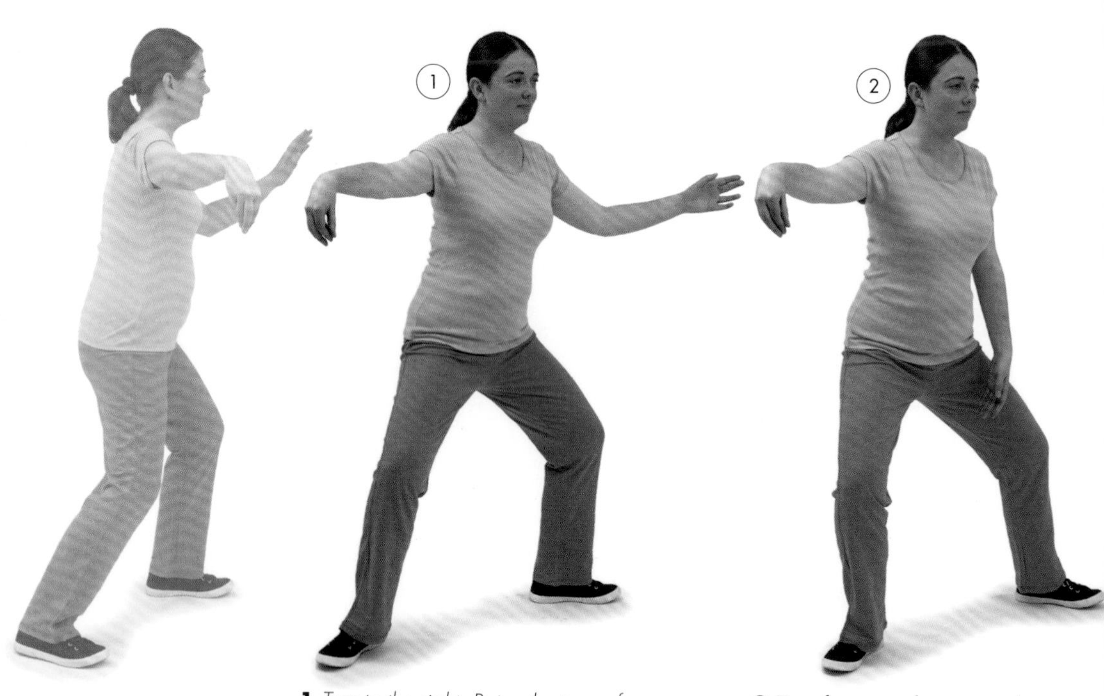

1 *Turn to the right. Raise the toes of your right foot from the ground and turn your foot through a 135-degree angle so that the toes are pointing northeast. At the same time, turn the palm of your left hand to the right, while the right hand remains in its beak position with the right arm out to the side.*

2 *Transfer most of your weight onto your right leg, sinking toward the ground as you draw your left arm back and then downward, fingers pointing toward the ground. As you do so, turn in the toes of your left foot a little.*

flexibility to get down low without pulling your spine out of alignment, then adapt the move. Tai chi is not about creating particular shapes with your body but is more about the internal process of energy flow, relaxation, and stability.

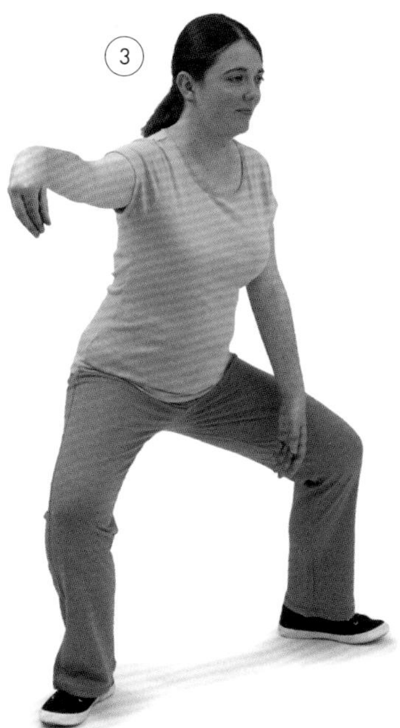

3 *Continue sinking downward with the weight mostly on your right leg without overreaching with the knee or tensing the back or shoulders.*

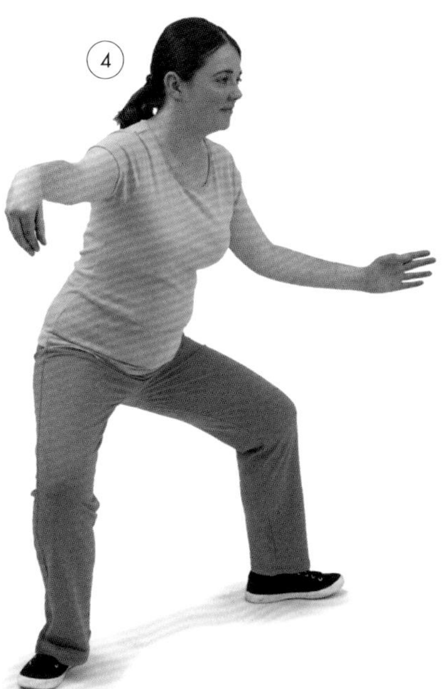

4 *Lower your left elbow to point the fingers forward, relaxing the shoulders as you do so to avoid leaning, then turn the toes of your left foot back to the west and shift forward so that 60 percent of your weight is on your left leg. This is Descending Single Whip.*

STEP FORWARD TO THE SEVEN STARS

In this sequence, you move up from the low stance of Descending Single Whip, transferring your weight onto the left leg so that you are free to step forward with the right. Be sure

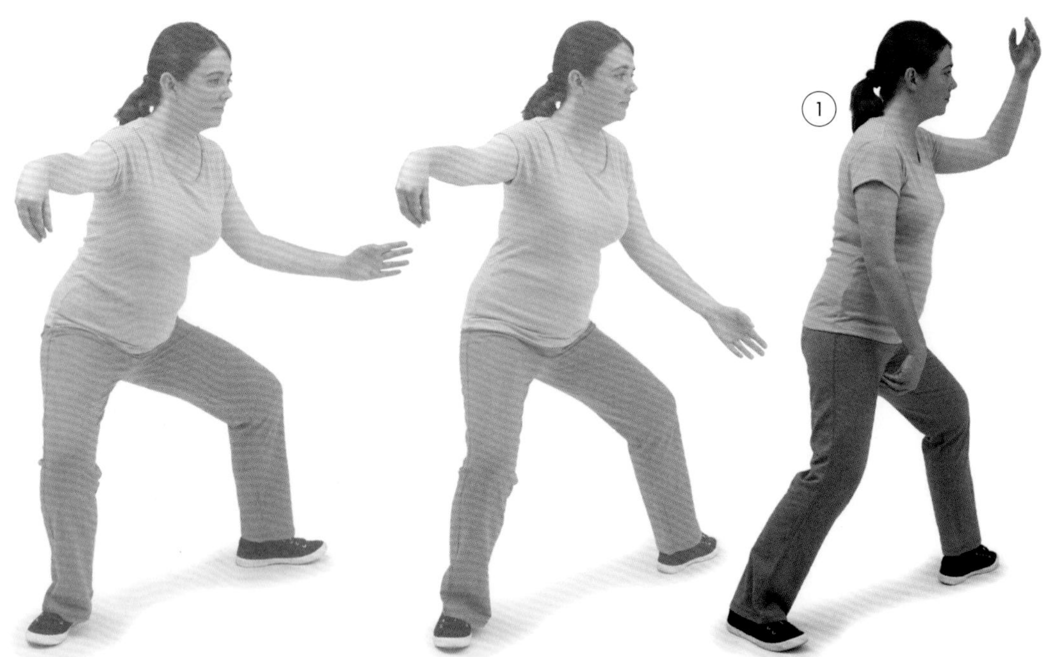

1 *Start to shift your weight to your left leg, rotating the heel of your left foot to turn the foot 45 degrees so that it faces southwest. Finish putting all your weight on your left foot as your left hand rises to shoulder height.*

to shift all the weight before you start to step to ensure that your base remains stable. In the final posture, the right foot remains empty, in Toe Stance (see page 76).

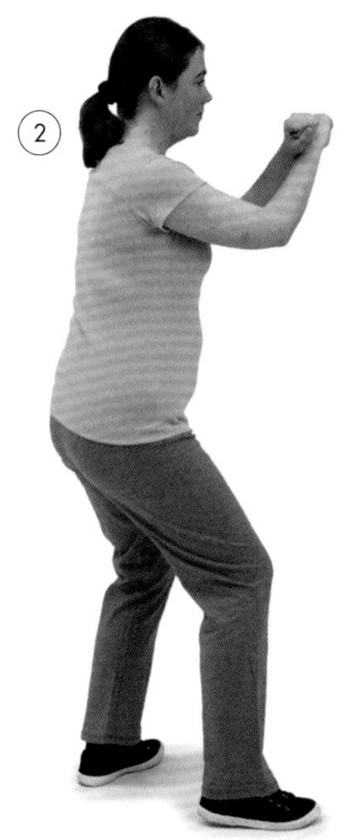

2 *Keeping your weight on your left foot, step forward with your right foot into Toe Stance. As you do so, close both hands into Tai Chi Fists (see page 115) and cross them at the wrists, right hand to the outside, at about chest height. Relax your shoulders.*

Take Your Time

As you move toward the final movements, be aware of any urge to hurry through them in order to finish the form. Try to maintain the same pace and mindful awareness throughout the whole of the form.

The Final Part of the Form

After the beautifully named Step Forward to the Seven Stars comes the equally evocative Step Back to Ride the Tiger. The name may be inspired by an old Chinese proverb about "riding on the back of a tiger without being able to get off," signifying a difficult situation that you cannot get out of and so must be dealt with to its conclusion. The tiger motif is referenced at several points in the form (more often than any other animal) and is a significant animal in Chinese mythology. It is considered the king of beasts, and represents masculine energy, courage, and power. In martial art terms, this sequence involves a step backward (seemingly a move of retreat) followed by an attack.

Sweep the lotus

Near the end of the form is a posture that most people find the most difficult of all, Turn and Sweep the Lotus, in which you turn the body through a full circle and then lift up the right leg into a sweeping heel kick.

Experienced practitioners perform the turn in one smooth movement, but you can do it in stages to make it easier. As you swivel around, it is tempting to rise upward, so try to keep a sense of sinking throughout this sequence. The waist should remain loose and relaxed both during the turn and the subsequent lotus kick, which is led by the waist.

With the kick, the right leg comes up into a heel kick and traces a circle in the air, slapping the foot against the fingertips of the outstretched hands. This takes skill and great flexibility, and therefore is adapted for beginner level. Be sure to keep the knee of the kicking leg softly bent.

The closing movements

The tiger makes a final appearance in Draw a Bow to Shoot the Tiger, the last new posture to learn in the form. The familiar postures that follow—Step Forward, Deflect, Intercept, and Punch, and Withdraw and Push—lead to the closing sequence, which brings you back to face north and almost mirrors the starting point. You can then choose to end your practice, or to continue with another run-through of the form.

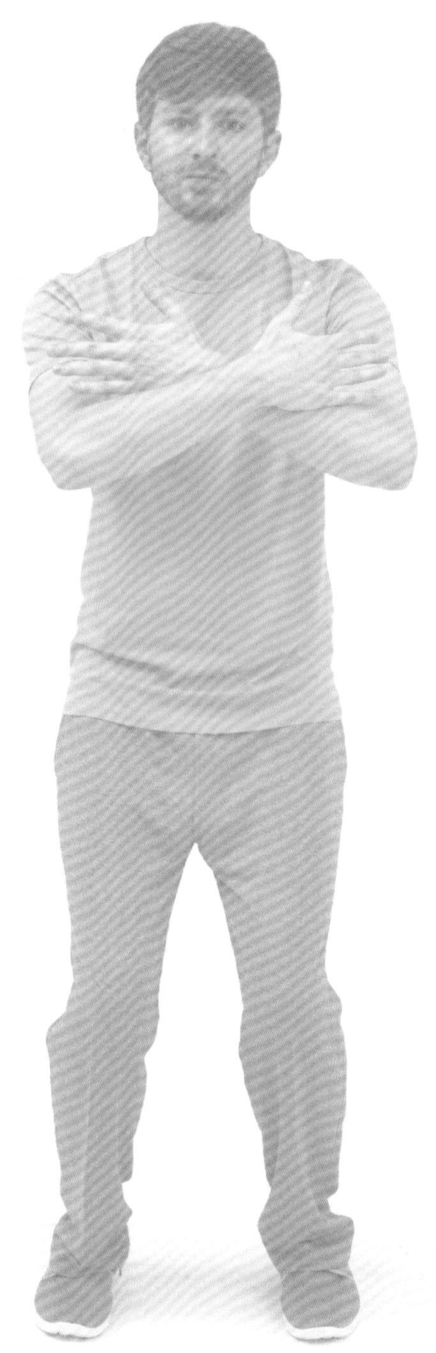

STEP BACK TO RIDE THE TIGER In this sequence, you turn away and step backward—as if retreating from an opponent—before turning back to face him or her and bringing the right arm up as if to strike. Sink deeply into your right leg to help power the move, and make sure that your arm rises in conjunction with the waist turn.

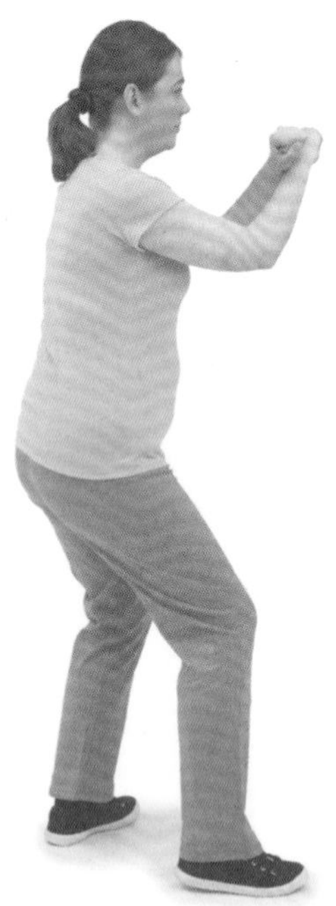

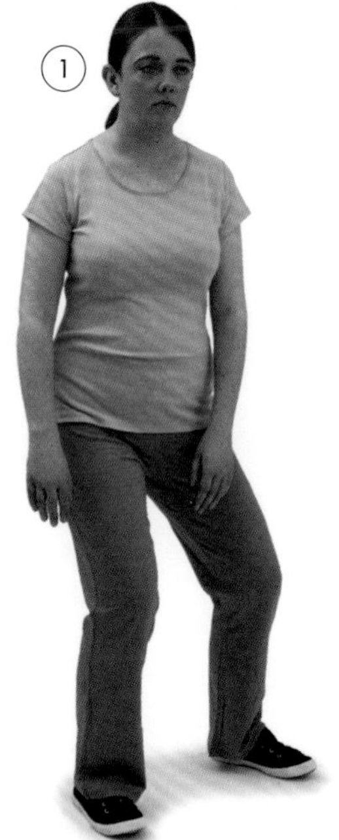

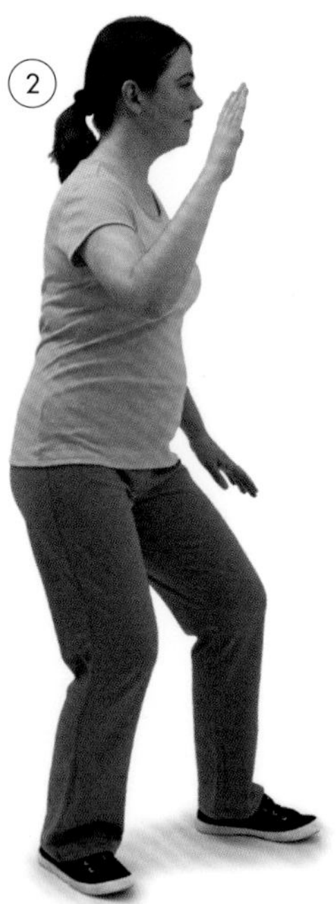

1 *Release both fists while stepping backward with your right foot, placing the toes down first to face northwest and shifting your weight onto your right leg as you turn. At the same time, release your arms so that they hang down either side of your right thigh.*

2 *Turn your body to the west, keeping your right hip relaxed while adjusting your left foot into Toe Stance. This movement creates the momentum to bend your right elbow so that the palm of your right hand faces forward, while the palm of your left hand brushes over your left thigh.*

TURN & SWEEP THE LOTUS

In this complex sequence, you complete a 360-degree turn to the right followed by a sweeping kick. You begin by first turning left to help create the momentum for the clockwise turn, using the right foot as a pivot. Keep your waist relaxed as you turn.

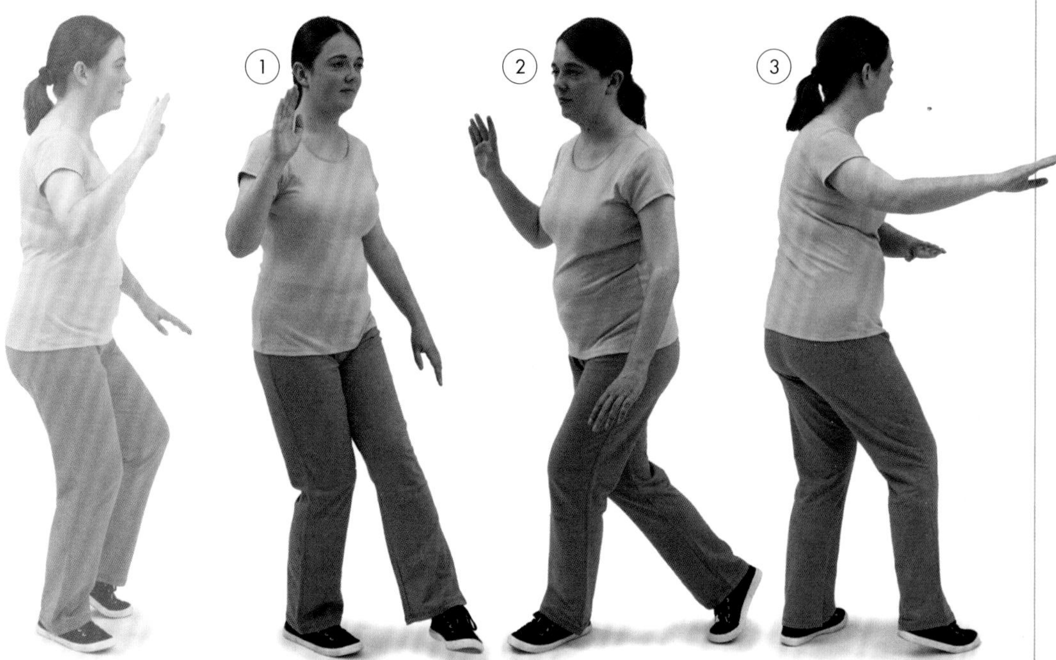

1 *Swing your left leg back from the knee and then forward. As it swings forward, bring it around to the right, using the momentum to spin on the ball of your right foot, carrying your arms with you.*

2 *At the end of the spin, your momentum should enable you to step across with your left leg so that your feet are aligned east–west with the toes pointing northeast.*

3 *Turn to the west on the balls of both feet. As you do so, softly point both hands, palms down, to the right, with your left hand in front of your body. Keep your weight on your left leg, while your right foot rests on the toes ready to kick.*

Continued overleaf

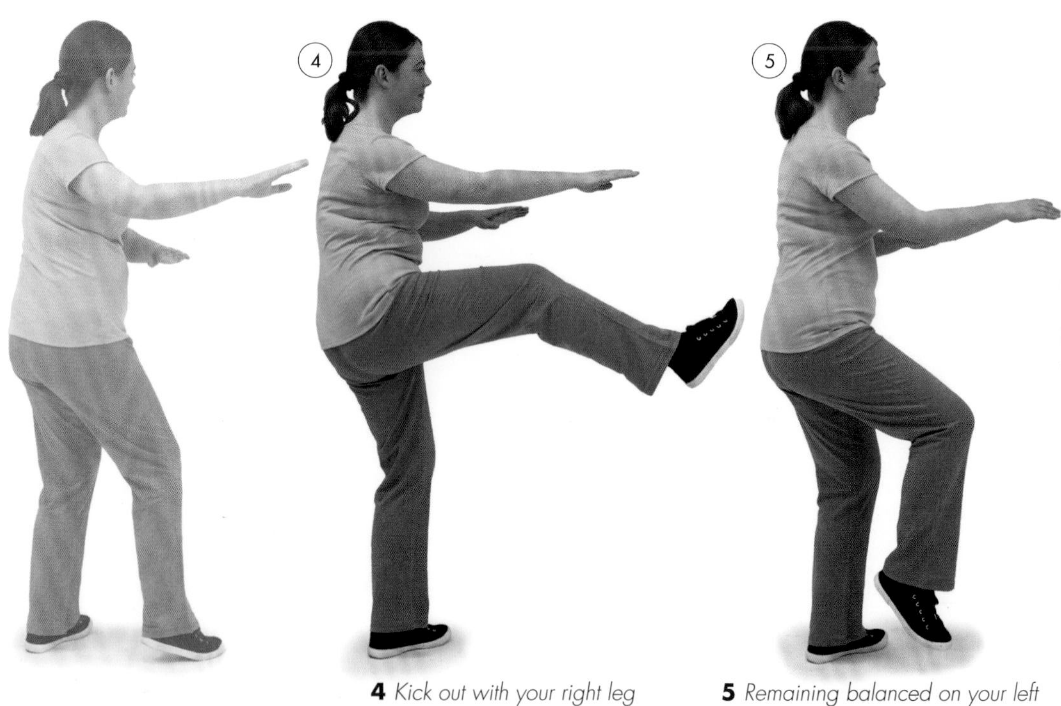

4 *Kick out with your right leg as close to waist height as is comfortable, with the toes drawing an arc from left to right. As you do so, pass your hands leftwards.*

5 *Remaining balanced on your left leg, finish by relaxing your right leg so that it descends with the toes close to the ground (touch the ground with your toes if it helps you to balance).*

DRAW A BOW TO SHOOT THE TIGER

This is a powerful move in which you punch high with the right hand and low with the left. Make sure that your hands follow the turn of the waist. Keep the right elbow dropped, the shoulders relaxed, and the body upright.

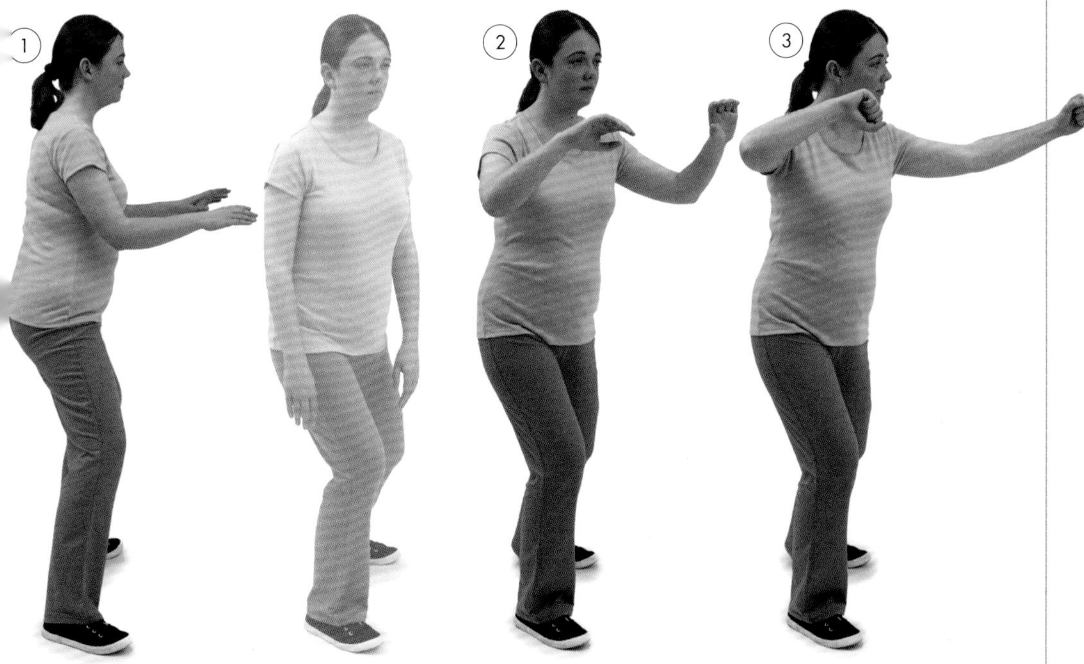

1 *Step to the north with your right heel, toes pointing northwest.*

2 *Transfer your weight onto your right leg, using the momentum generated by this shift to first swing the arms to either side of your right thigh. Continue to move your arms so that your hands float up to around shoulder height.*

3 *Form your hands into Tai Chi Fists (see page 115), then turn your head to face west without moving the rest of your body. Keeping your shoulders relaxed, extend your left arm out to the west and bring your right fist close to your face. The backs of both fists should be facing to the left.*

STEP FORWARD, DEFLECT, INTERCEPT & PUNCH

This sequence appears in the first section, and is repeated here as part of the final movements of the form. It is not exactly the same because you start from the right side rather than the left.

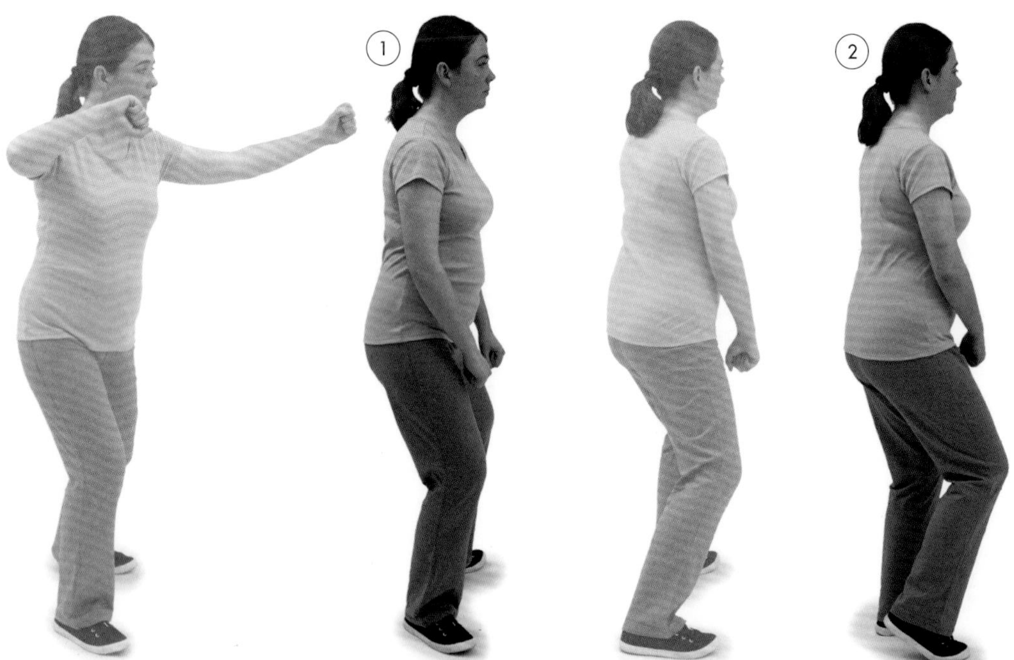

1 *First release the neck, then pivot on the ball of your left foot to turn the heel in. Relax the arms so that they hang down by your thighs.*

2 *Shift your weight onto your left leg in Bow Stance (see page 74), releasing and opening your left-hand fist but maintaining your right-hand fist, then draw the toes of your right foot in to your left ankle.*

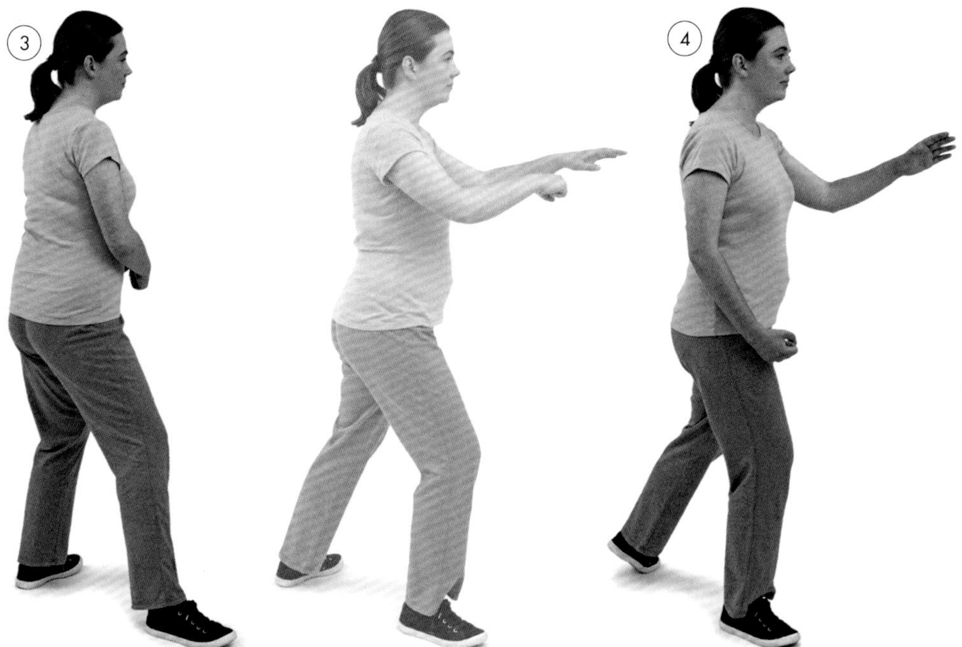

3 *Step forward with your right foot, placing it heel first and with the toes pointing comfortably toward the northwest.*

4 *Transfer your weight onto your right leg, bringing your arms up, then as you turn to the right, leave the left arm in place with the palm facing forward while dropping the right-hand fist to outside your right thigh.*

Continued overleaf

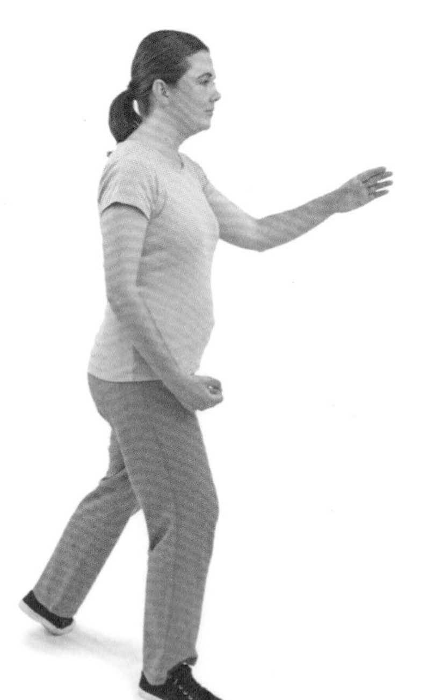

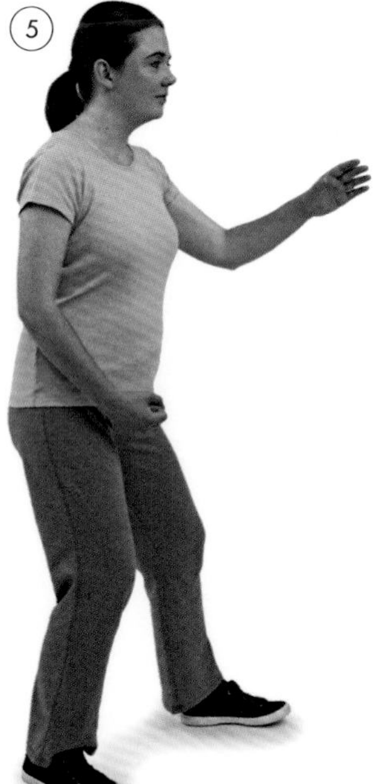

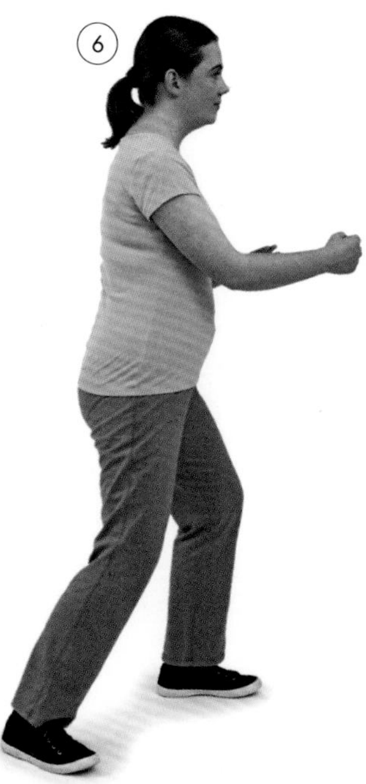

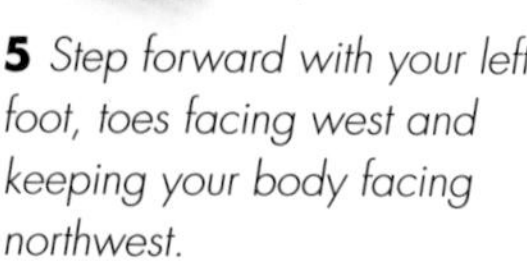

5 *Step forward with your left foot, toes facing west and keeping your body facing northwest.*

6 *Transfer 70 percent of your weight onto your left leg (Bow Stance—see page 74). At the same time, bring your right-hand fist up and forward, rotating it through a quarter turn to the left (counterclockwise) and then delivering the Punch. Keep your left hand in its protective position, palm facing your right forearm at the end of the movement.*

WITHDRAW & PUSH

This posture is also known as Apparent Close, because you seemingly retreat before pushing forward again. These moves succeed Intercept and Punch, and lead into Cross Hands (see page 214).

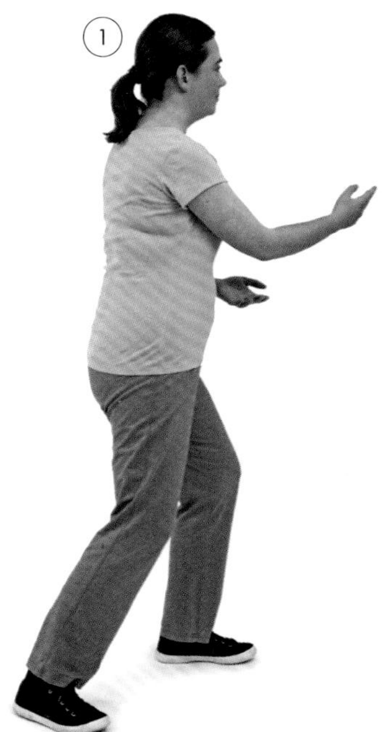

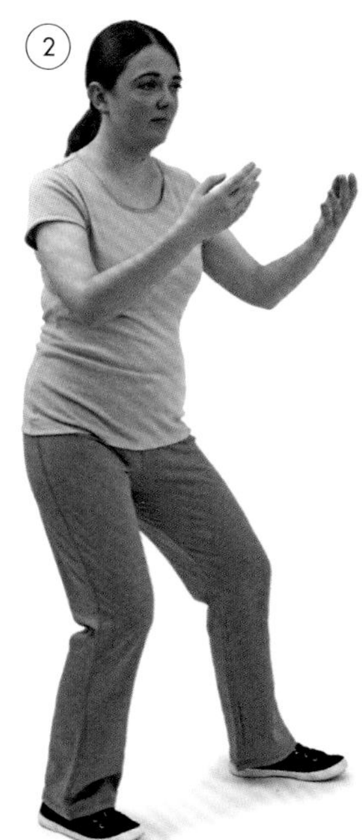

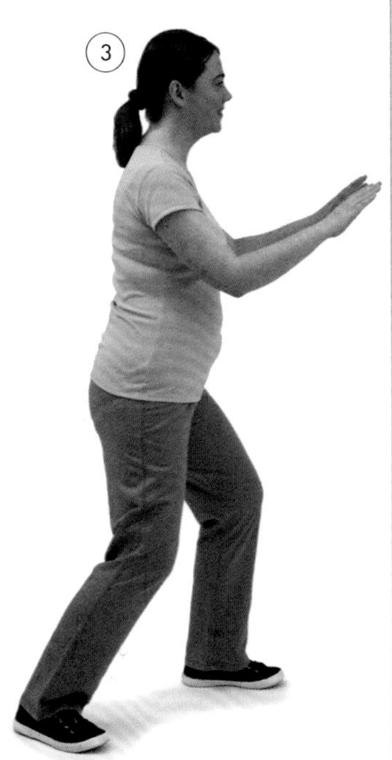

1 *Turn the upper body slightly to the left, maintaining the position of the feet and the 70/30 weight distribution between your left and right legs. Release your right hand from its fist as you drop your right elbow and your right hand rises. Lower your left hand and turn the palm upward, as if cupping your right elbow.*

2 *Sink your weight into your right leg as you turn back to the right and face northwest, with both hands in front, palms upward.*

3 *Turn the palms outward as you transfer about 70 percent of your weight onto your left leg, turning back to the left to face west (Bow Stance again—see page 74). This is Push.*

CROSS HANDS

This sequence brings you back to facing north again. Have a sense of gathering in energy as you bring the hands in before they move downward in the final Completion (see page 216). As before, the weight distribution between

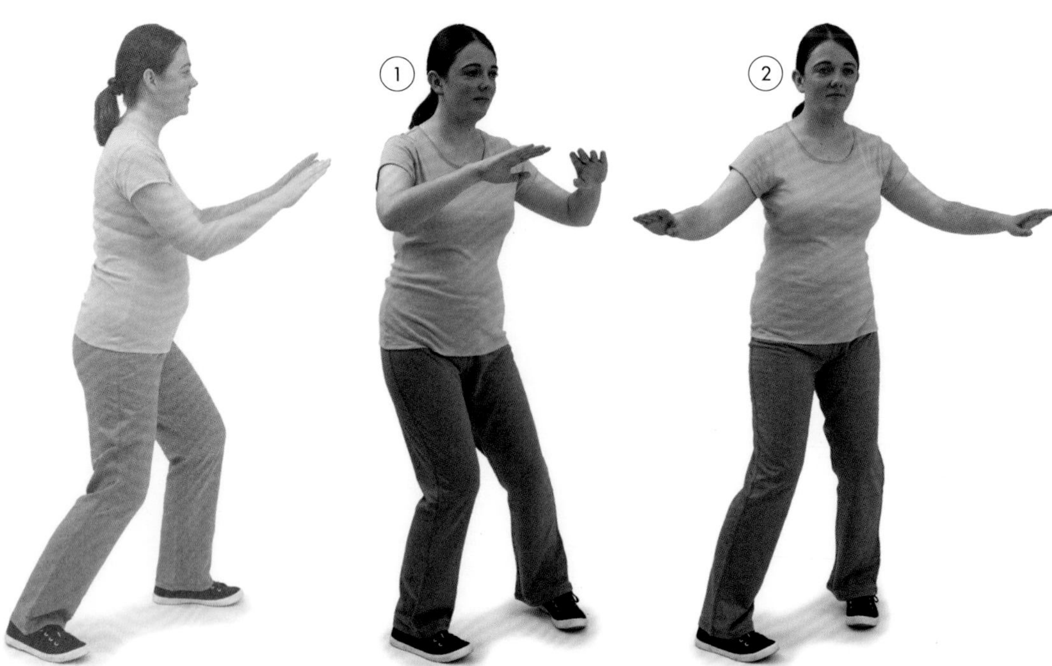

1 *Sink your weight back into your right leg, carrying your arms comfortably with you. Turn your left toes in as close to north as is comfortable.*

2 *Turn out your left heel slightly and transfer some weight to your left leg, moving your arms apart and outward at waist height.*

your left and right legs at the end of Cross Hands is 60/40, although some practitioners prefer to have it evenly distributed.

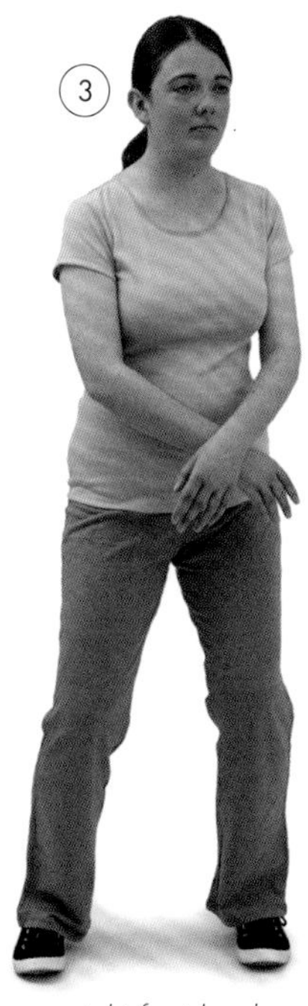

3 *Step your right foot back so that it is a shoulder-width distance from your left foot and parallel to it. Circle your hands in, crossing your left wrist over your right wrist in front of your navel, palms facing inward.*

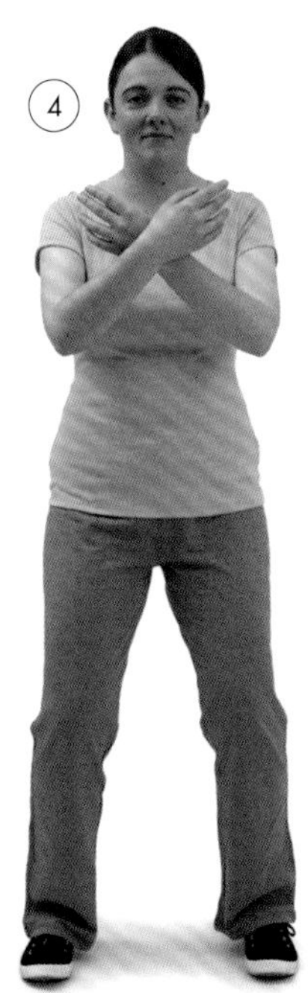

4 *Shift about 40 percent of your weight onto your right leg, leaving 60 percent on your left leg, while you float your hands up until they are in front of your chest, palms facing inward, so that the right hand is now on the outside.*

COMPLETION The movements in the completing form bring you back to your starting point, ending the cycle of the form—and, of course, enabling you to move into another cycle if you so wish. Try to treat this sequence with reverence as you ground your energy and enjoy the stillness of your mind.

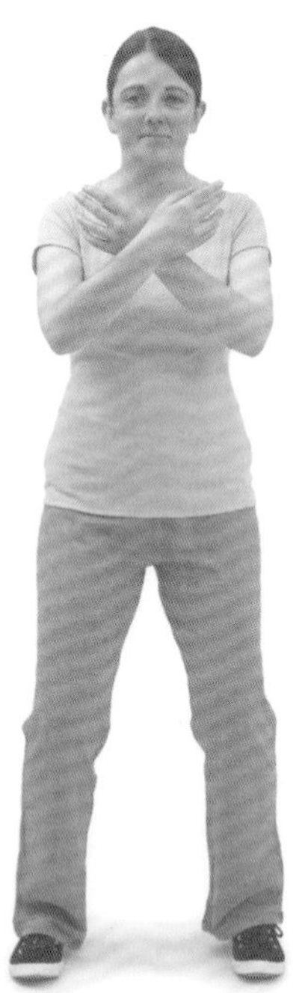

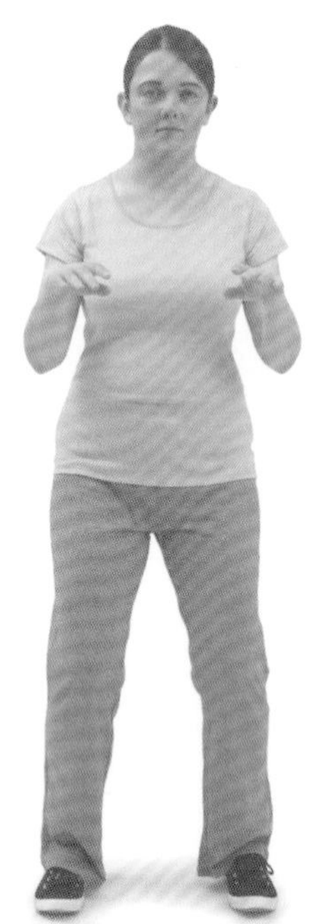

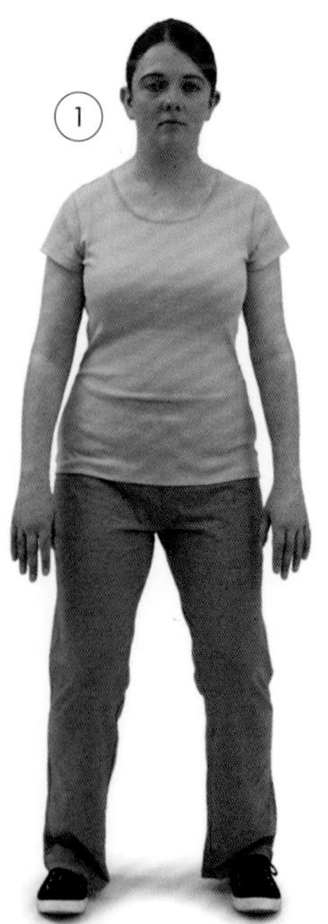

1 *From Cross Hands, let your hands float forward. Turn your hands so that the palms face downward and let them float down as your body rises up.*

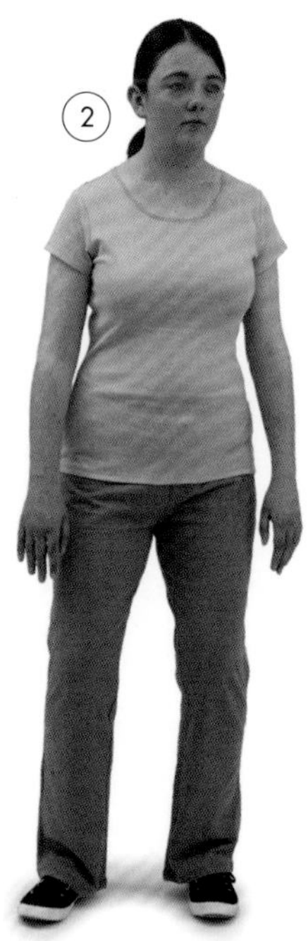

2 *To close, shift some weight onto your left leg, turn your hips, and turn in the heel of your right foot.*

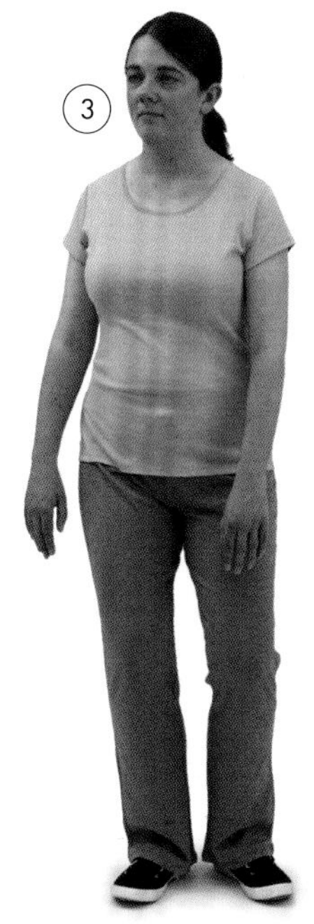

3 *Shift some weight onto your right leg, turn your hips, and turn in the heel of your left foot.*

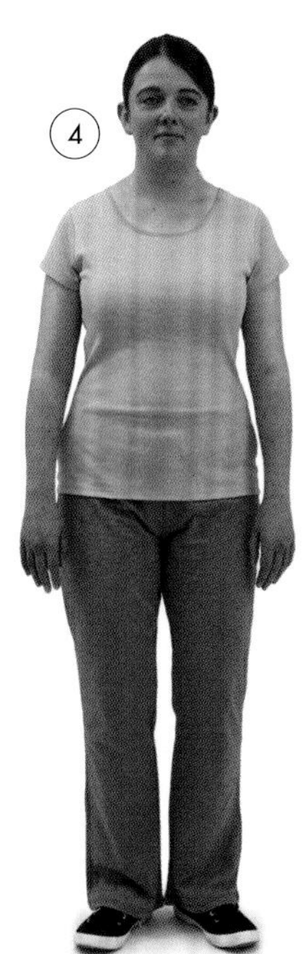

4 *Settle in the center as you were at the start of the form, release again, and breathe.*

Check In

At the end of the form, spend a few moments checking through the key points of the tai chi posture, breathing calmly. Take this calm grounded sense of yourself with you as you leave your practice, and let it inform your day.

1 Head and spine straight.

2 Chin tucked in.

3 Shoulders relaxed and slightly rounded.

4 Space under the armpits.

5 Tongue on hard palette.

6 Knees softly bent.

7 Feet fully connected with the ground.

GLOSSARY

Cheng Man Chung Influential twentieth-century teacher. He shortened and simplified the Yang style long form into the 37-posture form used in this book.

chi Often defined as life force, *chi* flows through everything in the universe. The practice of tai chi is intended to replenish and regulate the flow of *chi* within the body.

dantien The *dantiens* are three centers of energy in the body; the term "dantien" is also used specifically for the lower dantien, which is sited a short distance beneath the navel and within the abdomen.

empty and full In tai chi, you are constantly shifting weight from one foot to another, as if pouring water from one vessel to another. When your weight is entirely on one foot, it is "full" and the weightless foot is "empty."

form A collection of tai chi moves linked together to make one flowing sequence.

push hands Two-person training routines; practitioners face each other and practice yielding and pushing movements with the hands. Push hands exercises are a good way of gaining feedback about your tai chi practice.

rooting Creating a strong connection between the body and the ground, through the feet. This is partly a physical action, ensuring the entire foot is in contact with the floor, and part mental focus.

sinking Mentally directing the chi in the upper body down to the dantien.

style There are five major branches, or styles, of tai chi; all of them draw on the same basic principles. They are named for the families who originated them. Some teachers incorporate elements of different styles in their classes—combination-style tai chi.

yin and yang The opposing, yet complementary forces of *chi*: yin is yielding, soft, feminine energy, while yang is dynamic, hard masculine energy. Tai chi movements are constantly shifting from yin to yang and back again; this is believed to create balance in the body.

FURTHER INFORMATION

BOOKS

Cheng Man Ch'ing, translated by Benjamin Pang Jeng Lo and Martin Inn. *Cheng Tzu's Thirteen Treatises on T'ai Chi Chu'an*
Blue Snake Books, 1993

Barbara Davis, Benjamin Lo et al. *Cheng Man-ch'ing and T'ai Chi*
Via Media Publishing Company, 2014

Angus Clark. *Illustrated Elements of Tai Chi*
Element 2002

Peter M. Wayne PhD with Mark L. Fuerst. *The Harvard Medical School Guide to Tai Chi*
Shambala Publications, 2013

Waysun Liao. *Tai Chi Classics*
Shambala, 2001

ORGANIZATIONS

Simon Robins—The School of Tai Chi Chuan and Internal Arts
www.taichiandinternalarts.com

The Taijiquan and Qigong Federation for Europe
www.tcfe.org

American Tai Chi and QiGong Association
2465 J-17 Centreville Road, #150
Herndon
Virginia 20171
USA
www.americantaichi.org

Tai Chi for Health Institute
6 Fisher Place
Narwee
NSW 2209
Australia
www.taichiforhealthinstitute.org

WEBSITES

www.beginnerstaichi.com
Overview of the different styles of tai chi, with useful tips, warm-ups, and analysis of key moves.

www.americantaichi.net
Online journal run by the American Tai Chi and QiGong Association.

www.everyday-taichi.com
Useful website on all aspects of tai chi and chi kung.

INDEX

a

accessing the *dantien* 24-5, 41
acupuncture 8, 22
ankle circles 66-7
Apparent Close see Withdraw & Push
art of discipline 48-9
attitude 33, 36

b

back pain 18
backward stepping 122, 137
balance 18, 22, 26, 38, 153
Beautiful Hands 27, 128, 142
Beginning 84-5
benefits of tai chi 8, 13, 15, 18, 36, 39, 46, 122
Bow Stance 72, 74-5, 91, 96, 115
brain 18, 153
breathing 18, 52, 82-3, 117
  abdominal 8, 18, 20-1, 38, 72, 142
  accessing the *dantien* 24-5, 38, 41
  Horse Stance 72
Brush Left Knee & Punch Downward 168-9
Brush Left Knee & Push 108-9, 111, 164-5
Brush Right Knee & Push 166-7

c

cardiac fitness 18
check & sink 38
Chen family 12, 14
Chen style 13, 14
Cheng Man Ching 15, 26, 27, 32, 78, 86, 122, 178
chi 8, 22, 23, 26, 27, 44, 104, 122
chi kung 22
chi walking 36
circles 32
classes 50-1
clothing 28, 44
Cloud Hands see Wave Hands Like Clouds
Commencement 84
Completion 216-17
consciousness 33
cranes 12, 86, 104
Cross Hands 72, 118-19, 214-15

d

daily routine 38
dantien 24, 25, 26
  accessing 24-5, 38, 41
Daoism see Taoism
Deflect 112-15, 204, 210-12
Deflect Downward 112-15
Descending Single Whip 150, 154-5, 180, 200-1
Diagonal Flying 140-1
discipline 48-9
Draw a Bow to Shoot the Tiger 204, 209
duality 10

e

early closing 119
Embrace Tiger, Return to Mountain 122, 124-5
emotions 18
empty foot/leg 26, 31, 72
empty stances 72
endurance 18
energize the arms 60-3

f

Fair Lady Weaves the Shuttle 180, 182-9
falls 18
feet
  ankle circles 66-7
  backward stepping 122, 137
  contact with the earth 83
  empty foot/leg 26, 31, 72
  full foot/leg 26, 72
  lifting the toes 165
  position 72
  slide the foot 155
feng shui 22

fist 112, 115
Fist Under Elbow 122, 132-3
flexibility 18, 22, 41
footwear 28, 44
Four Corners *see* Fair Lady Weaves the Shuttle
full foot/leg 26, 72

g
Golden Rooster Stands on One Leg 77, 150, 152-3, 156-7
Grasp the Sparrow's Tail 86-95, 180
group practice 49

h
hands
  Beautiful Hands 27, 128, 142
see also punches
head, safe movement 57
health benefits 8, 13, 15, 18, 36, 39, 46, 122
Heel Stance 72, 77, 102
high blood pressure 18
hippocampus 18
history of tai chi 12
Hold the Ball 68-71, 87, 192
holding an egg 85
Horse Stance 72, 74

i
imperial guard 14, 15
integrated movements 41
Intercept & Punch 112-15, 204, 210-12

k
kicks 104, 152
  Left Toe Kick 160-1
  Right Toe Kick 158-9
  Turn & Kick with Left Heel 162-3
  Turn & Sweep the Lotus 204, 207-8
knees
loosening 53
raising 156
kung fu 14

l
Left Toe Kick 160-1
Lifting Hands 102
lifting the toes 165
lineage 51
loosening the knees 53

m
martial art 8, 12, 18, 86, 204
  Chen style 14
  defensive moves 92, 180
  retreat 122
  Toe Stance 104
meditation 38
meridians 24
mindfulness 33, 153, 203
minimum effort 41
motivation 48
moving from the waist 26, 92
muscle tone 18

n
nature 12, 22, 36, 44, 86
neck, relaxing 54-7
neurons 18
New Yang Style 15
Newton, Isaac 10
no forcing/no tension 26

o
one-legged stance 77
opposing pairs 10, 107
origins of tai chi 12
outdoors 36, 44

p
points of the compass 81
posture 18, 21
  straight spine 26, 38, 169, 170
  tai chi posture 28-9, 38, 72
practise space 44, 49

pregnancy 46
Preparation 80, 82-3
preparing for the form 54-67
Press & Push 86, 94-5, 127-8, 173-4, 195, 196
principles of tai chi 32-3
  foundation principles 26-31
proprioception 18
punches
  Brush Left Knee & Punch Downward 168-9
  Intercept & Punch 112-15, 204, 210-12
  tai chi fist 112, 115
Push Hands 86

q

qigong *see* chi kung

r

raise the knee 156
regular practice 44, 48-9
reiki 22
relaxation 21, 80
relaxation/sinking 26, 32, 38
relaxed attitude 33
relaxing the neck 54-7
relaxing the shoulders 58-9
respiratory fitness 18
resting 36
Right Toe Kick 158-9
Rollback 86, 92-3, 126, 172, 194
rooting 32

s

safe head movement 57
seasons 22
separating weight 26, 72, 74, 83
Shaolin monastery 14
shiatsu 22
shoes 28, 44
Shoulder Stroke 103
shoulder-width apart 73
shoulders, relaxing 58-9
Single Whip 86, 96-101, 129-31, 148-9, 175-7, 196-9
  Descending 150, 154-5, 180, 200-1
sinking 26, 32, 38, 152
Sit Stance 72, 75
sitting 38
slide the foot 155
slow movement 32
smooth movement 109
Snake Creeps Down 152
speed 32, 203
squatting 152
stable posture 115
stamina 22
Step Back to Repulse Monkey 122, 134-9
Step Back to Ride the Tiger 204, 206
Step Forward, Deflect, Intercept & Punch 112-15, 204, 210-12
Step Forward to the Seven Stars 180, 202-3
straight spine 26, 38, 169, 170
strength 18, 22, 41
stress 18, 36
Strum the Lute 103, 110-11
styles of tai chi 13, 14-15
  choosing a style 13
Sun style 13
Sweep the Lotus 204, 207-8
swimming in air 32, 178
swing the legs and arms 66-7

t

T-Stance 103
Taoism 10, 12, 13, 22
tension 26, 41, 165
theory of tai chi 22-3
tigers 122, 204
Toe Stance 72, 76, 77, 104, 106
transferring weight 30-1, 38, 41

Turn & Kick with Left Heel 162-3
Turn & Sweep the Lotus 204, 207-8

w

waist
- moving from 26, 92
- waist turns 64-5

walking
- backward walking 122
- chi walking 36
- tai chi walking 34-5

Ward Off Left 86, 88-9, 190-1
Ward Off Right 86, 90-1, 170-1, 192-3
warming up 52-3
Wave Hands Like Clouds 122, 142-7
weight
- empty/full foot 26, 31, 72
- separating weight 26, 72, 74, 83
- testing 31
- transferring 30-1, 38, 41

wellbeing 8, 13, 18, 36, 39, 122
Western mode of thought 13
White Crane Spreads Its Wings 104-7
whole-body movement 33, 139
wholeness 10, 13
Withdraw & Push 116-17, 204, 213
Wu style 13, 15

y

Yang Lu Chan 14, 15
Yang Short Form 15, 72, 78, 80
Yang style 13, 14-15, 80
yielding 10, 14, 86
yin & yang 22, 104
- embracing the yin 36
- symbol 10
- yang energy 44
- yin energy 44

yoga 13, 16

z

Zhang San Feng 12

ACKNOWLEDGMENTS

Every effort has been made to trace copyright holders and obtain permission. The publishers apologize for any omissions and would be pleased to make any necessary changes at subsequent printings.

Alamy/World History Archive: 11; Mawardi Bahar: 49.

Shutterstock/Dragon Images: 17; Irina oxilixo Danilova: 12; KUCO: 8; Marzolino: 23; MicroOne: 81; Monkey Business Images: 47; nullplus: 37; patrimonio designs: 12; Pranee Chaiyadam: 19; Rawpixel.com: 43; TonyV3112: 9; vanhurck: 45.